Advances in Veterinary Oncology

Advances in Veterinary Oncology

Edited by Emilia Farrell

SYRAWOOD
PUBLISHING HOUSE

New York

Published by Syrawood Publishing House,
750 Third Avenue, 9th Floor,
New York, NY 10017, USA
www.syrawoodpublishinghouse.com

Advances in Veterinary Oncology
Edited by Emilia Farrell

International Standard Book Number: 978-1-64740-256-3 (Hardback)

Cataloging-in-Publication Data

Advances in veterinary oncology / edited by Emilia Farrell.
    p. cm.
Includes bibliographical references and index.
ISBN 978-1-64740-256-3
1. Veterinary oncology. 2. Tumors in animals. 3. Veterinary medicine. I. Farrell, Emilia.
SF910.T8 A38 2022
636.089 699 4--dc23

TABLE OF CONTENTS

Permissions

List of Contributors

Index

PREFACE

The subspecialty within veterinary medicine which deals with the diagnosis of cancer in animals as well as its treatment is known as veterinary oncology. Due to a large number of deaths in pet animals being caused by cancer, veterinary oncology is an important field of study within veterinary medicine. Many animals such as cats and dogs suffer from similar cancers as humans. Thus, advances in veterinary oncology and human cancer research complement each other in a way which benefits both animals and humans. There are various treatments which are used to cure and control cancer in animals such as surgery, chemotherapy and radiation therapy. This book includes contributions of experts and scientists which will provide innovative insights into this field. It provides significant information of this discipline to help develop a good understanding of veterinary oncology and the advances which have been made in it.

After months of intensive research and writing, this book is the end result of all who devoted their time and efforts in the initiation and progress of this book. It will surely be a source of reference in enhancing the required knowledge of the new developments in the area. During the course of developing this book, certain measures such as accuracy, authenticity and research focused analytical studies were given preference in order to produce a comprehensive book in the area of study.

This book would not have been possible without the efforts of the authors and the publisher. I extend my sincere thanks to them. Secondly, I express my gratitude to my family and well-wishers. And most importantly, I thank my students for constantly expressing their willingness and curiosity in enhancing their knowledge in the field, which encourages me to take up further research projects for the advancement of the area.

Editor

Effects of epidermal growth factor receptor kinase inhibition on radiation response in canine osteosarcoma cells

Fernanda B. Mantovani[1], Jodi A. Morrison[2] and Anthony J. Mutsaers[1,2]*

Abstract

Background: Radiation therapy is a palliative treatment modality for canine osteosarcoma, with transient improvement in analgesia observed in many cases. However there is room for improvement in outcome for these patients. It is possible that the addition of sensitizing agents may increase tumor response to radiation therapy and prolong quality of life. Epidermal growth factor receptor (EGFR) expression has been documented in canine osteosarcoma and higher EGFR levels have been correlated to a worse prognosis. However, effects of EGFR inhibition on radiation responsiveness in canine osteosarcoma have not been previously characterized. This study examined the effects of the small molecule EGFR inhibitor erlotinib on canine osteosarcoma radiation responses, target and downstream protein expression in vitro. Additionally, to assess the potential impact of treatment on tumor angiogenesis, vascular endothelial growth factor (VEGF) levels in conditioned media were measured.

Results: Erlotinib as a single agent reduced clonogenic survival in two canine osteosarcoma cell lines and enhanced the impact of radiation in one out of three cell lines investigated. In cell viability assays, erlotinib enhanced radiation effects and demonstrated single agent effects. Erlotinib did not alter total levels of EGFR, nor inhibit downstream protein kinase B (PKB/Akt) activation. On the contrary, erlotinib treatment increased phosphorylated Akt in these osteosarcoma cell lines. VEGF levels in conditioned media increased after erlotinib treatment as a single agent and in combination with radiation in two out of three cell lines investigated. However, VEGF levels decreased with erlotinib treatment in the third cell line.

Conclusions: Erlotinib treatment promoted modest enhancement of radiation effects in canine osteosarcoma cells, and possessed activity as a single agent in some cell lines, indicating a potential role for EGFR inhibition in the treatment of a subset of osteosarcoma patients. The relative radioresistance of osteosarcoma cells does not appear to be related to EGFR signalling exclusively. Angiogenic responses to radiation and kinase inhibitors are similarly likely to be multifactorial and require further investigation.

Keywords: Osteosarcoma, Dog, Canine, Erlotinib, Epidermal growth factor receptor (EGFR), Radiation, Vascular endothelial growth factor (VEGF), Radiosensitization

Background

Osteosarcoma (OSA) is the most common primary bone tumor of the domestic dog, occurring predominantly in large breeds, and accounting for up to 85 % of skeletal tumors in this species [1]. Local tumor growth causes severe pain and lameness secondary to bone lyses, proliferation or both, and eventual metastasis from OSA to the lungs and other locations occurs in the vast majority of cases [1]. Surgical removal of the primary tumor, either by amputation of the affected limb or by limb-sparing surgery, followed by adjuvant chemotherapy is considered the standard of care for canine OSA. However, surgery may be contraindicated in dogs with preexisting orthopedic or neurologic disease, may not be elected by owners, or may not be feasible in cases of tumors affecting the axial skeleton. Thus, there is increasing interest in treating the primary tumor by utilizing external beam radiation therapy (RT) for dogs with OSA. Radiation therapy has mainly been applied in palliative settings to

* Correspondence: mutsaers@uoguelph.ca
[1]Department of Clinical Studies, Ontario Veterinary College, University of Guelph, Guelph, Ontario, Canada
[2]Department of Biomedical Sciences, Ontario Veterinary College, University of Guelph, Guelph, Ontario, Canada

provide analgesia and improve quality of life for canine OSA patients. Most reports in the veterinary literature describe radiation protocols consisting of two to four treatments (fractions), delivering total doses of 16 to 32 Gray (Gy) [2]. Although pain control is achieved in approximately 70–90 % of treated dogs, responses seen with palliative RT protocols are transient, with clinical improvement lasting approximately 2 to 4 months [2]. Treatment failure is associated with recurrent primary tumor growth and therefore novel strategies to improve the response to RT for canine OSA may translate into better clinical outcomes for these patients. Pre-clinical work conducted in vitro using cell lines has indicated that canine OSA is a moderately radioresistant tumor, with a high mean surviving fraction after treatment with 2 Gy [3]. Increasing the sensitivity of OSA cells to ionizing radiation could enhance the effects of RT, possibly improving patient outcomes.

Advances in molecular biology have resulted in the identification of several pathways involved in the pathogenesis and progression of cancer, which can be utilized as therapeutic targets. The epidermal growth factor receptor (EGFR) is a transmembrane receptor tyrosine kinase (RTK) involved in signaling for cell growth, proliferation, invasion and survival [4]. Over-expression and constitutive activation of EGFR have been found in numerous human cancers, including breast, lung and head and neck carcinomas [5]. In veterinary oncology, EGFR expression has been identified in various epithelial malignancies, including canine lung, nasal, mammary and transitional cell carcinoma, and feline squamous cell carcinoma (SCC) [6–11]. Additionally, higher expression levels of EGFR have been associated with more aggressive cancer behavior [6–11]. The role of aberrant activation of EGFR in the pathogenesis of mesenchymal tumors, such as OSA, is less well defined. Expression of EGFR has been documented in human [12, 13] and canine OSA [14], and correlated with a worse prognosis, indicating that EGFR may play a role in OSA tumor biology and therefore EGFR pathway inhibition could represent a viable treatment option for OSA. In vitro targeting of EGFR with RTK inhibitors has been reported in the veterinary literature, with successful inhibition of cell proliferation and growth of canine mammary carcinoma and OSA cell lines [15, 16], further supporting EGFR inhibition as a possible treatment approach for canine OSA.

The combining of RT with cytotoxic chemotherapy and/or more targeted cancer therapeutics has been widely investigated in human oncology, with the goal of improving the effectiveness of radiation (radiosensitization) [4]. Targeting the EGFR pathway is an attractive approach for radiosensitization for multiple reasons. EGFR inhibitors commonly produce a cytostatic effect

with arrest in the G1 phase of the cell cycle, which can prevent tumor cell repopulation post-radiation [17, 18]. Additionally, exposure of tumor cells to ionizing radiation can activate EGFR independently from ligands, contributing to tumor radioresistance [4, 19, 20]. Therefore, neutralizing this tumor response to radiation by inhibiting EGFR signaling could maintain tumor sensitivity. Erlotinib is a selective inhibitor of EGFR tyrosine kinase, which blocks cell cycle progression at the G1 phase and induces apoptosis of select human carcinoma cells in vitro [21]. Erlotinib has been used in the treatment of several human malignancies, and is approved for the treatment of non-small-cell lung cancer (NSCLC) and advanced pancreatic cancer in the United States. In human oncology, the use of erlotinib as a radiosensitizer has been successful in pre-clinical work [22–24], and has shown promising results in phase I/II clinical trials for head and neck SCC and NSCLC [25–27].

The effects of EGFR activation are exerted via subsequent activation of multiple downstream intracellular signaling pathways, including the phosphatidylinositol-3-kinase (PI3K) signaling cascade that culminates with activation of the serine/threonine kinase Protein kinase B (PKB/Akt). Upon stimulation of EGFR, PI3K is activated and generates phosphatidylinositol-3,4,5-trisphosphate (PIP3), which in turn acts as a second messenger for activation of Akt. Upon activation, Akt phosphorylates numerous downstream cytoplasmic and nuclear substrates, ultimately resulting in enhanced cell survival, proliferation, and inhibition of apoptosis [28, 29]. Radiation treatment may lead to enhancement of this signaling pathway in cancer cells as a response to treatment. Exposure of human carcinoma and glioblastoma cells to radiation in vitro activated Akt, and promoted increased cell survival and proliferation [28–30], through activation of EGFR via a ligand-independent mechanism. In these studies, increased levels of phosphorylated-Akt (p-Akt) were found within 4 h of RT, and inhibition of Akt enhanced radiosensitivity of tumor cells [28–30]. It is possible that similar EGFR activation and secondary increases in p-Akt levels could be seen following RT of canine OSA. Furthermore, evaluating the PI3K/Akt pathway could potentially serve as a surrogate biomarker for inhibition of upstream receptor targets like EGFR after treatment with erlotinib or other agents.

This study investigated the effects of erlotinib alone and in combination with RT on canine OSA cell lines. Therapeutic effects were evaluated by clonogenic survival, cell viability, and the expression of target and downstream proteins. Finally, because one of the mechanisms of action for both radiation and EGFR inhibition has been shown to be inhibition of angiogenesis, we investigated the impact of treatment on levels of the potent angiogenesis factor vascular endothelial growth factor (VEGF) secreted by OSA cells into conditioned media. Dose dependent erlotinib single agent activity was observed in all cell lines. Erlotinib provided enhancement of radiation effects on Dharma OSA cells at 2, 4 and 6 Gy doses, which are lower doses than the commonly used 8 Gy per fraction dose utilized in most palliative radiation protocols for osteosarcoma. Erlotinib increased VEGF levels in conditioned media and this effect was particularly evident with combination treatment.

Methods
Cell culture
Canine osteosarcoma cell lines D17, Abrams and Dharma were used. D17 cells were obtained from Sigma-Aldrich/ European Collection of Cell Cultures (ECACC). Abrams cells were a generous gift from Mike Huelsmeyer at the University of Wisconsin. Both D17 and Abrams cell lines have been utilized on several published studies and have been characterized as canine OSA cells based on morphology and xenograft analysis [31]. Dharma cells were isolated and adapted to culture from a clinical case by Dr. Anthony Mutsaers, and validated as OSA by histopathology evaluation of tumors produced from successful xenograft outgrowth after implantation in immunocomprised (nude) mice. All cells were grown in Dulbecco's modified Eagle's media (Hyclone DMEM - Fisher Scientific- Ottawa, ON, Canada) supplemented with 10 % fetal bovine serum (Life Technologies, Burlington, ON, Canada) and 1 % penicillin/streptomycin (BioWhittaker, Mississauga, ON, Canada). All cell cultures were maintained at 37 °C and 5 % CO_2 in a humidified incubator.

Radiation therapy
Cell culture plates were irradiated at ambient temperature and pressure, at a rate of 400 monitor units/min utilizing a 6-MV linear accelerator (Clinac IX System, Varian Medical Systems, Inc., Palo Alto, CA, USA). Cell culture dishes were placed between two solid water-equivalent plates, with thickness of 4.5 cm on top and 5 cm on the bottom. The dose distribution for this set up was medical physicist verified. Control cell culture plates were transported to the radiation therapy area but kept outside the radiation vault during treatments.

Clonogenic survival
Cells were seeded into six-well plates (D17 and Abrams at 500 cells/well, and Dharma at 1,500 cells/well) with 3 ml of media. After 24 h, the media of all wells was replaced and erlotinib (SelleckChem, Houston, TX, USA) at 10 μM was added to treatment group wells. Erlotinib was diluted in dimethyl sulfoxide (DMSO) resulting in a final concentration of 0.04 % DMSO in each well. After incubation for 4 to 6 h, doses of 0, 2, 4, 6, 8 and 10 Gy

of radiation were administered to individual plates. Colony formation was monitored daily and the experiment stopped after 10 to 14 days, before the control colonies became confluent. Cells were stained with 0.5 % crystal violet in 20 % methanol for 30 minutes, then washed gently twice with tap water [32]. Colonies were visualized by light microscopy and counted. A colony was defined as an aggregate of ≥ 50 cells. The cell surviving fraction, normalized for plating efficiency, was determined for each radiation dose. All experiments were repeated three times.

Cell viability
To assess cell viability, Resazurin Cell Viability Kit (Sigma-Aldrich, Oakville, ON, Canada) was used at a concentration of 5.0 mg/ml. Cells were seeded into 96-well plates (D17 and Abrams at 500 cells/well, and Dharma at 2,000 cells/well), and settled for 24 h at 37 °C and 5 % CO_2 [33]. Erlotinib was administered at 10 μM and 40 μM, plates were incubated for 4 to 6 h, and doses of 0, 2, 4, 6, 8 and 10 Gy of radiation were delivered to individual plates. After 72 h, 100 μl of Resazurin solution was pipetted into each well. After the solution in wells changed in color, absorbance readings were obtained from a Synergy 2 spectrophotometer (BioTek, Winooski, VT, USA), at an excitation wavelength of 570 nm and emission wavelength of 600 nm. Relative viable cell number was assessed by means of sextuplicate wells for each erlotinib concentration and corresponding control group, and each experiment was repeated three times. Absorbance values were corrected for media only readings in sextuplicate wells.

Protein detection
Cells were seeded into six-well plates (D17 and Abrams at 150,000 cells/well, and Dharma at 200,000 cells/well) and settled for 24 h at 37 °C and 5 % CO_2. The media of all wells was replaced to divide groups into erlotinib at 10 μM or control, followed by incubation for 4 to 6 h. Plates were irradiated with a 2 Gy dose or kept in the radiation control room during treatment. Cells were lysed in ice cold buffer (Cell Signaling technology, Whitby, ON, Canada) containing aprotinin, phenylmethanesulfonyl fluoride and a phosphatase inhibitor cocktail, and collected 0.25, 0.5, 1, 2, 24 and 48 h post radiation, and placed immediately on ice. Cell lysis buffer additives were obtained from Sigma-Aldrich (Oakville, ON, Canada). Equal amounts of protein were separated by SDS polyacrylamide gel electrophoresis and transferred to a polyvinyl difluoride membrane (Roche Diagnostics Corporation, Indianapolis, IN, USA). Membranes were hybridized to an appropriate primary antibody and horseradish peroxidase (HRP) conjugated secondary antibody, then visualized using the Bio-Rad Chemi-Doc

system (Universal Hood III). Primary antibody against β-actin, EGFR, Akt and p-Akt were purchased from Cell Signaling Technology (Whitby, ON, Canada). The secondary antibodies, HRP-conjugated goat anti-rabbit IgG were obtained from Santa Cruz Biotechnology Inc. (Dallas, TX, USA).

VEGF levels

Conditioned media was collected and pooled from sextuplicate wells treated with erlotinib at 10 μM, with or without radiation treatment at 2 Gy and 8 Gy at 72 h. Levels of VEGF were quantified using the Quantikine Canine VEGF ELISA Kit (R&D Systems, Minneapolis, MN, USA), following the manufacturer's instructions [33]. The optical density of the standard solutions was plotted against their corresponding concentrations to generate a standard curve and allow determination of sample VEGF concentrations. Absorbance was read at 450 nm and corrected by subtracting readings at 540 nm, as per manufacturer recommendation.

Statistical analysis

Statistical analyses were performed with Graph-Pad Prism 5 software (GraphPad Software, Inc., La Jolla, CA, USA). For clonogenic survival and cell viability assays, a two-way analysis of variance (ANOVA) with Sidak method for multiple comparisons was used to determine whether erlotinib treatment had an effect in clonogenic survival and cell viability compared to radiation only treatment groups. For VEGF levels, a one-way ANOVA was used to determine whether treatment with erlotinib and/or radiation had an effect on VEGF concentrations compared to control groups. To account for changes in cell number that may influence VEGF levels, readings were normalized to cell viability of respective wells, as measured by Resazurin assay. Overall significance was set at $p < 0.05$.

Results
Effects of erlotinib and radiation on clonogenic survival

Erlotinib showed single agent activity through reduction in clonogenic survival in 2 out of 3 cell lines: $p < 0.0001$ for Dharma and $p = 0.0003$ for D17 (Fig. 1). No effect was seen in Abrams cells. Radiation administered at doses ranging from 2 to 10 Gy demonstrated a dose dependent reduction in clonogenic survival, as expected, in all 3 OSA cell lines examined (Fig. 2). Treatment with erlotinib four to six hours prior to radiation therapy resulted in a significant reduction in clonogenic survival of Dharma OSA cells for the lower radiation doses of 2 Gy ($p < 0.0001$), 4 Gy ($p < 0.0001$) and 6 Gy ($p = 0.0127$). This effect was lost at the higher radiation doses that resulted in a lower survival fraction from radiation treatment alone. In this cell line the shape of the survival curve for the "erlotinib" group had a

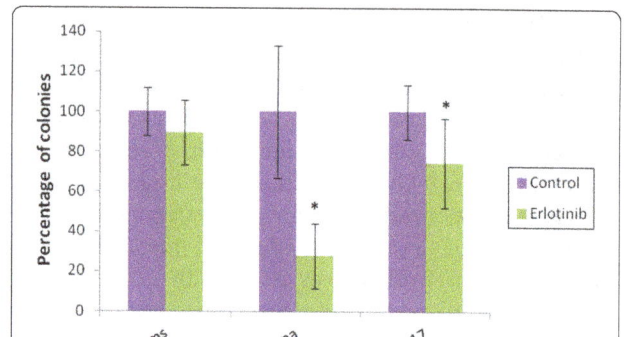

Fig. 1 Effects of single agent erlotinib on clonogenic survival. Canine OSA cells treated with erlotinib at 10 μM for 4-6 h ("erlotinib"). Experiments were repeated three times and average of results are shown. Erlotinib showed single agent activity through reduction in clonogenic survival in 2 out of 3 cell lines. * $p < 0.05$ indicates statistical significant reduction in clonogenic survival compared to control

more narrow shoulder compared to the "control" curve (Fig. 2), indicating the potential for reduced sublethal damage repair in these erlotinib treated cells. Enhancement of radiation effects was not observed in D17 ($p = 0.39$) and Abrams ($p = 0.71$) OSA cells.

Effects of erlotinib and radiation on cell viability

Cell viability assays were assessed 72 h post-radiation (Fig. 3). Radiation administered at doses ranging from 2 to 10 Gy demonstrated dose dependent reductions in cell viability for 2 out of 3 OSA cell lines. The viability of Dharma cells was less impacted by radiation but interestingly, these cells were more sensitive to single agent erlotinib on cell viability assays, with statistically significant reductions in cell viability for all erlotinib treated groups ($p < 0.0001$), as shown in Fig. 3. Given the lack of response seen in 2 cell lines with erlotinib at 10 μM, a higher dose of 40 μM was tested. The viability of all 3 cell lines was reduced by this higher, but clinically/pharmacologically less relevant concentration of erlotinib. Addition of erlotinib at 40 μM resulted in decreased cell viability compared to radiation alone for all cell lines, however these effects were not statistically significant for Abrams cells at radiation doses above 4 Gy ($p = 0.14$). Treatment with erlotinib at the lower 10 μM dose further decreased viability in radiated Dharma cells ($p ≤ 0.0002$), but failed to provide enhancement of radiation effects for Abrams ($p = 0.25$) and D17 cells ($p = 0.38$).

Expression of target proteins

Western blot analyses detected endogenous expression of EGFR, total Akt and p-Akt in all three OSA cell lines investigated. Treatment with erlotinib, with or without radiation, increased levels of p-Akt in Dharma and D17 cells at 0.25, 0.5, 1, 2 and 24 h after radiation treatment (Fig. 4). Levels of p-Akt showed

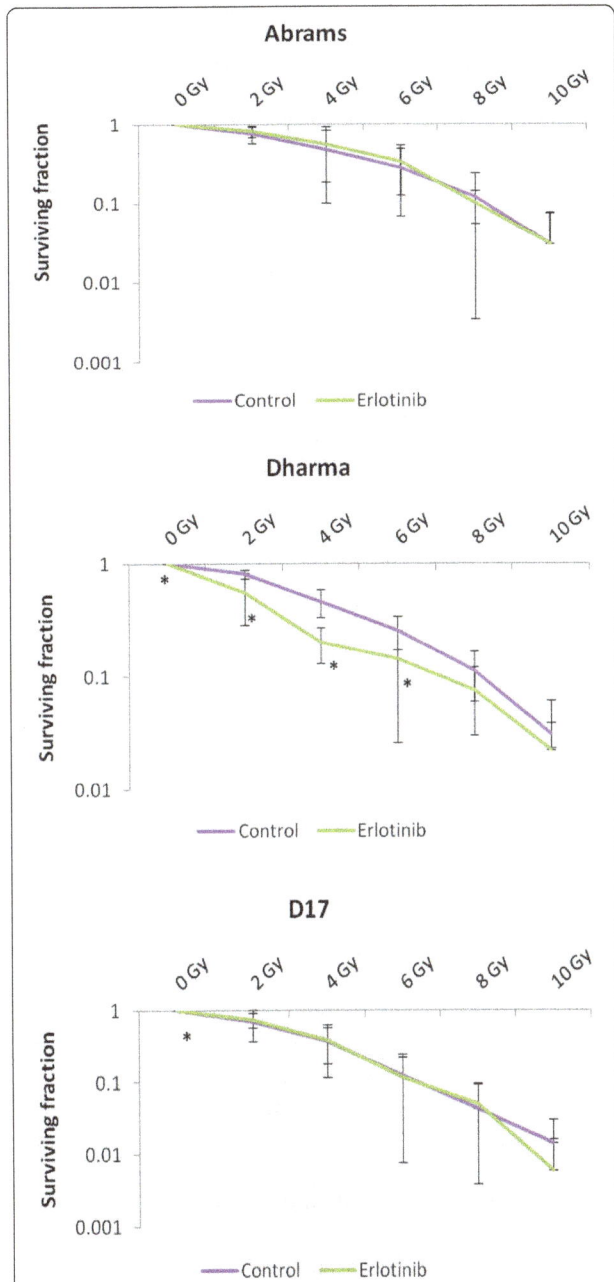

Fig. 2 Clonogenic survival curves. Canine OSA cells were treated with radiation only ("control") or in combination with erlotinib at 10 μM ("erlotinib") given 4-6 h before radiation. Experiments were repeated three times and average of results are shown. Survival fractions are plotted on a log-scale. Erlotinib treatment resulted in statistically significant reduction in cell survival of Dharma cells for radiation doses of 0, 2, 4 and 6 Gy, and statistically significant reduction in cell survival for D17 cells at 0 Gy, but did not promote enhancement of radiation effects for D17 or Abrams cell lines. *$p < 0.05$ indicates statistical significant reduction in clonogenic survival compared to [1]control at the corresponding radiation dose

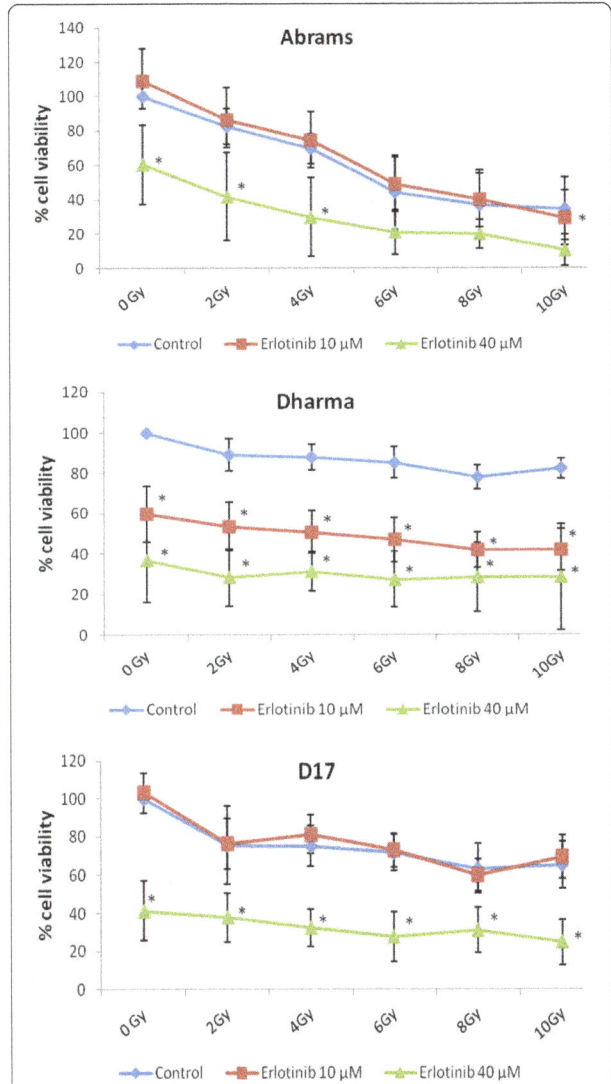

Fig. 3 Cell viability assays 72 h post-radiation. Cells were treated with either radiation only ("control"), or radiation plus erlotinib at 10 μM or 40 μM. Experiments were repeated three times and average of results are shown. Addition of erlotinib resulted in statistically significant decreases in cell viability for Dharma cells at 10 μM, and for all cell lines at 40 μM dose. Enhancement of radiation effects were less pronounced at 10 μM, as seen in Dharma cells. *$p < 0.05$ indicates statistically significant reduction in percentage of viable cells compared to control group at the corresponding radiation dose

minimal variation among treatment groups in Abrams cells. Total Akt and EGFR were detected in all cell lines at all time points and treatment combinations, with no consistent variations seen among treatment groups.

Effects of erlotinib and radiation on VEGF levels

Secreted VEGF was detected in the conditioned media from all three canine OSA cell lines investigated (Table 1). Changes in VEGF levels compared to control occurred more consistently after combination treatment with radiation doses of 2 and 8 Gy (Fig. 5, Table 2). Interestingly, conditioned media from Dharma and

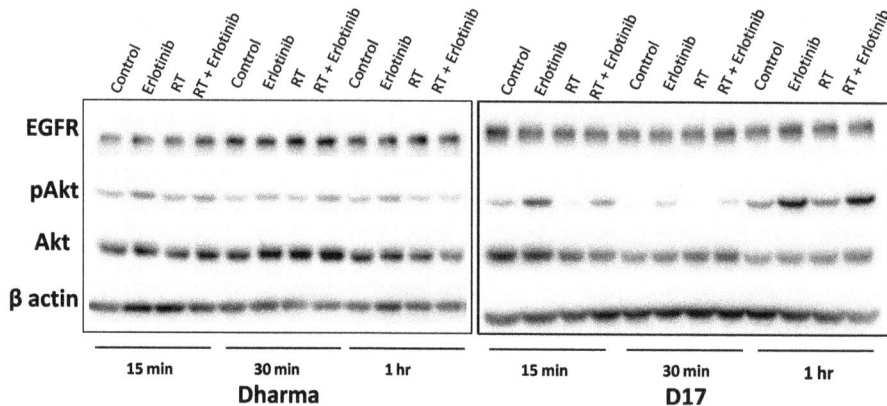

Fig. 4 Western blot analysis of EGFR and downstream proteins. EGFR, total Akt and p-Akt were detected in all OSA cell lines investigated. Higher levels of p-Akt were seen after treatment with erlotinib, with or without radiation, in Dharma and D17 cells at 0.25, 0.5, 1, 2 and 24 hours

Abrams cells showed increases in VEGF levels, whereas D17 cells showed decreases. Exposure to radiation at 8 Gy provided a significant reduction in VEGF levels for D17 cells ($p < 0.09$), but no other statistically significant changes were observed.

Discussion

The interaction of ionizing radiation with cells promotes both direct and indirect effects. Energy absorption can induce direct damage of molecules, however most of the energy deposited within cells is absorbed by water, generating free radicals. These are highly reactive molecules that can cause breakage of deoxyribonucleic acid (DNA) strands. If damaged DNA is not successfully repaired, either cell death or chromosomal aberrations may occur upon cell division [34]. With the exception of a few cell types, such as lymphocytes, that undergo apoptosis shortly after radiation exposure, most cell death secondary to irradiation takes place by mitotic catastrophe [34]. Rapidly proliferating cells have a high rate of cell division, and will therefore be more sensitive to radiation effects, or at least manifest the consequences of radiation damage sooner than slower dividing cell populations. However, cells that are proficient in DNA repair will be more resistant to radiation cytotoxicity.

Table 1 Median VEGF concentration in conditioned media 72 h post-radiation (pg/mL)

	Abrams	Dharma	D17
Control	57.8 ± 36.4	476.7 ± 177.2	143.7 ± 60.1
Erlotinib	144.1 ± 63.4	413.9 ± 204.6	157.6 ± 91.4
2Gy	34.8 ± 20.4	465.8 ± 181.1	139.2 ± 57.1
8Gy	21.1 ± 7.7	447.3 ± 162.9	135.5 ± 37.8
2Gy + Erlotinib	130.4 ± 55.6	490.9 ± 225.3	148.9 ± 73.3
8Gy + Erlotinib	52.8 ± 15.9	398.8 ± 92	163.4 ± 54.9

After irradiation, cells may continue to be metabolically active (which is detectable in viability assays), but they may lose the capacity to undergo normal cell division and maintain continued reproductive ability [34]. Clonogenic survival assays after RT assess a cell's ability to survive treatment, preserve cell division and repopulate the tumor, and therefore these assays provide an important in vitro assessment of potential therapeutic success. Radiation dose-response cell survival curves based on colony formation assays represent the total cumulative clonogenic outgrowth. The shoulders of these curves illustrate the capability of cells to repair sublethal DNA damage, and a wider shoulder indicates more efficient repair and subsequent repopulation, keeping clonogenic survival high. Cell survival curves in this current study were in agreement with previously reported RT dose-response curves for canine OSA cells, displaying a wide shoulder and moderate radioresistance [3]. Treatment with erlotinib provided statistically significant reductions in cell survival of Dharma cells at doses of 2, 4 and 6 Gy compared to control groups (Fig. 2). The radiosensitization effects of erlotinib are proposed to be, at least in part, secondary to cell cycle arrest in the G1 phase [4, 17, 18]. Cells in G1 phase are less radiosensitive than cells in G2 or M phases of the cell cycle, which makes radiosensitization by EGFR inhibitors appear counterintuitive. However, arrest in G1 also provides a cytostatic effect that prevents tumor cell repopulation between fractions of RT, still potentially enhancing the efficacy of a radiation protocol [4, 17, 18, 34]. It is possible that the sequence of treatment with a targeted EGFR inhibitor may play a role in radiosensitization. In this study cells were pre-treated with erlotinib 4 h prior to radiation, and drug treatment only after radiation was not investigated. Figure 2 also illustrates a narrowing of the shoulder in the cell survival curve for Dharma cells, indicating that decreased repopulation may have contributed to enhancement of radiation effects seen in this cell line. Colony

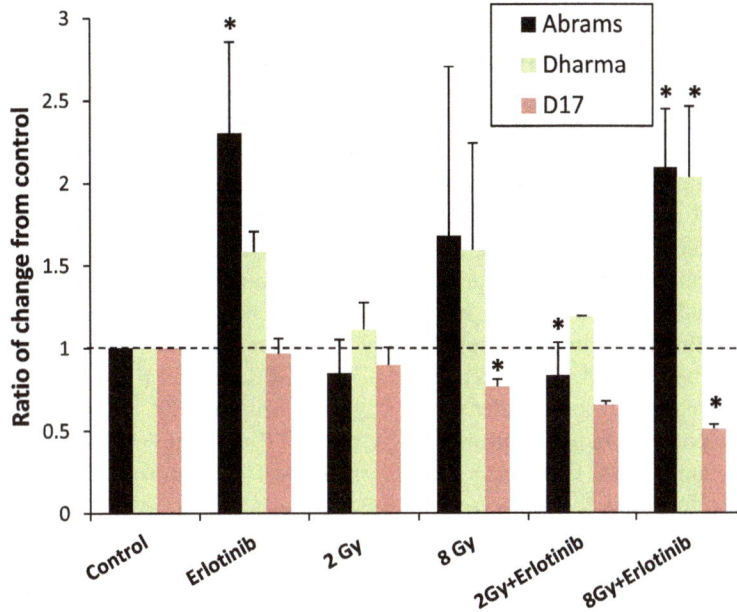

Fig. 5 Concentration of VEGF in conditioned media 72 h post-radiation. VEGF levels are expressed as a ratio of change from control. *$p < 0.05$ indicates statistical significant change. Changes in VEGF levels were variable among cell lines, but significant changes occurred most consistently with combination RT plus erlotinib treatment

formation assays in the present study showed no radiosensitizing effects of erlotinib on Abrams or D17 cells. Finally, it is also unknown whether Abrams cells, which appear to be more inherently resistant to erlotinib based on the results of Fig. 1, fail to undergo any G1 arrest after treatment with this drug.

Cell viability assays, such as the Resazurin assay, rely on bioreduction of the reagent dye by metabolically active cells, providing an indirect determination of cell viability. Such assays may not reflect the later death following cell divisions that is reflected in clonogenic survival assay results. Nevertheless, cell viability was assessed in the present study to investigate possible radiation enhancing effects of erlotinib by multiple mechanisms (Fig. 3). Abrams cells showed marked radiation dose-dependent reduction of cell viability, but moderate radioresistance on clonogenic survival assays. This discrepancy could potentially be explained by efficient repopulation. Abrams cells are very fast growing with a

Table 2 Median VEGF concentration 72 h post-radiation normalized to cell viability (pg/mL) * indicates significant change from control ($p < 0.05$)

	Abrams	Dharma	D17
Control	0.57	4.76	0.76
Erlotinib	1.22*	7.66	0.75
2Gy	0.37	5.22	0.61
8Gy	0.44	5.67	0.49*
2Gy + Erlotinib	1.32*	9.96	0.56
8Gy + Erlotinib	1.14*	9.32*	0.38*

doubling time of approximately 17 h. Therefore at 72 h post-radiation, multiple cell divisions would likely have occurred, with consequent mitotic deaths, and corresponding low cell viability on Resazurin assays. Any surviving clones would have then undergone repopulation, resulting in the cell survival curves shown in Fig. 2. It could be concluded that erlotinib failed to prevent repopulation of Abrams cells, at least at the 10 μM dose. These findings were in contrast to Dharma cells, which showed less pronounced dose-dependent effects of radiation on cell viability assays, yet radiation demonstrated consistent suppression of clonogenic survival. Dharma cells have a doubling time of 34 h. Thus, after only 72 h the cytotoxic effects of RT may have been undetectable, as a significant proportion of cells have not yet undergone mitosis. D17 cells showed moderate radiation dose-response sensitivity on cell viability assays, which was more pronounced on clonogenic survival assays. Interestingly, the doubling time of D17 cells is 23 h, which is longer than Abrams cells but shorter than Dharma cells.

Erlotinib treatment promoted cytotoxic effects as a single agent at 10 μM for Dharma and D17 cells, and at 40 μM for all three cell lines investigated. Additionally, enhancement of radiation effects was seen at the 40 μM dose for all cell lines on cell viability assays. In addition to dosing, the order of treatment and period of exposure can influence the effects of combination therapy. In this study erlotinib was administered to cells 4 to 6 h prior to RT, and remained in the media until the end of experiments, in an effort to mimic how RTK inhibitors are used clinically. It is possible that a more prolonged period of erlotinib exposure prior to RT would have promoted enhancement of RT effects on D17 and Abrams cells. Nevertheless, the cytotoxic and radiation enhancing effects of erlotinib demonstrated in this current study support in vivo evaluation of EGFR inhibition as a possible treatment strategy for a subset of canine OSA cases. As erlotinib-induced enhancement of RT effects on cell viability were more pronounced at RT doses of 2 and 4 Gy, it can be expected that EGFR inhibition might be more effective in potentiating the effects of hyperfractionated curative protocols as opposed to the currently used palliative RT protocols. Further investigations of the ideal dosing, timing of drug exposure and RT protocol, utilizing additional OSA cells, xenograft models and other EGFR inhibitors is recommended to improve our understanding of potential radiosensitization effects of EGFR targeting in canine OSA. Given that not all patients are likely to benefit from this therapy, evaluation of EGFR expression and pathway activation for individual tumors could be investigated further as potential biomarkers of treatment response.

Protein analysis by Western blot confirmed EGFR expression in all three cell lines, with no variation in levels among treatment groups consistently throughout the time points examined. In contrast to antibody therapeutics such as cetuximab that can impact receptor trafficking, the small molecule kinase inhibitor erlotinib may not be expected to cause decreased total EGFR with signaling inhibition. The protein Akt was evaluated as a potential downstream indicator of EGFR kinase signaling inhibition. Activation of Akt post-radiation has been documented in human carcinoma and glioblastoma cells in vitro [28–30]. In the current study, increased levels of p-Akt post RT were not observed. It is possible that RT treatment does not activate the EGFR pathway in canine OSA cells as it occurs with human carcinoma and glioblastoma cells [28–30]. Interestingly however, increased levels of p-Akt were observed after erlotinib was used as a single agent or in combination with RT in D17 and Dharma cells. Increased levels of p-AKT may contribute to cell survival, and this was an unexpected finding with erlotinib treatment. These findings in the context of EGFR inhibitor use suggest that the EGFR pathway may not be exclusively responsible for the radioresistance of canine OSA, and illustrate that signaling responses after molecular targeting agents may be multifaceted. Other signaling cascades downstream of EGFR not investigated herein, such as the mitogen-activated protein kinases (MAPK/erk) pathway, could also be involved in the cytotoxic effects of erlotinib. Further evaluation of signaling events post RT and EGFR inhibition for canine OSA cells are warranted, as such studies could shed more light on the potential mechanisms involved in this treatment and improve targeted therapeutic strategies for this cancer.

The amount of VEGF secreted by OSA cells constitutively and after treatment with RT, erlotinib and combinations was quantified in this study. Increased serum VEGF levels in dogs with OSA has been correlated with decreased disease free intervals [35], and constitutive VEGF levels have previously been observed in canine OSA cells [33]. Dose-dependent increases in VEGF levels after RT have been documented in human glioblastoma cells and in lung cancer mouse xenografts [36, 37], and proposed to be associated with radioresistance. In the veterinary literature, RT up-regulated VEGF production in a melanoma cell line in a dose-dependent manner [38], but no changes in VEGF levels post-radiation were seen in a mast cell tumor cell line [39]. There are also correlations between the EGFR and VEGF pathways, as these share parallel and reciprocal downstream signaling mechanisms, and exert direct and indirect effects on tumor cells that contribute to cancer progression [40]. Additionally, epidermal growth factor, an important ligand for EGFR, also drives VEGF expression, and an overactive VEGF pathway plays a role in tumor resistance to treatment with EGFR inhibitors [40, 41]. Treatment with gefitinib, a selective EGFR RTK, resulted in decreased cell proliferation and decreased microvascular density and VEGF levels in murine renal cell carcinoma [42].

In the present study, VEGF production was not up-regulated after RT, and statistically significant decreased levels were seen by D17 cells after 8 Gy. Treatment with RTK inhibitors can modulate VEGF levels in an off-target manner. Increased VEGF levels have been found in vitro after canine OSA cells were treated with masitinib, a RTK inhibitor targeting c-Kit and platelet-derived growth factor receptor [33]. In our study, statistically significant changes in VEGF levels occurred more consistently after combination therapy. Additionally, D17 cells showed decreases whereas Dharma and Abrams cells had increases in VEGF production. This variability in VEGF levels post tyrosine kinase inhibitor treatment and RT illustrates the complexity of responses of individual cancers to cytotoxic stimuli, and the need for further investigation of angiogenic responses to anti-cancer therapeutics.

Conclusions

Erlotinib treatment promoted modest enhancement of radiation effects in canine OSA cells, and showed activity as a single agent, indicating a possible role of EGFR inhibition in the treatment of a subset of OSA patients. Radioresistance of OSA cells does not appear to depend exclusively on EGFR signaling. Expanding research into signaling cascade alterations and angiogenic responses to combinations of RT with RTK inhibitors are worthy of further investigation.

Abbreviations

Akt, Serine/threonine kinase, also known as protein kinase B; DNA, Deoxyribonucleic acid; EGFR, Epidermal growth factor receptor; MAPK, mitogen-activated protein kinase, also known as erk; NSCLC, Non-small-cell lung cancer; OSA, Osteosarcoma. p-Akt, Phosphorylated Akt; PI3K, Phosphatidylinositol-3-kinase; PIP3, Phosphatidylinositol-3,4,5-trisphosphate; RT, Radiation therapy; RTK, Receptor tyrosine kinase; SCC, Squamous cell carcinoma; VEGF, Vascular endothelial growth factor

Acknowledgements

The authors would like to thank the radiation therapists from the Ontario Veterinary College, Laura Furness, Maria Helena Hartono and Kim Stewart for their contribution to irradiation of cells throughout the study period, radiation oncologist Valerie Poirier, and medical physicist Andre Fleck from the Grand River Cancer Centre for verification of dose distribution. The authors thank Dr. Arata Matsuyama for his input regarding statistical analysis.

Funding

This project was supported by the OVC Department of Biomedical Sciences, OVC Dean's office, and a memorial donation through the University of Guelph Alumni Affairs and Development.

Author's contributions

FM carried out clonogenic and cell viability assays, protein analysis, analyzed the data and drafted the manuscript. JM performed Western blots and ELISA analyses, conducted replicates of cell viability experiments and assisted with data analysis. AJM conceived the study, participated in its design and coordination, and revised the manuscript. All authors read and approved the final manuscript.

Competing interests

The authors declare that they have no competing interests.

Consent for publication

Not applicable.

References

1. Ehrhart NP, Ryan SD, Fan TM. Tumors of the skeletal system. In: Withrow SJ, Vail DM, Page RL, editors. Withrow and MacEwen's Small Animal Clinical Oncology. St Louis, Missouri: Saunders; 2013. p. 463–531.
2. Coomer A, Farese J, Milner R, Liptak J, Bacon N, Lurie D. Radiation therapy for canine appendicular osteosarcoma. Vet Comp Oncol. 2009;7(1):15–27.
3. Fitzpatrick CL, Farese JP, Milner RJ, Salute ME, Rajon DA, Morris CG, et al. Intrinsic radiosensitivity and repair of sublethal radiation-induced damage in canine osteosarcoma cell lines. Am J Vet Res. 2008;69(9):1197–202.
4. Nyati MK, Morgan MA, Feng FY, Lawrence TS. Integration of EGFR inhibitors with radiochemotherapy. Nat Rev Cancer. 2006;6(11):876–85.
5. Hynes NE, Lane HA. ERBB receptors and cancer: The complexity of targeted inhibitors. Nat Rev Cancer. 2005;5(5):341–54.
6. Gama A, Gartner F, Alves A, Schmitt F. Immunohistochemical expression of epidermal growth factor receptor (EGFR) in canine mammary tissues. Res Vet Sci. 2009;87(3):432–7.
7. Hanazono K, Fukumoto S, Kawamura Y, Endo Y, Kadosawa T, Iwano H, et al. Epidermal growth factor receptor expression in canine transitional cell carcinoma. J Vet Med Sci. 2015;77(1):1–6.
8. Yoshikawa H, Ehrhart EJ, Charles JB, Thamm DH, Larue SM. Immunohistochemical characterization of feline oral squamous cell carcinoma. Am J Vet Res. 2012; 73(11):1801–6.
9. Shiomitsu K, Johnson CL, Malarkey DE, Pruitt AF, Thrall DE. Expression of epidermal growth factor receptor and vascular endothelial growth factor in malignant canine epithelial nasal tumours. Vet Comp Oncol. 2009;7(2):106–14.
10. Sabattini S, Marconato L, Zoff A, Morini M, Scarpa F, Capitani O, et al. Epidermal growth factor receptor expression is predictive of poor prognosis in feline cutaneous squamous cell carcinoma. J Feline Med Surg. 2010;12(10):760–8.
11. Sabattini S, Mancini FR, Marconato L, Bacci B, Rossi F, Vignoli M, et al. EGFR overexpression in canine primary lung cancer: Pathogenetic implications and impact on survival. Vet Comp Oncol. 2014;12(3):237–48.
12. Lee JA, Ko Y, Kim DH, Lim JS, Kong CB, Cho WH, et al. Epidermal growth factor receptor: Is it a feasible target for the treatment of osteosarcoma? Cancer Res Treat. 2012;44(3):202–9.
13. Wen YH, Koeppen H, Garcia R, Chiriboga L, Tarlow BD, Peters BA, et al. Epidermal growth factor receptor in osteosarcoma: Expression and mutational analysis. Hum Pathol. 2007;38(8):1184–91.
14. Selvarajah GT, Verheije MH, Kik M, Slob A, Rottier PJ, Mol JA, et al. Expression of epidermal growth factor receptor in canine osteosarcoma: Association with clinicopathological parameters and prognosis. Vet J. 2012;193(2):412–9.
15. Kennedy KC, Qurollo BA, Rose BJ, Thamm DH. Epidermal growth factor enhances the malignant phenotype in canine mammary carcinoma cell lines. Vet Comp Oncol. 2011;9(3):196–206.
16. McCleese JK, Bear MD, Kulp SK, Mazcko C, Khanna C, London CA. Met interacts with EGFR and Ron in canine osteosarcoma. Vet Comp Oncol. 2013;11(2):124–39.
17. Di Gennaro E, Barbarino M, Bruzzese F, De Lorenzo S, Caraglia M, Abbruzzese A, et al. Critical role of both p27KIP1 and p21CIP1/WAF1 in the antiproliferative effect of ZD1839 ('Iressa'), an epidermal growth factor receptor tyrosine kinase inhibitor, in head and neck squamous carcinoma cells. J Cell Physiol. 2003; 195(1):139–50.
18. Kriegs M, Gurtner K, Can Y, Brammer I, Rieckmann T, Oertel R, et al. Radiosensitization of NSCLC cells by EGFR inhibition is the result of an enhanced p53-dependent G1 arrest. Radiother Oncol. 2015;115(1):120–7.
19. Schmidt-Ullrich RK, Mikkelsen RB, Dent P, Todd DG, Valerie K, Kavanagh BD, et al. Radiation-induced proliferation of the human A431 squamous carcinoma cells is dependent on EGFR tyrosine phosphorylation. Oncogene. 1997;15(10): 1191–7.
20. Todd DG, Mikkelsen RB, Rorrer WK, Valerie K, Schmidt-Ullrich RK. Ionizing radiation stimulates existing signal transduction pathways involving the activation of epidermal growth factor receptor and ERBB-3, and changes of intracellular calcium in A431 human squamous carcinoma cells. J Recept Signal Transduct Res. 1999;19(6):885–908.
21. Moyer JD, Barbacci EG, Iwata KK, Arnold L, Boman B, Cunningham A, et al. Induction of apoptosis and cell cycle arrest by CP-358,774, an inhibitor of epidermal growth factor receptor tyrosine kinase. Cancer Res. 1997;57(21):4838–48.
22. Gonzalez JE, Barquinero JF, Lee M, Garcia O, Casaco A. Radiosensitization induced by the anti-epidermal growth factor receptor monoclonal antibodies cetuximab and nimotuzumab in A431 cells. Cancer Biol Ther. 2012;13(2):71–6.
23. Tsai YC, Ho PY, Tzen KY, Tuan TF, Liu WL, Cheng AL, et al. Synergistic blockade of EGFR and HER2 by new-generation EGFR tyrosine kinase inhibitor enhances radiation effect in bladder cancer cells. Mol Cancer Ther. 2015;14(3):810–20.
24. Zhang HH, Yuan TZ, Li J, Liang Y, Huang LJ, Ye JC, et al. Erlotinib: An enhancer of radiation therapy in nasopharyngeal carcinoma. Exp Ther Med. 2013;6(4): 1062–6.
25. Gilbert J, Rudek MA, Higgins MJ, Zhao M, Bienvenu S, Tsottles N, et al. A phase I trial of erlotinib and concurrent chemoradiotherapy for stage III and IV (M0) squamous cell carcinoma of the head and neck. Clin Cancer Res. 2012;18(6):1735–42.
26. Iyengar P, Kavanagh BD, Wardak Z, Smith I, Ahn C, Gerber DE, et al. Phase II trial of stereotactic body radiation therapy combined with erlotinib for patients with limited but progressive metastatic non-small-cell lung cancer. J Clin Oncol. 2014;32(34):3824–30.
27. Lilenbaum R, Samuels M, Wang X, Kong F, Jänne P, Masters G, et al. A phase II study of induction chemotherapy followed by thoracic radiotherapy and erlotinib in poor-risk stage III non-small-cell lung cancer: results of CALGB 30605 (alliance)/RTOG 0972 (NRG). J Thorac Oncol. 2015;10(1):143–7.
28. Li HF, Kim JS, Waldman T. Radiation-induced Akt activation modulates radioresistance in human glioblastoma cells. Radiat Oncol. 2009;4:43.
29. Yip PY. Phosphatidylinositol 3-kinase-AKT-mammalian target of rapamycin (PI3K-akt-mTOR) signaling pathway in non-small cell lung cancer. Transl Lung Cancer Res. 2015;4(2):165–76.
30. Contessa JN, Hampton J, Lammering G, Mikkelsen RB, Dent P, Valerie K, et al. Ionizing radiation activates erb-B receptor dependent akt and p70 S6 kinase signaling in carcinoma cells. Oncogene. 2002;21(25):4032–41.

31. Legare ME, Bush J, Ashley AK, Kato T, Hanneman WH. Cellular and phenotypic characterization of canine osteosarcoma cell lines. J Cancer. 2011;2:262–70.

32. London CA, Bernabe LF, Barnard S, Kisseberth WC, Borgatti A, Henson M, et al. Pre-clinical evaluation of the novel, orally biaoavailable Selective Inhibitor of Nuclear Export (SINE) KPT-335 in spontaneous canine cancer: results of a phase I study. BMC Vet Res. 2014;10:160.

33. Fahey CE, Milner RJ, Kow K, Bacon NJ, Salute ME. Apoptotic effects of the tyrosine kinase inhibitor, masitinib mesylate, on canine osteosarcoma cells. Anticancer Drugs. 2013;24(5):519–26.

34. Harding SM, Hill RP, Bristow RG. Molecular and cellular basis of radiotherapy. In: Tannock IF, Hill RP, Bristow RG, Harrington L, editors. The basic science of oncology. New York: McGraw-Hill Education LLC; 2013. p. 333–55.

35. Thamm DH, O'Brien MG, Vail DM. Serum vascular endothelial growth factor concentrations and postsurgical outcome in dogs with osteosarcoma. Vet Comp Oncol. 2008;6(2):126–32.

36. Chen YH, Pan SL, Wang JC, Kuo SH, Cheng JC, Teng CM. Radiation-induced VEGF-C expression and endothelial cell proliferation in lung cancer. Strahlenther Onkol. 2014;190(12):1154–62.

37. Hovinga KE, Stalpers LJ, van Bree C, Donker M, Verhoeff JJ, Rodermond HM, et al. Radiation-enhanced vascular endothelial growth factor (VEGF) secretion in glioblastoma multiforme cell lines - a clue to radioresistance? J Neurooncol. 2005;74(2):99–103.

38. Flickinger I, Rütgen B, Gerner W, Calice I, Tichy A, Saalmüller A, et al. Radiation up-regulates the expression of VEGF in a canine oral melanoma cell line. J Vet Sci. 2013;14(2):207–14.

39. Sekis I, Gerner W, Willmann M, Rebuzzi L, Tichy A, Patzl M, et al. Effect of radiation on vascular endothelial growth factor expression in the C2 canine mastocytoma cell line. Am J Vet Res. 2009;70(9):1141–50.

40. Tabernero J. The role of VEGF and EGFR inhibition: implications for combining anti-VEGF and anti-EGFR agents. Mol Cancer Res. 2007;5(3):203–20.

41. Li H, Takayama K, Wang S, Shiraishi Y, Gotanda K, Harada T, et al. Addition of bevacizumab enhances antitumor activity of erlotinib against non-small cell lung cancer xenografts depending on VEGF expression. Cancer Chemother Pharmacol. 2014;74(6):1297–305.

42. Oh HY, Kwon SM, Kim SI, Jae YW, Hong SJ. Antiangiogenic effect of ZD1839 against murine renal cell carcinoma (RENCA) in an orthopic mouse model. Urol Int. 2005;75(2):159–66.

2

Canine intrathoracic sarcoma with ultrastructural characteristics of human synovial sarcoma

SER Lovell[1], RK Burchell[2], PJ Roady[3], RL Fredrickson[3] and A Gal[2]* (iD)

Abstract

Background: Canine joint sarcomas, designated synovial sarcomas, are uncommon malignant mesenchymal neoplasms that occur in the large joints of the extremities of middle-aged, large-breed dogs. We report the diagnosis of an intrathoracic sarcoma with ultrastructural characteristics reminiscent of human synovial sarcoma in a dog.

Case presentation: A 7-year-old female spayed Tibetan terrier crossbred dog was presented for acute severe labored breathing and diagnosed with an intrathoracic neoplastic mass. The neoplasm resulted in the accumulation of substantial amounts of viscous pleural fluid that led to dyspnea. The neoplastic mass consisted of interweaving bundles of large pleomorphic mesenchymal cells, supported by an alcian blue positive myxomatous matrix. The neoplastic cells were immunohistochemically negative for cytokeratin and CD18. Transmission electron microscopy indicated that the neoplastic cells had desmosome junctions, short microvilli-like structures and ample amounts of rough endoplasmic reticulum resembling type B-like synoviocytes and synovial sarcoma as reported in people. Despite complete surgical excision of the neoplastic mass, clinical signs recurred after a month and led to the euthanasia of the dog.

Conclusion: Currently, there are no immunohistochemical markers specific for synovial sarcoma. Canine neoplasms with transmission electron microscopy characteristics resembling type B-like synoviocytes should be considered similar to the human sarcomas that carry the specific translocations between chromosomes X and 18.

Keywords: Dog, Synovial sarcoma, Thoracic neoplasm, Transmission electron microscopy

Background

The normal synovial membrane consists of two cell types. The spindloid histiocytic type-A synoviocytes are phagocytic round cells that express the histiocytic immunohistochemical marker CD18. The epitheloid type-B synoviocytes produce the synovial fluid. Currently, there are no immunohistochemical markers specific for the epitheloid type-B synoviocytes [1]. Ultrastructurally, the spindloid histiocytic type-A synoviocytes have many lysosomes, large empty vacuoles, pinocytotic vesicles, prominent Golgi apparatus, and small amounts of rough endoplasmic reticulum [1]. In contrast, the epitheloid type-B synoviocytes have an epithelium-like arrangement with desmosome junctions and basement membrane-like structures [1]. The epitheloid type-B synoviocytes have a large indented nucleus, and small amounts of the cellular cytoplasm containing ample amounts of rough endoplasmic reticulum, limited numbers of vacuoles and vesicles, and a less developed Golgi apparatus. The cytoplasm of type-B synoviocytes also contains microfilaments and intermediate filaments. However, these cells do not consistently stain for the immunohistochemical marker cytokeratin [1].

Pathologists classify synovial sarcomas histologically as monophasic or biphasic if the neoplasms consist of one cell type or both, respectively [2]. However, there is debate as to whether a subset of joint sarcomas are true synovial sarcomas that arise from type-A and type-B synoviocytes. The debate is because of the inability to demonstrate the true origin of the neoplastic cells in the absence of specific immunohistochemical markers for synoviocytes, and also because of the assumption that these neoplasms develop from neoplastic transformation of blood-borne mesenchymal pluripotent cells [3]. To

* Correspondence: a.gal@massey.ac.nz
[2]Institute of Veterinary, Animal and Biomedical Sciences, Massey University, Private Bag 11-222, Palmerston North 4442, New Zealand
Full list of author information is available at the end of the article

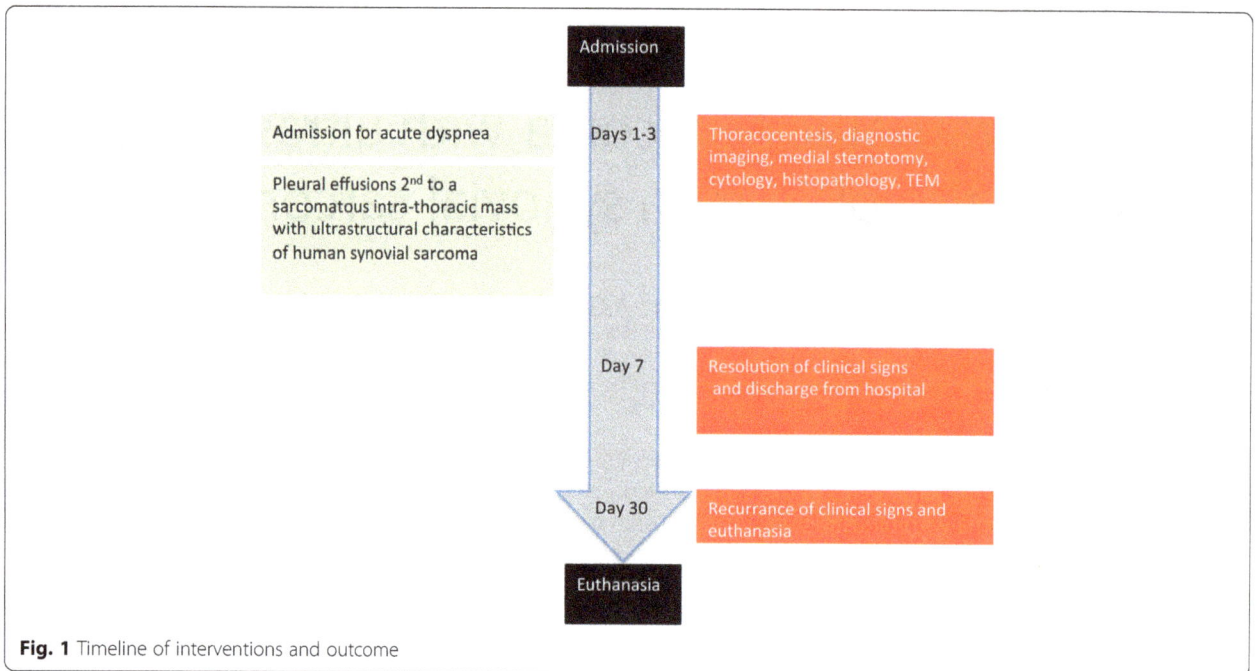

Fig. 1 Timeline of interventions and outcome

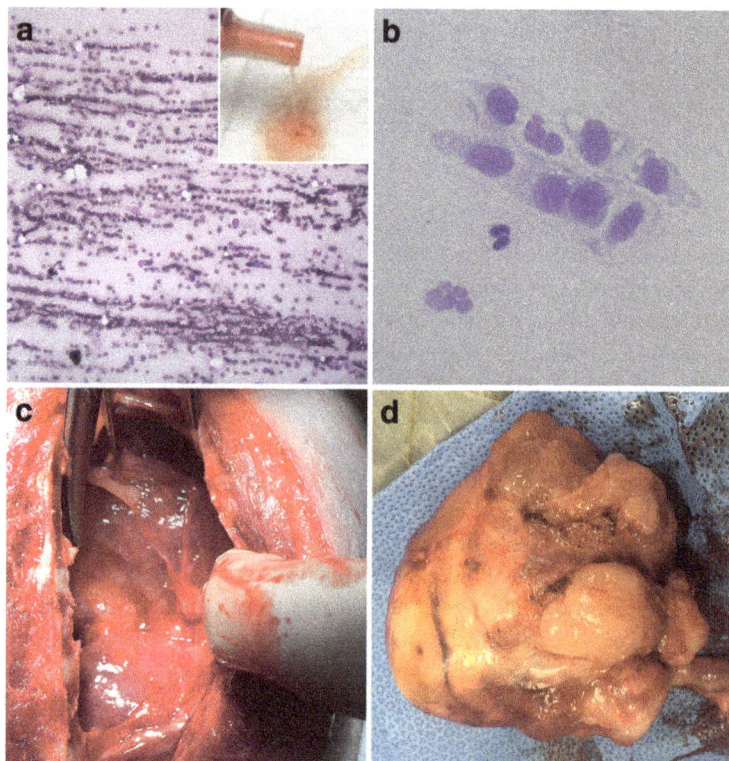

Fig. 2 Presumptive intrathoracic synovial sarcoma, dog, gross and cytological characteristics. **a**, windrowing of the neoplastic cells in a viscous proteinaceous background. Inset, gross characteristics of the pleural fluid. **b**, a small aggregate of neoplastic cells in a pale pink proteinaceous background. The neoplastic cells exhibiting few criteria of malignancy that include high nucleus to cytoplasmic ratio, karyomegaly, anisocytosis and anisokaryosis, and fine chromatin. **c**, intraoperative view of the neoplastic mass. **d**, gross appearance of the neoplastic mass

the authors' knowledge, there are no previous reports of a canine sarcoma with ultrastructural characteristics similar to the human neoplasm designated synovial sarcoma.

Case presentation

The Massey University Pet Emergency Center admitted a 7-year-old female spayed Tibetan terrier crossbred dog in acute respiratory distress (Fig. 1). An emergency thoracocentesis yielded small amounts of highly viscous fluid from the thoracic cavity (Fig. 2a inset). The fluid was thick and sticky, with a nucleated cell count of six cells/µl. The fluid had aggregates of nucleated cells exhibiting 'windrowing' in a coarsely stippled magenta background (Fig. 2a). Differential cell count indicated 64% large mononuclear cells, 30% small mononuclear cells, and 6% neutrophils. The high viscosity of the fluid did not permit the determination of the fluid's protein content. Diagnostic imaging of the chest included thoracic radiographs, thoracic ultrasound, and thoracic computed tomography (Fig. 3). Radiologically, large amounts of pleural fluid expanded the pleural space and severely collapsed the lungs (i.e., pulmonary atelectasis). The left ventral thorax contained a 13 cm long, 7.8 cm tall and 6.4 cm wide complexed cystic mass that extended from the diaphragm to the thoracic inlet and predominantly had peripheral contrast enhancement and variable disorganized contrast enhancing tissue. The mass severely compressed the left caudal lobar bronchus and displaced the trachea. Ultrasonographically, the mass had heterogeneous echogenicity and large amounts of anechoic pleural fluid surrounded the mass. Ultrasound-guided fine needle aspirates were inconclusive. The aspirates contained a few oval cells of a predominantly medium size admixed within a light blue background. The cells had homogenous basophilic cytoplasm and a single large round to oval nucleus with fine chromatin and pin-point sized nucleoli (Fig. 2b). These cells had a high nucleus to cytoplasmic ratio, and moderate anisocytosis and anisokaryosis. To establish a definitive diagnosis, the owner consented to surgery. The thorax was approached via a median sternotomy, and the mass was removed in toto (Fig. 2c, d). The dog recovered uneventfully and was discharged after a week.

Grossly, the mass was pale red to tan, large, firm, and slippery due to copious amounts of viscous fluid that oozed out (Fig. 2d). The cut surface had multifocal depressed soft areas. Histologically, the mass was nonencapsulated and poorly circumscribed, multinodular, densely cellular, and invasive. The neoplastic mesenchymal cells

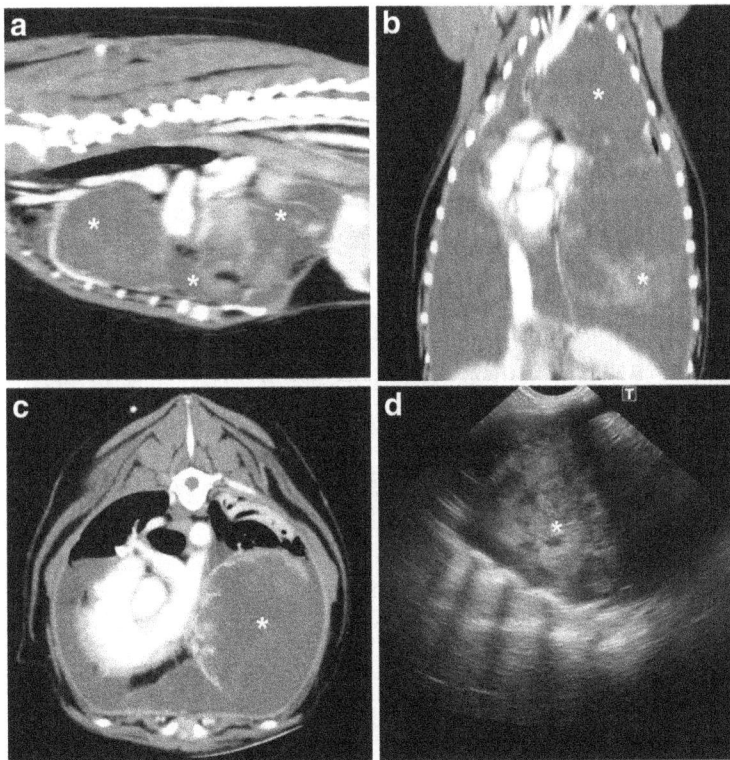

Fig. 3 Presumptive intrathoracic synovial sarcoma, dog, CT. **a**, sagittal plane, post intravenous contrast. **b**, dorsal plane, post intravenous contrast. **c**, transverse plane, post intravenous contrast. **d**, thoracic ultrasonography. A large neoplastic mass of heterogeneous echogenicity is surrounded by pleural anechoic fluid. White asterisks represent the neoplastic mass

formed interlacing bundles, streams (Fig 4a), occasional large perivascular whorls (Fig. 4b), and lined caverns with empty spaces. A dense collagenous mucinous matrix supported the neoplastic cells. The neoplastic cells were large, oval to spindloid, with poorly defined cytoplasmic borders and small amounts of pale eosinophilic to amphophilic cytoplasm. Most neoplastic cells had a single large, round to oval nucleus with vesicular chromatin and 1–3 small basophilic round nucleoli. Occasionally, there were bi-, tri-, and multinucleated neoplastic cells (Fig. 4c). The neoplastic cells had marked anisocytosis, anisokaryosis, and karyomegaly. There were no mitotic figures in ten, 400× fields. Multifocal blood vessels contained intraluminal fibrin thrombi, and there were multifocal areas of hemorrhage and necrosis. The neoplastic matrix stained light blue-green with the histochemical stain alcian blue (pH 2.5)(Fig. 4d). Immunohistochemistry for cytokeratin and CD18 did not stain any of the neoplastic cells.

Transmission electron microscopy indicated that the neoplastic cells had sharply defined ovoid nuclei, with narrow, dense rims of chromatin, small amounts of cytoplasm (Fig. 5a) with large numbers of rough endoplasmic reticulum (Fig. 5b), microfilaments (5–6 nm in diameter), desmosome junctions (Fig. 5c), short microvilli-like structures on the cytoplasmic membrane (Fig. 5d), and intermittent basal membrane.

Based on the combination of the findings above the final diagnosis was presumptive synovial sarcoma of the thoracic cavity, and the long-term prognosis was poor due to high likelihood of recurrence or regrowth of neoplasia and return of clinical signs. One month after the initial presentation, the dog developed severe dyspnea due to recurrence of pleural effusion and was euthanized. The owners opted not to pursue a necropsy.

To the authors' knowledge, this report represents the first case of a presumptive synovial sarcoma with ultrastructural characteristics similar to the human neoplasm designated synovial sarcoma. The neoplastic mass developed within the thorax of an adult small breed dog. The authors based this diagnosis on a combination of supportive evidence. The physical characteristics of the pleural fluid resembled synovial fluid. The cytology of the mass revealed mesenchymal cells in a mucinous background. Histopathology indicated a sarcoma. Histochemistry confirmed the presence of mucin production. The immunohistochemistry ruled out a histiocytic sarcoma or poorly differentiated carcinoma that were the top differential diagnoses. Transmission electron

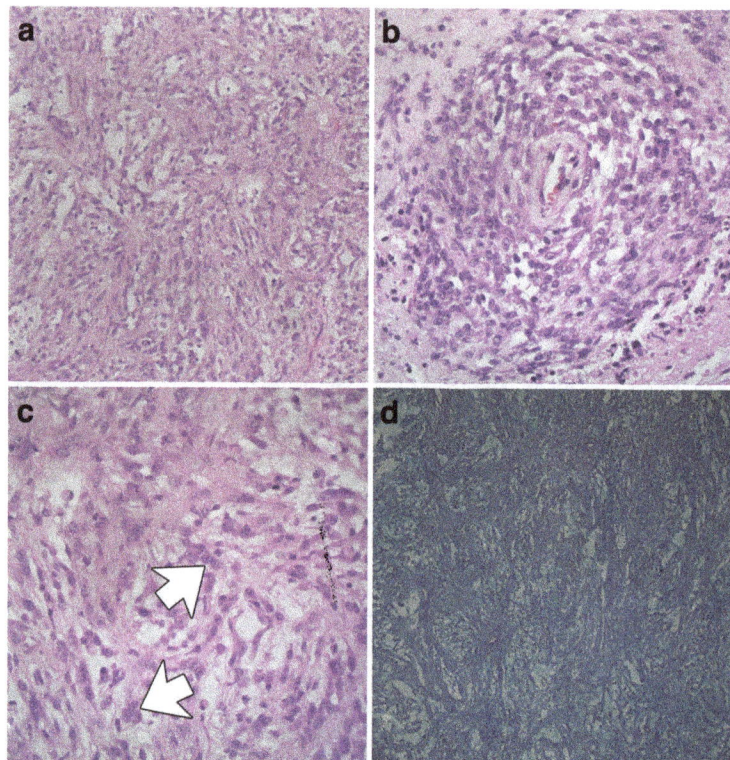

Fig. 4 Presumptive intrathoracic synovial sarcoma, dog, HE and alcian blue (pH 2.5). **a**, the neoplastic cells are arranged in interweaving bundles, 20X magnification. **b**, The neoplastic cells whorls around small blood vessels, 20X magnification. **c**, the neoplastic cells are spindloid to polygonal, have indistinct cytoplasmic borders and a single round nucleus with a prominent nucleolus. Occasional neoplastic cells are multinucleate (white arrows). 40X magnification. **d**, An alcian blue positive blue green stroma supports the neoplastic cells, 20X magnification

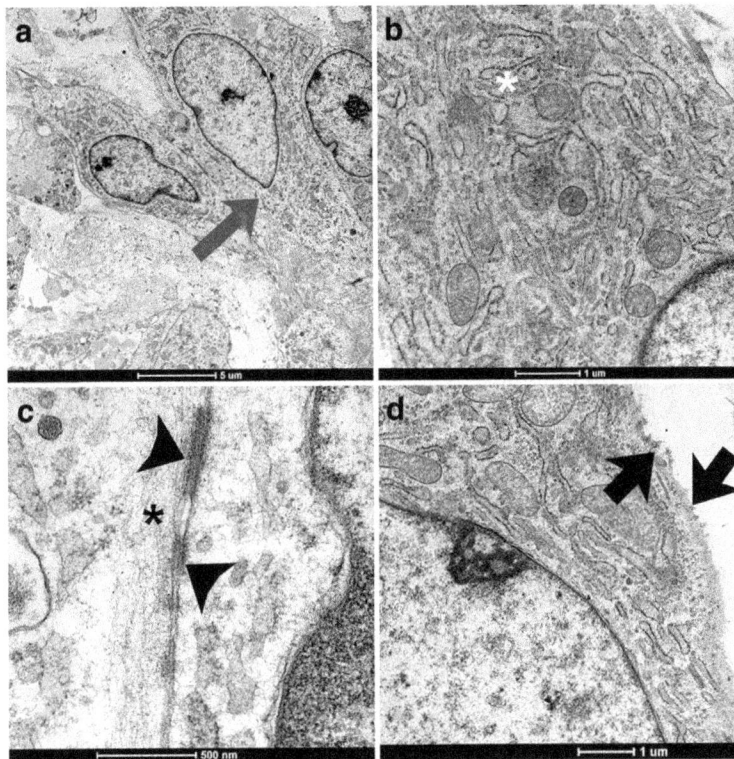

Fig. 5 Presumptive intrathoracic synovial sarcoma, dog, TEM. **a**, a small cluster of cohesive neoplastic cells with a basal membrane between cells (grey arrow). Bar = 5 µm. **b**, the neoplastic cells have large numbers of rough endoplasmic reticulum (white asterisk). Bar = 1 µm. **c**, the neoplastic cells have desmosome junctions (black arrowheads) and microfilaments (black asterisk). Bar = 500 nm. **d**, the neoplastic cells have microvilli-like structures on the cell membrane (black arrows). Bar = 1 µm

microscopy demonstrated cells with ultrastructural features that are consistent with synovial sarcoma in people. These included large numbers of rough endoplasmic reticulum, desmosome junctions, short microvilli-like structures on the cytoplasmic membrane, and a basal membrane (Fig. 5) [4–6].

The subset of joint sarcomas, previously designated synovial sarcomas, are malignant mesenchymal neoplasms that typically occur in the stifle, carpus, and tarsus of the extremities of middle-aged, large-breed dogs [7]. In a retrospective study, synovial sarcomas constituted five out of the 35 of canine synovial tumors [7]. Previous cases of synovial sarcomas include the left elbow of a Rottweiler [8] and the right hindlimb of a cat [9]. To our knowledge, there is only one case report of a synovial sarcoma occurring in non-joint tissue, which was in the subcutaneous region of the left mandible of a dog [10].

The description of intrathoracic sarcomas, designated as synovial sarcomas, has been well documented in the human medical literature [4–6]. Common presenting symptoms include dyspnea, chest pain, cough, and lethargy [4]. The cases from the human medical literature have the same histopathologic and ultrastructural features of the tumor described here [4–6].

In the human medical literature, it is postulated that sarcomas, designated synovial sarcomas, originate from pluripotential mesenchymal cells capable of partial or aberrant epithelial differentiation [3, 5]. If the sarcomas, designated synovial sarcomas, originate from pluripotential mesenchymal cells, it would explain how they could arise in areas such as the thoracic cavity. In the veterinary literature, the development of synovial sarcomas from pluripotential mesenchymal cells is uncertain [11].

In the human pathology literature, sarcomas, designated synovial sarcomas, have monophasic (spindle) and biphasic (spindle and epithelial) forms [3]. The spindle and epithelial components of biphasic synovial sarcomas resemble type A-like and type B-like synoviocytes. In the veterinary field, type A-like synoviocytes are immunohistochemically positive for the CD18 antigen [11]. In contrast, there is no immunohistochemical marker that identifies type B-like synoviocytes [11]. The neoplastic cells, in this case, had ultrastructural characteristics of type B-like synoviocytes and produced viscous fluid with physical characteristics of synovial fluid. Therefore it is plausible that they are derived from pluripotential mesenchymal that differentiated to type B-like synoviocytes.

In people, sarcomas, designated synovial sarcoma, are associated with a specific translocation between chromosomes X and 18 leading to a fusion of the SYT gene on chromosome 18 to the SSX1, SSX2 or SSX4 genes on chromosome X [3, 12]. This translocation occurs in over 90% of synovial sarcomas in people [12]. In situ hybridization detects this specific chromosomal translocation and is considered the gold standard for the diagnosis in people [12]. We did not attempt to perform in situ hybridization in this case, and it remains to be determined if similar translocations occur in dogs.

Conclusion
In conclusion, we describe a spontaneous, aggressive, intrathoracic sarcoma. The neoplasm had cytological, histological and ultrastructural characteristics that are similar to the human sarcomas that carry the specific translocations between chromosomes X and 18. This report contributes to expanding the body of knowledge on these sarcomas in dogs.

Abbreviations
CD: Cluster of differentiation

Acknowledgements
The authors would like to thank Dr. Sandra Forsyth for the evaluation and interpretation of the cytologic specimens, Dr. Bob Bahr for evaluation of the CT images, Dr. Jon Bray for performing the surgery, and Miss Jordan Taylor who performed the transmission electron microscopy.

Funding
The authors declare that any funding did not support this study.

Authors' contributions
All authors read and approved the final manuscrip t. SER-L This author wrote the manuscript, and managed the case. RK-B This author wrote and critically reviewed the manuscript, and had critical input in the case management. PJ-R This author performed and the immunohistochemistry and helped writing the manuscript. RL-F This author performed and the immunohistochemistry. A-G This author wrote the manuscript, managed the case, and read the histopathology, histochemistry, and transmission electron microscopy.

Consent for publication
Not applicable

Competing interests
The author(s) declared no potential conflicts of interest with respect to the research, authorship, and publication of this article.

Author details
[1]Animal Referral Centre, Auckland, New Zealand. [2]Institute of Veterinary, Animal and Biomedical Sciences, Massey University, Private Bag 11-222, Palmerston North 4442, New Zealand. [3]Veterinary Diagnostic Laboratory, University of Illinois at Urbana-Champaign, Springfield, IL, USA.

References
1. Iwanaga T, Shikichi M, Kitamura H, Yanase H, Nozawa-Inoue K. Morphology and functional roles of synoviocytes in the joint. Arch Histol Cytol. 2000;63(1):17–31.
2. Fox DB, Cook JL, Kreeger JM, Beissenherz M, Henry CJ. Canine synovial sarcoma: a retrospective assessment of described prognostic criteria in 16 cases (1994-1999). J Am Anim Hosp Assoc. 2002;38(4):347–55.
3. Thway K, Fisher C. Synovial sarcoma: defining features and diagnostic evolution. Ann Diagn Pathol. 2014;18(6):369–80.
4. Essary LR, Vargas SO, Fletcher CD. Primary pleuropulmonary synovial sarcoma: reappraisal of a recently described anatomic subset. Cancer. 2002;94(2):459–69.
5. Suster S, Moran CA. Primary synovial sarcomas of the mediastinum: a clinicopathologic, immunohistochemical, and ultrastructural study of 15 cases. Am J Surg Pathol. 2005;29(5):569–78.
6. Hirano H, Kizaki T, Sashikata T, Maeda T, Yoshii Y, Mori H. Synovial sarcoma arising from the pleura: a case report with ultrastructural and immunohistological studies. Med Electron Microsc. 2002;35(2):102–8.
7. Craig LE, Julian ME, Ferracone JD. The diagnosis and prognosis of synovial tumors in dogs: 35 cases. Vet Pathol. 2002;39(1):66–73.
8. Loukopoulos P, Heng HG, Arshad H. Canine biphasic synovial sarcoma: case report and immunohistochemical characterization. J Vet Sci. 2004;5(2):173–80.
9. Cazzini P, Frontera-Acevedo K, Garner B, Howerth E, Torres B, Northrup N, Sakamoto K. Morphologic, molecular, and ultrastructural characterization of a feline synovial cell sarcoma and derived cell line. J Vet Diagn Investig. 2015;27(3):369–76.
10. Takimoto N, Suzuki K, Ogawa T, Segawa R, Hara S, Itahashi M, Kimura M, Iwasaki N, Nishifuji K, Shibutani M. A non-joint tissue biphasic synovial sarcoma in a dog. J Comp Pathol. 2014;150(2–3):204–7.
11. Craig LE, Dittmer KE, Thompson KG. Bones and joints. In: Maxie MG, editor. Pathology of domestic animals. 6th ed. St. Louis, MO: Elsevier; 2016. p. 159.
12. Eilber FC, Dry SM. Diagnosis and management of synovial sarcoma. J Surg Oncol. 2008;97(4):314–20.

3

Significance of EZH2 expression in canine mammary tumors

Hyun-Ji Choi[1,2], Sungwoong Jang[1,2], Jae-Eun Ryu[1,2], Hyo-Ju Lee[1,2], Han-Byul Lee[1,2], Woo-Sung Ahn[1], Hye-Jin Kim[2], Hyo-Jin Lee[2], Hee Jin Lee[2], Gyung-Yub Gong[2] and Woo-Chan Son[1,2]*

Abstract

Background: Current studies report that aberrations in epigenetic regulators or chromatin modifications are related to tumor development and maintenance. EZH2 (Enhancer of zeste homolog 2) is one of the catalytic subunits of Polycomb repressive complex 2, a crucial epigenetic regulator. EZH2 has a master regulatory function in such processes as cell proliferation, stem cell differentiation, and early embryogenesis. In humans, EZH2 is linked to oncogenic function in several carcinomas, including breast cancer, and dysregulation of EZH2 has been particularly associated with loss of differentiation and the development of poorly differentiated breast cancer. In our present study, we were interested in determining whether EZH2 is increased in canine mammary tumors, which show similarities to human breast cancer.

Results: Investigation of the expression of EZH2 in canine mammary tumors revealed that EZH2 protein was overexpressed in canine mammary carcinomas, as in human breast cancer. In addition, the immunohistochemical expression level of EZH2 was associated with the degree of malignancy in canine mammary carcinoma. This is the first report to describe EZH2 expression in canine mammary tumors.

Conclusions: Because the expression of EZH2 was similar in canine mammary carcinoma and human breast cancer, spontaneous canine mammary tumors may be a suitable model for studying EZH2 and treatment development.

Keywords: Dog, Canine mammary tumor, EZH2, Comparative oncology

Background

Breast cancer is expected to be the most common malignancy among women in the United States in 2015 [1]. Although several prognostic markers in human breast cancer have been investigated, only a small number of markers are in clinical use, possibly because of a poor correlation between the findings of animal studies and clinical trials. Therefore, there is a need for more appropriate therapeutic targets and additional models to improve the understanding and biological characterization of human breast cancer and therapeutic development.

EZH2 is a catalytic subunit of the epigenetic regulator Polycomb repressive complex 2 (PRC2). PRC2, which includes EZH2, suppressor of zeste 12 (SUZ12), and embryonic ectoderm development (EED), trimethylates

histone 3 lysine residue 27 (H3K27) and leads to silencing of genes involved in processes such as stem cell maintenance and tumor progression without DNA sequence modification [2–4]. Recently, overexpression or mutation of EZH2 have been found in a wide range of human tumors, including breast, prostate, urinary bladder, ovarian, lung, gastric cancer, renal cell carcinoma, and glioblastoma [5–12]. The evidence indicates that EZH2 plays a role in the initiation, development, progression, and metastasis of cancer and drug resistance [13]. In particular, EZH2 has been connected to the aggressiveness of breast cancer [14, 15]. In addition, EZH2 has been reported to be an adverse prognostic marker for breast cancer and an index of an unfavorable tamoxifen outcome [16–18]. A correlation between loss of differentiation and deregulated expression of EZH2 has also been proposed in human breast cancer [19]. Recent evidence implicates EZH2 in transcriptional activation, but the mechanisms are not clearly defined [20].

* Correspondence: wcson@amc.seoul.kr
[1]Asan Institute for Life Sciences, Asan Medical Center, Seoul, Republic of Korea
[2]Department of Pathology, University of Ulsan College of Medicine, Asan Medical Center, 88 Olympic-ro 43-gil, Songpa-gu, Seoul 138-736, South Korea

In order to investigate the feasibility of an additional animal model to improve our understanding of EZH2, we collected and investigated naturally occurring canine mammary tumors (CMTs). Mammary tumors are the most commonly diagnosed neoplasms in female dogs and nearly 50 % are malignant [21, 22]. One study has found an annual incidence of mammary tumors of 16.8–47.7 % (benign) and 47.5 % (malignant) [23]. This incidence is greater than that of human breast cancers. Dog and human lineages are similar in terms of both nucleotide divergence and rearrangements [24] and dogs have been suggested as additional tumor models [25, 26]. Although histomorphological features may differ between human breast cancer and CMTs, they share many similarities in terms of age of onset, risk factors, molecular marker expression, behavior, and prognosis [27–30]. In addition, the incidence of CMTs is sufficiently high to secure proper number of subjects in clinical trials and the size of dogs makes multimodality protocols feasible [31]. Therefore, it is expected that the study of cancer using mammary tumors of domesticated dog might provide new insights into cancer understanding and therapy development.

The purpose of our present study was to investigate EZH2 in CMTs. We found that EZH2 is overexpressed in clinical samples of canine mammary carcinomas.

Results

Histological evaluation

The clinical and morphologic features of the 74 mammary gland cases were identified (Table 1). There were five non-neoplastic lesions including lobular hyperplasia and duct ectasia. Sixty-nine CMT cases showed benign morphological features (3 cases, 4 %) and malignant features (66 cases, 96 %) such as carcinoma with simple tubular or tubulopapillary type, complex type, mixed type, solid type, anaplastic and inflammatory carcinoma, mucinous carcinoma, lipid-rich carcinoma, and comedo-carcinoma (Fig. 1). The most common type of carcinoma identified was the complex type (26 cases, 39 %), followed by mixed type (18 cases, 27 %) and simple tubular type (12 cases, 18 %). Canine mammary carcinomas exhibited a malignancy ranging from 1–3 as follows: 1 (38 cases, 58 %), 2 (18 cases, 27 %), and 3 (10 cases, 15 %).

Immunohistochemistry

We were interested in determining whether EZH2 is dysregulated in CMTs, which are similar to human breast cancers. In immunohistochemical analyses, there was negative or weak nuclear staining in normal (Fig. 2a) and non-neoplastic mammary tissues. Clear nuclear staining for EZH2 could be observed in CMTs (Fig. 2b-f). The intensity of nuclear pattern was especially strong in comedocarcinoma (Fig. 2e), anaplastic carcinoma (Fig. 2f), and solid carcinoma. Carcinomas showed higher EZH2 expression level than hyperplastic lesions (Fig. 3). High expression of EZH2 was found to be associated with mammary carcinoma malignancy (Table 2, Fig. 4). We sorted each grade of carcinomas according to the expression level of EZH2 to clarify the association between grade of malignancy and EZH2 expression. Malignancy grade 1 was found in 2 cases (5 %) of EZH2 score 0,19 (50 %) of EZH2 score 1, 16 (42 %) of EZH2 score 2, and 1 (3 %) of EZH2 score 3. Malignancy grade 2 was seen in 3 cases (17 %) of EZH2 score 1, 7

Table 1 Demographics of canine mammary cases

Type	Non-neoplastic lesion			Benign tumor	Malignant tumor					
	Hyperplasia	Ectasia	Total	Adenoma	Complex type	Mixed type	Tubular type	Anaplastic carcinoma	Comedo-carcinoma	Total
Total	4	1	5	3	26	18	12	3	2	61
Mean age, year	8	14	9	6	11	10	10	12	10	11
Malignancy grade, no.										
1	-	-	-	-	15	15	7	0	0	37
2	-	-	-	-	9	1	4	1	0	15
3	-	-	-	-	2	2	1	2	2	9
Mean	-	-	-	-	1.5	1.3	1.5	2.7	3	1.5
EZH2 score, no.										
0	1	1	2	0	0	1	0	0	0	1
1	2	0	2	2	8	9	4	0	0	21
2	1	0	1	1	12	6	4	2	0	24
3	0	0	0	0	6	2	4	1	2	15
Mean	1	0	0.8	1.3	1.9	1.5	2	2.3	3	1.9

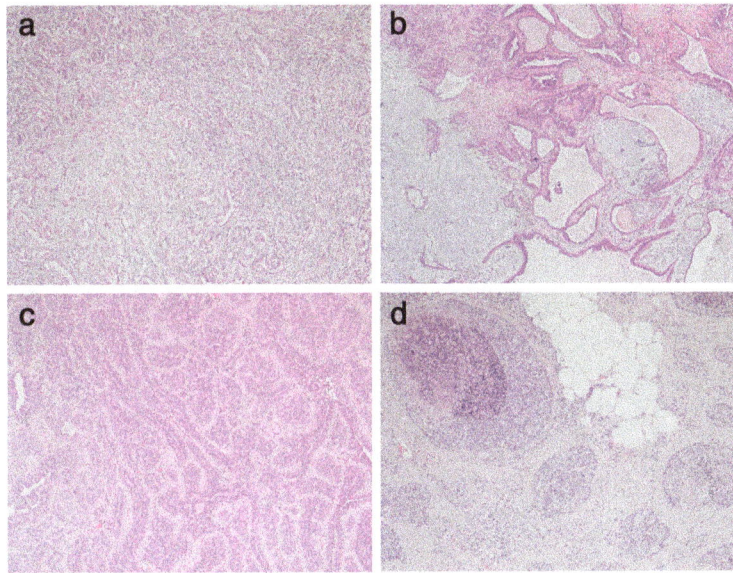

Fig. 1 Representative mammary carcinoma tissues with H&E staining. **a** Carcinoma complex type with a malignant epithelial component and a benign myoepithelial component. **b** Carcinoma mixed type with a malignant epithelial component and a benign mesenchymal component (cartilage). **c** Carcinoma, tubular type. The tumor cells are predominantly arranged in a tubular pattern. **d** Comedocarcinoma. There are necrotic areas within the center of neoplastic cell aggregates

(39 %) of EZH2 score 2, and 8 (44 %) of EZH2 score 3. Malignancy grade 3 was present in no cases of EZH2 score 1, 2 (20 %) of EZH2 score 2, and 8 (80 %) of EZH2 score 3. According to these criteria, 99 % cases of CMTs had elevated EZH2 expression. It did not show any relationship within the most frequent three carcinoma types (Complex, mixed and tubular type) of this study (Fig. 5).

Western blotting

We used immunoblotting to compare our immunohisto-chemistry and molecular data and further investigate the correlations between the grade of malignancy and the expression levels of EZH2. Western blot analysis showed an increase in the expression of EZH2 in the CMT tissues compared with control non-neoplastic mammary tissues. Grade 3 carcinomas showed higher expression of EZH2 than grades 1 and 2 (Fig. 6, Table 3).

Discussion

Although increased expression of EZH2 has been observed in aggressive solid tumors in humans, the mechanism involved in the mediation of tumor aggressiveness by EZH2 remains unclear. In our current study, we characterized the expression pattern of EZH2 in CMTs by immunohistochemical staining and immunoblot analysis of CMTs and non-neoplastic mammary tissues. We found that EZH2 protein is increased in CMTs when compared with non-neoplastic mammary tissues. In our immunohistochemical analysis, tumor cells exhibited a

clear nuclear staining pattern with various expression levels. When we compared EZH2 expression level with the tumor malignancy grade, type of carcinoma, and type of lesion (hyperplasia/adenoma/carcinoma) respectively, only carcinoma malignancy was found to have statistically significant association with EZH2 expression. The proportion of positive EZH2 staining increased as the malignancy grade increased. Furthermore, there was strong nuclear staining in anaplastic carcinoma, comedocarcinoma which are regarded as high malignant neoplasms between CMTs, and solid carcinoma which reveals poor differentiation. These results are consistent with a previous report that showed a correlation between the EZH2 expression level and aggressiveness or poor differentiation of human breast cancer [15, 19].

We compared the immunohistochemistry results with the immunoblotting results. EZH2 protein showed a higher expression level in grade 3 than grade 1 mammary cancers. There were some results that were inconsistent with the tendency for EZH2 expression to increase with malignancy. First, the number of cases was small and not enough to produce a powerful statistic. We also suspected that one of the reasons for these discrepancies is that there is usually prominent proliferation of the surrounding connective tissue or stroma in CMT tissue. Therefore, homogenization of a small portion of tissue does not always adequately represent the epithelial tumorous component. Nonetheless, there was a tendency for an increased expression of EZH2 with CMT malignancy evident in the immunoblotting

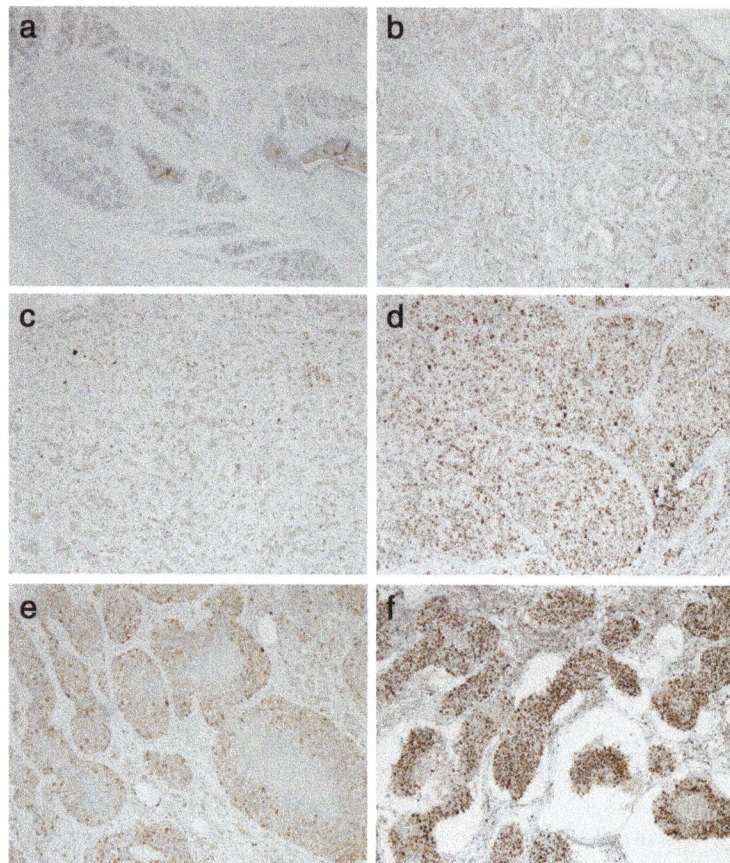

Fig. 2 Immunohistchemistry for EZH2. **a** Normal mammary gland. Immunohistchemistry for EZH2 showing negative staining of the mammary gland. **b** Adenoma. The intensity score of EZH2 is 1. **c** Carcinoma mixed type with malignancy grade 1. The intensity score of EZH2 is 1. **d** Carcinoma solid type with malignancy grade 3. Diffuse nuclear staining with the intensity score 3 of EZH2. **e** Comedocarcinoma. The intensity score of EZH2 is 3. **f** Anaplastic carcinoma. Note the strong nuclear staining of neoplastic cells with intensity score 3 of EZH2

results, which was consistent with the immunohisto-chemistry results. We found no correlation between the carcinoma type and the level of EZH2 expression, possibly due to the relatively small number of samples of each type of carcinoma.

Murine models such as xenograft and transgenic mouse models have been extremely useful tools in the study of human cancer and have provided valuable insights into cancer biology and biochemistry that could not be readily obtained with other models [32]. Despite the importance of these murine models, they have shown a few limitations with respect to some essential features of human cancer, including growth periods, immune function, genomic characterization, and the

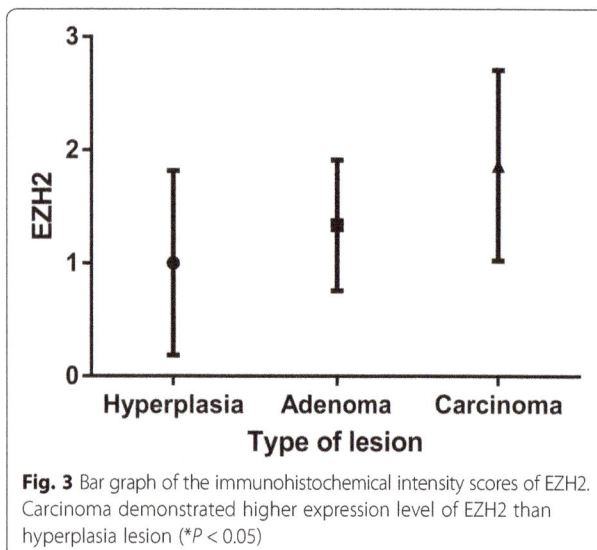

Fig. 3 Bar graph of the immunohistochemical intensity scores of EZH2. Carcinoma demonstrated higher expression level of EZH2 than hyperplasia lesion ($*P < 0.05$)

Table 2 Correlation between malignancy grade and EZH2 score

Malignancy grade	EZH2 score
1	1.4 ± 0.64
2	2.3 ± 0.77
3	2.8 ± 0.42

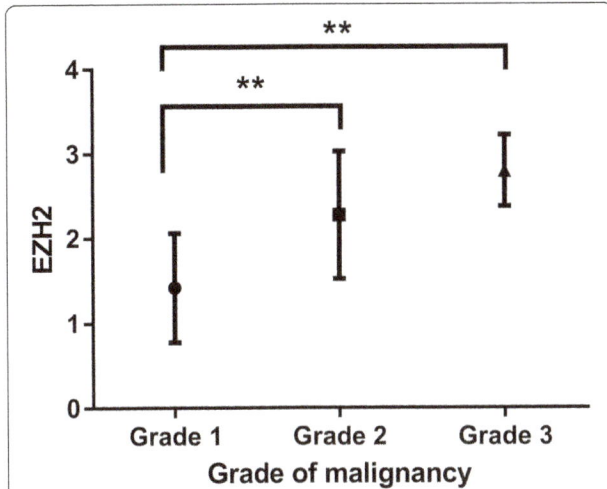

Fig. 4 Bar graph of the immunohistochemical intensity scores of EZH2. High malignancy grade tumor showed higher expression level of EZH2 than low grade tumor (**$P < 0.01$)

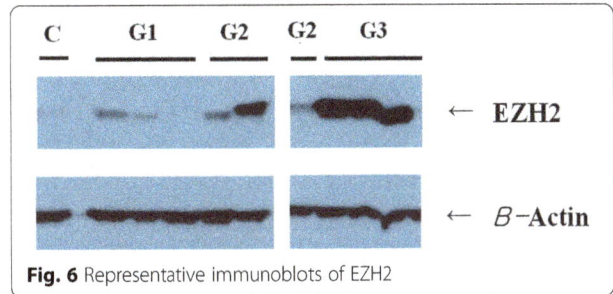

Fig. 6 Representative immunoblots of EZH2

significant heterogeneity of tumor cells and microenvironments. Even in recently developed patient-derived xenograft models, a higher mutation rate than would arise in the parent tumor, a variable transplantation failure rate, as well as increased costs are major challenges of this approach [33]. Accordingly, dogs with naturally occurring tumors are expected to provide an additional value to researchers.

As the CMTs in our current study in a canine model showed similarities to human breast cancers in terms of EZH2 expression, we suggest that dogs with naturally occurring CMTs could be used as animal models in future clinical trials. Canine tumor models may help to identify novel cancer-associated genes, further elucidate molecular pathways in tumors, and be used in the development of novel diagnostic, prognostic, and therapeutic tools [24].

No EZH2 inhibitors have been approved for the treatment of human cancers to date. The methyltransferase activity of EZH2 is not required for it to activate certain genes. Therefore, approaches based on disrupting the interaction between EZH2 and other factors might be potential therapeutic targets [2]. Because EZH2 plays a diverse role in cancers, insight into the regulation of its signaling would likely aid the development of EZH2-targeted therapeutics. EZH2 inhibitors are currently being developed and clinical trials for B cell lymphoma are ongoing [34, 35].

To our knowledge, our current study is the first to report on the expression of EZH2 in CMTs. Our results lend credence to the view that CMTs are a valuable model for EZH2 studies. However, we have only just begun to understand the biology and functional role of EZH2 in CMTs, and we look forward to studies aimed at further elucidating the mechanisms involved.

Conclusions

EZH2 is expressed in CMTs, and its levels correlate with carcinoma malignancy.

This leads to a possibility of CMT usage as a model for future EZH2 research and clinical trials on breast cancer.

Methods
Tissue samples

Mammary gland samples were collected from 74 female domestic dogs who had been seen at a veterinary clinic due to a mass in the mammary gland. The canine mammary tissues were surgically removed from these animals at a mean age of 12 years (7–15 years) and were submitted

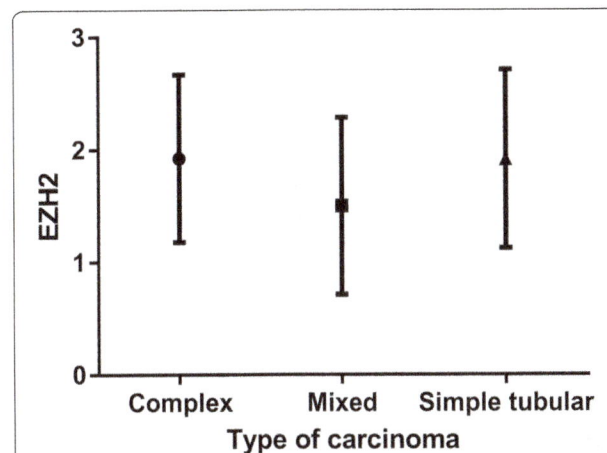

Fig. 5 Bar graph of the immunohistochemical intensity scores of EZH2. There is no significant difference between three types of carcinoma

Table 3 Semi-quantification of western blotting

Group	EZH2/β-actin
Control	1.0
Grade 1	1.4
Grade 2	2.0
Grade 3	2.7

to the University of Ulsan College of Medicine between June 2014 and May 2015. After microscopic examination, 5 samples were diagnosed as non-neoplastic lesions and 69 specimens were diagnosed as CMTs.

Histological evaluation

Slides were evaluated for growth pattern (ductular, papillary, or solid), invasion pattern (expansile, local, regional, nodal, or vascular), mitotic index, degree of necrosis, anaplasia, and inflammation. The morphologic diagnosis of CMT was based on the classification of Goldschidt et al. [36] Using this approach, the classification of benign mammary tumors includes adenoma simple, intraductal papillary adenoma, ductal adenoma, adenoma complex, benign mixed, fibroadenoma, and myoepithelioma. Malignant classifications include carcinoma simple, carcinoma complex, carcinoma mixed, anaplastic carcinoma, lipid-rich carcinoma, inflammatory carcinoma, mucinous carcinoma, and adenosquamous carcinoma. The carcinoma simple class has tubular, tubulopapillary, cystic-papillary, and cribriform subclasses. Tumors that were too poorly differentiated to be morphologically diagnosed were classified as solid carcinomas. Malignancy was evaluated using the following criteria: tumor type, tumor size, tubular formation pattern, significant nuclear and cellular pleomorphism, mitotic index (number of cells with mitotic figures per 10 high-power fields from the neoplastic area with mitotic activity), and presence of areas of necrosis [22]. All samples were also classified according to their morphologic origin. All microscopic evaluations were performed by two veterinary pathologists.

Immunohistochemistry

Sections (3 μm) from paraffin-embedded tissue blocks of canine mammary gland tumor tissues were mounted on glass slides. Immunohistochemistry was performed using an automated slide preparation system (Benchmark XT; Ventana Medical Systems Inc., Tucson, AZ). Deparaffinization, epitope retrieval, and immunostaining were performed according to the manufacturer's instructions with cell conditioning solutions (standard, for 60 min) and the BMK ultraVIEW diaminobenzidine detection system (Ventana Medical Systems). Tumor sections were stained with EZH2 (1:100, ab109398, Abcam, Cambridge, MA) for 36 min at 37 °C, followed by Ultraview HRP universal Multimer for 8 min at 37 °C. Positive signals were amplified using ultraVIEW copper, and sections were counterstained with hematoxylin and bluing reagent for 4 min respectively.

Immunohistochemical Evaluation of EZH2

EZH2 expression was evaluated on the slides using a semiquantitative scoring system described previously with some modifications [10]. Samples were evaluated for staining intensity (0, none; 1, weakly positive; 2, moderately positive; and 3, strongly positive).

SDS-PAGE and western blot

Approximately 10 mg of CMT tissue were prepared by TissueLyser II (Qiagen, Valencia, CA) and suspended in sample buffer (62 mmol/liter Tris-Cl, pH 6.8, 2 % SDS, 10 % glycerol, and 0.01 % bromophenol blue with 5 % 2-mercaptoethanol), incubated for 5 min at 100 °C, and then electrophoretically separated in a 12 % polyacrylamide mini-gel. Electrophoresis was performed in Tris-buffered saline (TBS) at a constant current of 60 mA for 2 h. Molecular weight standards (P8502-050; GenDEPOT) were run simultaneously. The gel was stained with Coomassie Blue. A parallel SDS-PAGE gel was run as described above, and the separated proteins were transferred directly by tank blotting onto a polyvinyl difluoride transfer membrane (Bio-Rad Corp, Hercules, CA) for 90 min at a constant current of 80 mA. After saturation of the nonspecific sites with 5 % nonfat milk/TBS overnight at 4 °C, the proteins were probed with a 1:500 dilution of rabbit anti-EZH2 antibody (ab186006; Abcam, Cambridge, MA) overnight at 4 °C. The blot was then washed in 20 mM Tris-HCl, pH 7.5, and 0.14 mM NaCl containing 0.5 % Tween 20 (TBS-Tween) and then incubated for 2 h in an anti-rabbit HRP-conjugated IgG antibody (SC-2004; Santa Cruz, Santa Cruz, CA) diluted 1:1000 in TBS-Tween at room temperature. The immunoblot was exposed to an enhanced chemiluminescence immunoassay substrate reagent (DG-WP250; DoGen, Seoul, Korea) for 1 min to detect signals and the membrane was exposed to X-ray film for 5 min. Band intensity on exposed film was semi-quantified using ImageJ software (National Institutes of Health, Bethesda, MD).

Statistical analysis

Data are expressed as the mean ± standard deviation of the mean. Since our data were not normally distributed in the Kolmogorov-Smirnov test, we compared the data with the Kruskal-Wallis test, which is a non-parametric method using the SPSS version 21 (IBM Corp., Armonk, NY). If significant, paired comparisons were done with the Mann Whitney test. A Bonferronic correction was applied to correct for multiple comparisons of the primary end point.

Abbreviations

CMTs, canine mammary tumors; EED, embryonic ectoderm development; EZH2, enhancer of zeste homolog 2; H3K27, histone 3 lysine residue 27; PRC2, polycomb repressive complex 2; SUZ12, suppressor of zeste 12

Acknowledgements

This study was supported by IICR (Institute for Innovative Cancer Research) and CACT (Center for Advancing Cancer Therapeutics).

Funding

This study was supported by grants from the Korean Health Technology Research and Development Project, Ministry of Health and Welfare, Republic of Korea (grant numbers: HI10C2014 and HI06C0868).

Authors' contributions

HC carried out the histopathological evaluation, immunohistochemistry and contributed to the drafting of the article. SJ performed immunohistochemistry and immunohistochemical evaluation. JR, HL1 (Hyo-Ju Lee) and HL2 (Han-Byul Lee) participated in the histopathological evaluation. WA carried out the western blot assay. HK, HL3 (Hyo-Jin Lee) assisted in experimental performance. HL4 (Hee Jin Lee), GG participated in the design of the study. WS conceived the study, and participated in its design and coordination, and contributed to the interpretation of the overall results. All authors read and approved the final manuscript.

Competing interests

The authors declare that they have no competing interests.

Consent for publication

Not applicable.

References

1. Siegel RL, Miller KD, Jemal A. Cancer statistics, 2015. CA Cancer J Clin. 2015;65(1):5–29.
2. Li LY. EZH2: novel therapeutic target for human cancer. Biomedicine (Taipei). 2014;4:1.
3. Chase A, Cross NC. Aberrations of EZH2 in cancer. Clin Cancer Res. 2011; 17(9):2613–8.
4. Volkel P, Dupret B, Le Bourhis X, Angrand PO. Diverse involvement of EZH2 in cancer epigenetics. Am J Transl Res. 2015;7(2):175–93.
5. Sun F, Chan E, Wu Z, Yang X, Marquez VE, Yu Q. Combinatorial pharmacologic approaches target EZH2-mediated gene repression in breast cancer cells. Mol Cancer Ther. 2009;8(12):3191–202.
6. Zhang JX, Chen LY, Han L, Shi ZD, Zhang JN, Pu PY, et al. EZH2 is a negative prognostic factor and exhibits pro-oncogenic activity in glioblastoma. Cancer Lett. 2015;356(2):929–36.
7. Xiao Y. Enhancer of zeste homolog 2: a potential target for tumor therapy. Int J Biochem Cell Biol. 2011;43(4):474–7.
8. Varambally S, Dhanasekaran SM, Zhou M, Barrette TR, Kumar-Sinha C, Sanda MG, et al. The polycomb group protein EZH2 is involved in progression of prostate cancer. Nature. 2002;419(6907):624–9.
9. Collett K, Eide GE, Arnes J, Stefansson IM, Eide J, Braaten A, et al. Expression of enhancer of zeste homologue 2 is significantly associated with increased tumor cell proliferation and is a marker of aggressive breast cancer. Clin Cancer Res. 2006;12(4):1168–74.
10. Bachmann IM, Halvorsen OJ, Collett K, Stefansson IM, Straume O, Haukaas SA, et al. EZH2 expression is associated with high proliferation rate and aggressive tumor subgroups in cutaneous melanoma and cancers of the endometrium, prostate, and breast. J Clin Oncol. 2006;24(2):268–73.
11. Wang H, Albadine R, Magheli A, Guzzo TJ, Ball MW, Hinz S, et al. Increased EZH2 protein expression is associated with invasive urothelial carcinoma of the bladder. Urol Oncol. 2012;30(4):428–33.
12. Li H, Cai Q, Godwin AK, Zhang RG. Enhancer of Zeste Homolog 2 promotes the proliferation and invasion of epithelial ovarian cancer cells. Mol Cancer Res. 2010;8(12):1610–8.
13. Yamaguchi H, Hung MC. Regulation and role of EZH2 in cancer. Cancer Res Treat. 2014;46(3):209–22.
14. Moore HM. The Role of EZH2 in Breast Cancer Progression and Metastasis: University of Michigan; 2013. PhD Thesis.
15. Kleer CG, Cao Q, Varambally S, Shen R, Ota I, Tomlins SA, et al. EZH2 is a marker of aggressive breast cancer and promotes neoplastic transformation of breast epithelial cells. Proc Natl Acad Sci U S A. 2003;100(20):11606–11.
16. Reijm EA, Jansen MP, Ruigrok-Ritstier K, van Staveren IL, Look MP, van Gelder ME, et al. Decreased expression of EZH2 is associated with upregulation of ER and favorable outcome to tamoxifen in advanced breast cancer. Breast Cancer Res Treat. 2011;125(2):387–94.
17. Reijm EA, Timmermans AM, Look MP, Meijer-van Gelder ME, Stobbe CK, van Deurzen CH, et al. High protein expression of EZH2 is related to unfavorable outcome to tamoxifen in metastatic breast cancer. Ann Oncol. 2014;25(11):2185–90.
18. Roh S, Park SY, Ko HS, Sohn JS, Cha EJ. EZH2 expression in invasive lobular carcinoma of the breast. World J Surg Oncol. 2013;11:299.
19. Raaphorst FM, Meijer CJ, Fieret E, Blokzijl T, Mommers E, Buerger H, et al. Poorly differentiated breast carcinoma is associated with increased expression of the human polycomb group EZH2 gene. Neoplasia. 2003;5(6):481–8.
20. Gonzalez ME, Moore HM, Li X, Toy KA, Huang W, Sabel MS, et al. EZH2 expands breast stem cells through activation of NOTCH1 signaling. Proc Natl Acad Sci U S A. 2014;111(8):3098–103.
21. Moe L. Population-based incidence of mammary tumours in some dog breeds. J Reprod Fertil Suppl. 2001;57:439–43.
22. Meuten DJ. Tumors in domestic animals. 4th ed. Ames, Iowa: Iowa State University Press; 2002.
23. Salas Y, Marquez A, Diaz D, Romero L. Epidemiological study of mammary tumors in female dogs diagnosed during the period 2002-2012: a growing animal health problem. PLoS One. 2015;10(5):e0127381.
24. Kung AL. Practices and pitfalls of mouse cancer models in drug discovery. Adv Cancer Res. 2007;96:191–212.
25. Macewen EG. Spontaneous tumors in dogs and cats - models for the study of cancer biology and treatment. Cancer Metastasis Rev. 1990;9(2):125–36.
26. Paoloni M, Khanna C. Translation of new cancer treatments from pet dogs to humans. Nat Rev Cancer. 2008;8(2):147–56.
27. Vinothini G, Balachandran C, Nagini S. Evaluation of molecular markers in canine mammary tumors: correlation with histological grading. Oncol Res. 2009;18(5-6):193–201.
28. Queiroga FL, Raposo T, Carvalho MI, Prada J, Pires I. Canine mammary tumours as a model to study human breast cancer: most recent findings. In Vivo. 2011;25(3):455–65.
29. Borge KS, Nord S, Van Loo P, Lingjaerde OC, Gunnes G, Alnaes GI, et al. Canine mammary tumours are affected by frequent copy number aberrations, including amplification of MYC and loss of PTEN. PLoS One. 2015;10(5):e0126371.
30. Strandberg JD, Goodman DG. Animal model of human disease: canine mammary neoplasia. Am J Pathol. 1974;75(1):225–8.
31. Ranieri G, Gadaleta CD, Patruno R, Zizzo N, Daidone MG, Hansson MG, et al. A model of study for human cancer: spontaneous occurring tumors in dogs. Biological features and translation for new anticancer therapies. Crit Rev Oncol Hematol. 2013;88(1):187–97.
32. Pinho SS, Carvalho S, Cabral J, Reis CA, Gartner F. Canine tumors: a spontaneous animal model of human carcinogenesis. Transl Res. 2012; 159(3):165–72.
33. Cook N, Jodrell DI, Tuveson DK. Predictive in vivo animal models and translation to clinical trials. Drug Discov Today. 2012;17(5-6):253–60.
34. Xu B, Konze KD, Jin J, Wang GG. Targeting EZH2 and PRC2 dependence as novel anticancer therapy. Exp Hematol. 2015;43(8):698–712.
35. Kuntz K, Keilhack H, Pollock R, Knutson S, Warholic N, Richon V, et al. The discovery and pre-clinical development of the first clinical stage EZH2-inhibitor, EPZ-6438 (E7438). Eur J Cancer. 2014;50:92.
36. Goldschmidt M, Pena L, Rasotto R, Zappulli V. Classification and grading of canine mammary tumors. Vet Pathol. 2011;48(1):117–31.

4

Diagnostic performance of the urinary canine calgranulins in dogs with lower urinary or urogenital tract carcinoma

Romy M. Heilmann[1,2*], Elizabeth A. McNiel[3,4], Niels Grützner[5,2], David J. Lanerie[2], Jan S. Suchodolski[2] and Jörg M. Steiner[2]

Abstract

Background: Onset of canine transitional cell carcinoma (TCC) and prostatic carcinoma (PCA) is usually insidious with dogs presenting at an advanced stage of the disease. A biomarker that can facilitate early detection of TCC/PCA and improve patient survival would be useful. S100A8/A9 (calgranulin A/B or calprotectin) and S100A12 (calgranulin C) are expressed by cells of the innate immune system and are associated with several inflammatory disorders. S100A8/A9 is also expressed by epithelial cells after malignant transformation and is involved in the regulation of cell proliferation and metastasis. S100A8/A9 is up-regulated in human PCA and TCC, whereas the results for S100A12 have been ambiguous. Also, the urine S100A8/A9-to-S100A12 ratio (uCalR) may have potential as a marker for canine TCC/PCA. Aim of the study was to evaluate the diagnostic accuracy of the urinary S100/calgranulins to detect TCC/PCA in dogs by using data and urine samples from 164 dogs with TCC/PCA, non-neoplastic urinary tract disease, other neoplasms, or urinary tract infections, and 75 healthy controls (nested case-control study). Urine S100A8/A9 and S100A12 (measured by species-specific radioimmunoassays and normalized against urine specific gravity [$S100A8/A9_{USG}$; $S100A12_{USG}$], urine creatinine concentration, and urine protein concentration and the uCalR were compared among the groups of dogs.

Results: $S100A8/A9_{USG}$ had the highest sensitivity (96%) and specificity (66%) to detect TCC/PCA, with specificity reaching 75% after excluding dogs with a urinary tract infection. The uCalR best distinguished dogs with TCC/PCA from dogs with a urinary tract infection (sensitivity: 91%, specificity: 60%). Using a $S100A8/A9_{USG} \geq 109.9$ to screen dogs ≥6 years of age for TCC/PCA yielded a negative predictive value of 100%.

Conclusions: $S100A8/A9_{USG}$ and uCalR may have utility for diagnosing TCC/PCA in dogs, and $S100A8/A9_{USG}$ may be a good screening test for canine TCC/PCA.

Keywords: Biomarker, Calprotectin, Diagnostic accuracy, S100A8/A9, S100A12, Transitional cell carcinoma

Background

Transitional cell carcinoma (TCC) is the most common naturally occurring lower urinary tract malignancy in dogs affecting a number of canine patients [1–3]. Several predisposing factors (including the use of certain drugs, chemicals, or preventive medications, breed, gender, and diet) have been evaluated (reviewed by Fulkerson et al.

[3]). Despite many advances in the management of dogs with TCC or prostatic carcinoma (PCA), early detection of these neoplasms is rare, and their onset is usually insidious with dogs presenting at an advanced stage of the disease (20–40% with metastasis) [1–4]. Thus, as with any cancer, a biomarker that can facilitate early detection of TCC/PCA (i.e., cancer screening) and improve patient survival would be a useful tool in clinical practice.

Urinary cytology as a test for TCC/PCA has been demonstrated to have a low sensitivity and specificity [3, 5]. The veterinary bladder tumor antigen (V-BTA)

* Correspondence: Romy.Heilmann@kleintierklinik.uni-leipzig.de
[1]College of Veterinary Medicine, University of Leipzig, An den Tierkliniken 23, DE-04103 Leipzig, Germany
[2]Gastrointestinal Laboratory, Texas A&M University, TAMU 4474, College Station, TX 77843-4474, USA
Full list of author information is available at the end of the article

test has been evaluated as a non-invasive screening tool for TCC in dogs and is currently the biomarker with the best diagnostic accuracy for non-invasive TCC diagnosis, but this test was shown to have a high false-positive rate (12–65%) [6–9]. Concentrations of urinary basic fibroblast growth factor was also increased in dogs with bladder cancer and to some extent discriminated dogs with TCC from dogs with a urinary tract infection (UTI) [10], but sensitivity and specificity of urinary basic fibroblast growth factor have not been reported in a larger population of dogs. A recent urine metabolomics study identified a metabolite signature that could discriminate dogs with TCC from healthy control dogs with a sensitivity of 86% and a specificity of 78% [11], and a mass spectrometry analysis of canine urine samples identified a multiplex biomarker model predicting the presence of TCC with 90% diagnostic accuracy [12]. However, the utility of these models as either a screening tool or a diagnostic test for canine TCC has not been evaluated to date.

S100A8/A9 (calgranulin A/B) and S100A12 (calgranulin C) are members of the S100/calgranulin family of Ca^{2+}-binding proteins, and both members are expressed by cells of the innate immune response [13]. Aside from its association with several inflammatory diseases [13, 14], the S100A8/A9 protein complex (also referred to as calprotectin) has been shown to be expressed by epithelial cells after malignant transformation [15–18] and to be involved in the regulation of cell proliferation [19] and metastasis [20, 21]. In humans, both S100A9 and S100A8 were found to be up-regulated in PCA and TCC [22–30], whereas studies on the expression of S100A12 in TCC/PCA have yielded ambiguous results [31, 32]. However, S100A12 has not been investigated extensively in cancer patients.

Similar to human urothelial carcinoma, the *S100A8/A9* gene has been shown to harbour an increased frequency of copy number gains in canine urothelial carcinoma [33], and pilot data by our group suggested that the urinary concentration of S100/calgranulins, particularly the S100A8/A9-to-S100A12 ratio (uCalR), may have potential as a diagnostic biomarker for TCC/PCA in dogs [34]. Thus, further evaluation of the urinary S100/calgranulins and uCalR in dogs is needed to determine their specificity for the diagnosis of TCC/PCA. This retrospective case-control study investigated urine S100A8/A9 and S100A12 concentrations as well as the uCalR in dogs with TCC/PCA (treated or treatment-naïve), dogs with other diseases of the urinary tract, dogs with neoplastic diseases not involving the urinary tract, and healthy control dogs. We hypothesized (1) that the concentration of S100/calgranulins in urine specimens is a useful screening test for TCC/PCA and (2) that the uCalR can distinguish dogs with TCC/PCA and UTI with high diagnostic accuracy.

Methods

Sampling population

A nested case-control study design was used. Urine samples from dogs with TCC/PCA that were treatment-naïve ($n = 22$) or receiving specific anticancer treatment at the time of sampling ($n = 40$), dogs with non-neoplastic diseases of the urinary tract ($n = 22$), dogs with other neoplasms ($n = 35$), dogs with a urinary tract infection (UTI; $n = 45$), and a group of healthy control dogs ($n = 75$) were used. The study design is summarized in the flow chart (Fig. 1). Cases were recruited at the Veterinary Medical Teaching Hospitals (VMTH) at Texas A&M University ($n = 99$), Michigan State University ($n = 62$) as part of another study [9], and three other North American universities ($n = 40$) as well as from seven Oncology referral practices located in five different US states ($n = 38$). Samples from some of the dogs (9 dogs with TCC/PCA, 9 dogs with a UTI, and 38 healthy dogs) had also been included in the assay validation study [34].

Complete patient information was extracted from the electronic medical records (for all VMTH cases) or a study questionnaire that had to be completed by the owner and/or the attending veterinary oncologist prior to patient enrolment (for all referral practice cases).

Sample collection and analyses

Urine samples were obtained by cystocentesis, urethral catheterization, or free-catch, and were prepared for analysis of S100A8/A9 and S100A12 as previously described [34]. Briefly, debris was separated from samples by centrifugation for three minutes at $1000 \times g$, and the supernatants were placed into cryovials and stored frozen at −80 °C until analyses. Urine samples were then thawed and diluted 1:2 in 0.05 M sodium phosphate, 0.02% sodium azide, and 0.5% bovine serum albumin (pH 7.5) [34].

Urine S100A8/A9 and S100A12 were measured in all samples using established and validated species-specific in-house radioimmunoassays [34]. Urine concentrations of S100A8/A9 and S100A12 were normalized against urine specific gravity[1] (S100A8/A9$_{USG}$ and S100A12$_{USG}$), urine creatinine concentration[2] (S100A8/A9$_{Cre}$ and S100A12$_{Cre}$), and urine protein concentration[3] (S100A8/A9$_{Prot}$ and S100A12$_{Prot}$) [34]. In addition, the S100A8/A9-to-S100A12 ratio (uCalR) was calculated for each sample [34].

Data analyses

Commercial statistical software packages[4,5] were used for all statistical analyses. Data were tested for the assumptions of normality and equality of variances using a Shapiro-Wilk and a Brown-Forsythe test, respectively. All parameters (S100A8/A9$_{USG}$, S100A8/A9$_{Cre}$, S100A8/A9$_{Prot}$, S100A12$_{USG}$, S100A12$_{Cre}$, S100A12$_{Prot}$, and uCalR) were

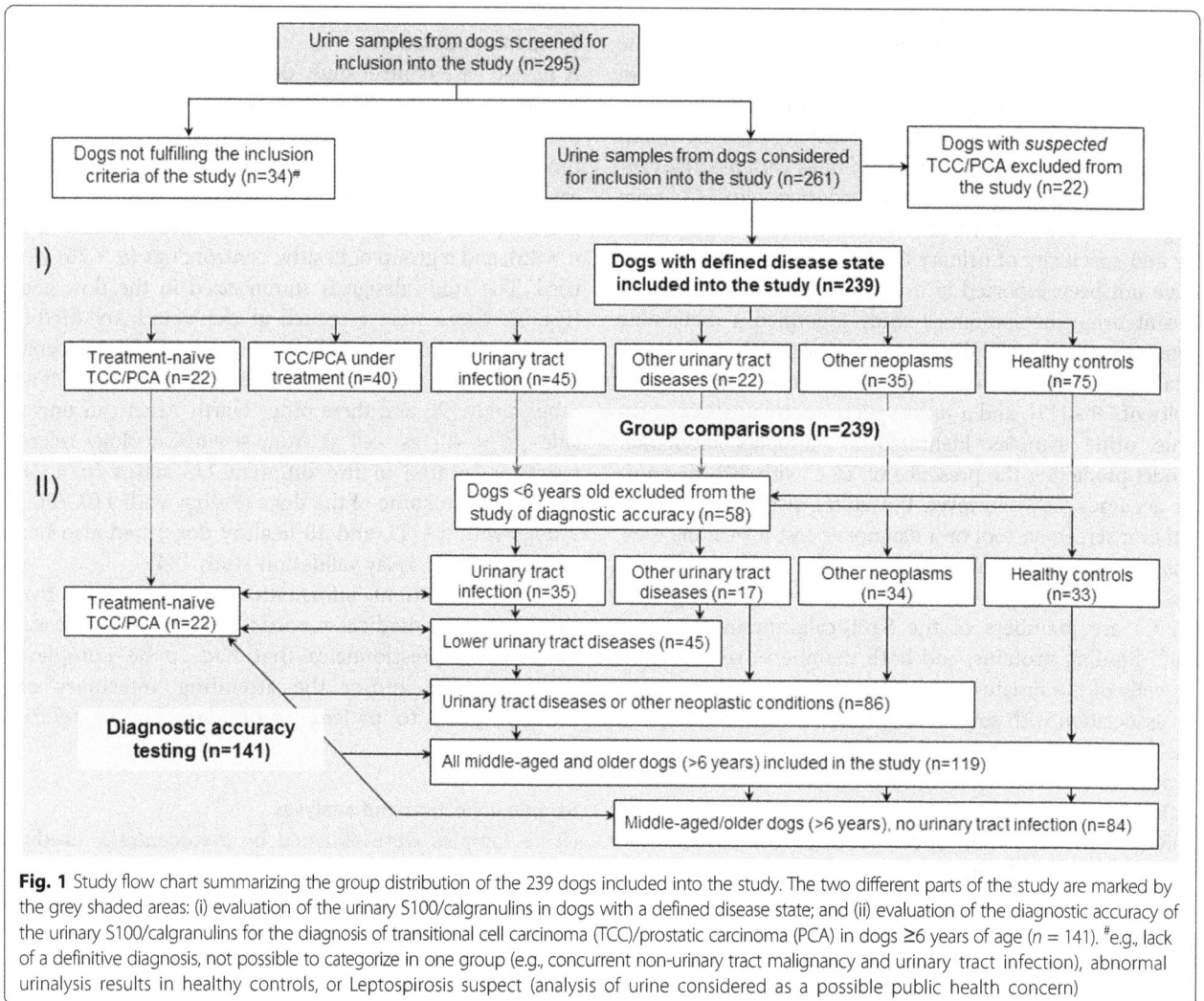

Fig. 1 Study flow chart summarizing the group distribution of the 239 dogs included into the study. The two different parts of the study are marked by the grey shaded areas: (i) evaluation of the urinary S100/calgranulins in dogs with a defined disease state; and (ii) evaluation of the diagnostic accuracy of the urinary S100/calgranulins for the diagnosis of transitional cell carcinoma (TCC)/prostatic carcinoma (PCA) in dogs ≥6 years of age (*n* = 141). #e.g., lack of a definitive diagnosis, not possible to categorize in one group (e.g., concurrent non-urinary tract malignancy and urinary tract infection), abnormal urinalysis results in healthy controls, or Leptospirosis suspect (analysis of urine considered as a possible public health concern)

tested among the six different groups of dogs using non-parametric multiple- (Kruskal-Wallis test followed by a Dunn's test for multiple comparisons) or two-group (Mann-Whitney U test) comparisons. Summary statistics are reported as medians and interquartile ranges (IQR).

Receiver operating characteristic (ROC) curves were constructed to determine the sensitivities and specificities of normalized urinary S100A8/A9, S100A12, and the uCalR to distinguish dogs with TCC/PCA from the other groups of dogs; the Youden index was used to establish the optimum cut-off values. Positive (PPV) and negative predictive values (NPV) were calculated for the best-performing markers; the prior probability for a diagnosis of TCC/PCA in middle aged to older dogs (defined as ≥6 years of age) was estimated at 0.7% [2], and in dogs older than 6 years after exclusion of a UTI and those with clinical signs of lower urinary tract disease

was estimated at 1% and 20%, respectively [8]. Significance was set at $P < 0.05$.

Results

Study population

Treatment-naïve TCC/PCA dogs

Breeds included Beagle (*n* = 3), Labrador Retriever (*n* = 3), Australian Cattle dog (*n* = 2), Scottish Terrier (*n* = 2), Shetland Sheepdog (*n* = 2), Australian Shepherd dog, Boston Terrier, Chow, Fox Terrier, Lhasa Apso (each *n* = 1), and mixed breed (*n* = 5). The most common tumor location was the urinary bladder (*n* = 15), followed by the urethra (*n* = 7), and the prostate (*n* = 5). The diagnosis was confirmed by histopathologic evaluation of a tissue biopsy (*n* = 7) or cytology (*n* = 15). A urine culture was performed in 12 dogs, 5 (42%) of which were positive for bacterial growth and the majority (80%) of positive samples were growing a single organism (*E. coli*,

Enterococcus sp., *Pseudomonas aeruginosa*, or *Streptococcus equisimilis*).

TCC/PCA dogs under treatment

Breeds included Beagle ($n = 5$), Shetland Sheepdog ($n = 4$), West Highland White Terrier ($n = 4$), Scottish Terrier ($n = 2$), American Spitz, Bichon Frise, English Springer Spaniel, Jack Russell Terrier, Labrador Retriever, Maltese, Miniature Pinscher, Miniature Schnauzer, Papillion, Poodle, Rat Terrier, Schipperke (each $n = 1$), and mixed breed ($n = 13$). Most common tumor site was the urinary bladder ($n = 33$), followed by the prostate ($n = 7$), and the urethra ($n = 6$). Treatment at the time of urine sample collection included non-steroidal anti-inflammatory drugs (NSAID; piroxicam: $n = 30$; carprofen: $n = 4$; firocoxib: $n = 2$; deracoxib: $n = 1$), chemotherapy (mitoxantrone: $n = 5$; cyclophosphamide: $n = 1$), a tyrosine kinase inhibitor (toceranib phosphate: $n = 3$), and/or surgical excision ($n = 2$). The diagnosis had been previously confirmed by histopathology or cytology. A urine culture was performed in 7 dogs, 3 (43%) of which were positive for bacterial growth and a single organism (*E. coli*, *Aerococcus* sp., *Mycoplasma canis*) being isolated in the majority (80%) of the dogs that had a positive urine culture.

Dogs with UTI

Breeds included Beagle ($n = 3$), Boston Terrier ($n = 3$), Labrador Retriever ($n = 3$), Pug ($n = 3$), Standard Schnauzer ($n = 3$), Bichon Frise ($n = 2$), Brittany Spaniel ($n = 2$), Dachshund ($n = 2$), Golden Retriever ($n = 2$), Australian Cattle dog, Boxer, Cocker Spaniel, English Bulldog, Fox Terrier, French Bulldog, Great Dane, Husky, Jack Russell Terrier, Lhasa Apso, Miniature Poodle, Miniature Schnauzer, Pembroke Welsh Corgi, Rat Terrier, Rottweiler, Shih Tzu, Swiss Mountain dog (each $n = 1$), and mixed breed ($n = 5$). Urine culture was positive in 44/45 (98%) dogs, and marked bacteriuria but a negative culture was seen in one dog. The isolated bacterial strains were documented in 38 dogs, 6 (16%) of which had a polymicrobial UTI. The most common isolate was *E. coli* ($n = 21$), followed by *Enterococcus* sp. ($n = 5$), *Klebsiella* ($n = 3$), *Proteus mirabilis* ($n = 6$), *Staphylococcus pseudintermedius* ($n = 2$), *Streptococcus canis* ($n = 2$), *Actinobacillus* sp., *Bacillus* sp., *Enterobacter* sp., *Pasteurella* sp., *Pseudomonas aeruginosa* (each $n = 1$). A recurrent UTI was seen in one dog and a resistant UTI in two dogs. One dog had concurrent bilateral ureteral ectopy and one dog had urolithiasis.

Dogs with non-neoplastic urinary tract diseases

Breeds included Miniature Schnauzer ($n = 3$), Beagle ($n = 2$), Maltese ($n = 2$), Australian Shepherd, Bichon Frise, Bloodhound, Chihuahua, Dalmatian, Golden Retriever, Labrador Retriever, Miniature Poodle, Standard Schnauzer, Soft Coated Wheaten Terrier, Shih Tzu, West Highland White Terrier, Yorkshire Terrier (each $n = 1$), and mixed breed ($n = 2$). Diseases included urolithiasis ($n = 11$), International Renal Interest Society (IRIS) stage I-IV chronic kidney disease ($n = 7$), detrusor sphincter dyssynergia, polypoid cystitis, urethral stricture, or urethral sphincter mechanism incompetence (each $n = 1$).

Dogs with non-urinary tract neoplasia

Breeds included Beagle ($n = 6$), Labrador Retriever ($n = 5$), Shetland Sheepdog ($n = 3$), West Highland White Terrier ($n = 3$), Golden Retriever ($n = 2$), Scottish Terrier ($n = 2$), Basset Hound, Bearded Collie, Boxer, Brittany Spaniel, Cockapoo, German Shorthaired Pointer, Greater Swiss Mountain dog, Rottweiler (each $n = 1$), and mixed breed ($n = 6$). Neoplastic diseases were: lymphoma ($n = 5$), mast cell tumor ($n = 5$), hepatocellular carcinoma ($n = 4$), appendicular osteosarcoma ($n = 3$), undefined adrenal masses ($n = 2$), undefined splenic masses with hemoabdomen ($n = 2$), thymoma ($n = 2$), adrenal carcinoma, hemangiosarcoma, hepatic carcinoma, oral soft tissue sarcoma, oral squamous cell carcinoma, perianal adenoma, plasma cell tumor, pulmonary carcinoma, renal adenocarcinoma, undefined intracranial neoplasia, undefined mandibular neoplasia, and undefined mesenchymal neoplasia (each $n = 1$). Oncologic therapy at the time or prior to urine sample collection for the study included surgery ($n = 12$), chemotherapy ($n = 8$), and/or radiation therapy ($n = 2$).

Healthy control dogs

Breeds included West Highland White Terrier ($n = 7$), Beagle ($n = 4$), Labrador Retriever ($n = 4$), Dachshund ($n = 3$), Scottish Terrier ($n = 3$), Shetland Sheepdog ($n = 3$), American Pitbull Terrier ($n = 2$), Giant Schnauzer ($n = 2$), Miniature Schnauzer ($n = 2$), Weimaraner ($n = 2$), Yorkshire Terrier ($n = 2$), Australian Shepherd, Basset Hound, Bichon Frise, Border Collie, Boston Terrier, Boxer, Chihuahua, Chinese Shar Pei, English Springer Spaniel, French Bulldog, Golden Retriever, Great Dane, Neopolitan Mastiff, Portuguese Water dog, Saint Bernard, Standard Poodle, White Shepherd dog (each $n = 1$), and mixed breed ($n = 17$); breed was not documented in 7 dogs. Urinalysis was unremarkable in 64 dogs and was not performed on the same urinalysis in 11 dogs (these dogs were determined to be healthy based on previous diagnostics). Age-related conditions (e.g., degenerative joint disease) not reported to affect the urinary tract were not considered as an exclusion criterion.

Among group comparisons

Patient characteristics, urine S100A8/A9 and S100A12 concentrations, and the uCalR are summarized in Table 1.

Table 1 Patient characteristics, normalized urine S100A8/A9 and S100A12 concentrations, and the urine S100A8/A9-to-S100A12 ratio (uCalR) in all dogs included in the study (n = 239)

Parameter	TCC/PCA, treatment-naïve	TCC/PCA, under treatment	Bacterial urinary tract infection	Non-neoplastic UT disease	Other, non-UT neoplasia	Healthy control dogs	P value[†]
Total number	22	40	45	22	35	75	–
Age[c], in years median [IQR]	10.2[A] [8.6–12.8]	11.1[A] [9.5–12.8]	8.8[A] [5.9–11.5]	10.0[A] [8.0–11.7]	9.4[A] [8.4–11.3]	5.5[B] [3.0–8.8]	**<0.0001**
Weight[a], in kg median [IQR]	18.2[A] [10.9–28.6]	13.7[A] [9.8–18.7]	12.7[A] [8.3–21.5]	9.8[A] [4.8–16.3]	21.8[A] [13.7–35.7]	18.1[b, A] [10.2–26.0]	**0.0006**
Sex male/female	9/13	20/20	12/33	9/13	17/18	40/32[b]	0.0618
S100A8/A9[c]$_{USG}$ median [IQR]	438.5[A] [199.8–8864.1]	196.3[A] [67.9–687.0]	310.7[A] [44.3–1384.5]	100.8[B] [28.4–290.1]	23.5[B] [13.4–97.6]	40.4[B] [15.3–145.3]	**<0.0001**
S100A8/A9[c]$_{Cre}$ median [IQR]	933.6[A] [353.8–11,600.2]	445.4[A] [145.5–1881.4]	956.3[A] [151.2–4242.0]	167.8[B] [42.4–606.6]	53.3[B] [29.6–225.7]	23.4[B] [4.5–123.6]	**<0.0001**
S100A8/A9$_{Prot}$ Median [IQR]	201.8[A] [43.6–2541.9]	81.7[A] [36.1–259.0]	176.0[A] [33.5–637.3]	37.8[B] [6.7–107.3]	16.4[B] [5.0–66.7]	151.5[A] [69.7–699.7]	**<0.0001**
S100A12[c]$_{USG}$ median [IQR]	12.4[A] [9.1–283.9]	5.0[A] [2.6–30.6]	44.5[A] [5.0–308.4]	2.8[B] [1.7–16.8]	1.9[B] [1.3–3.1]	4.5[B] [3.0–7.6]	**<0.0001**
S100A12[c]$_{Cre}$ median [IQR]	35.2[A] [14.7–803.6]	12.1[B] [4.2–61.5]	176.3[A] [11.2–1323.1]	4.9[B] [2.2–44.5]	3.9[B] [2.7–6.6]	6.1[B] [4.2–10.5]	**<0.0001**
S100A12$_{Prot}$ median [IQR]	7.5[A] [2.4–44.4]	3.0[A] [1.0–12.7]	41.3[A] [2.3–129.8]	2.4[B] [0.5–6.7]	1.6[B] [0.2–6.4]	10.9[A] [5.7–18.4]	**<0.0001**
uCalR[c] median [IQR]	14.7[A] [10.6–37.7]	29.9[A] [7.5–71.1]	6.9[B] [2.2–14.0]	14.2[A] [12.1–36.5]	12.1[A] [8.5–30.7]	10.6[A] [5.1–26.6]	**<0.0001**

TCC transitional cell carcinoma, PCA prostate gland carcinoma, UT urinary tract; [a]no significant differences detected when comparing individual groups with TCC/PCA group; [b]unknown in 3 dogs; [c]medians [IQR in brackets] within a row not sharing a common superscript (boldface) are significantly different from treatment-naïve TCC/PCA dogs at P < 0.05. [†]Global P value (boldface values indicate a significant difference at P < 0.05)

$S100A8/A9_{USG}$ (Fig. 2) and $S100A8/A9_{Cre}$ were numerically higher in dogs with untreated TCC/PCA than in dogs with TCC/PCA under treatment, but both differences did not reach significance ($P = 0.2587$ and 0.3715, respectively). No differences in $S100A8/A9_{USG}$ (Fig. 2) and $S100A8/A9_{Cre}$ were seen between treatment-naïve TCC/PCA dogs and those with a UTI ($P = 0.1763$ and 1.0000, respectively). Compared to treatment-naïve TCC/PCA dogs, urinary S100A12 concentrations were also lower in TCC/PCA dogs undergoing treatment, but the difference was only significant for $S100A12_{Cre}$ ($P = 0.0416$; $P = 0.0664$ for $S100A12_{USG}$), whereas dogs with a UTI had numerically higher (but not significant) $S100A12_{USG}$ and $S100A12_{Cre}$ (both $P = 1.0000$).

The uCalR did not differ between newly diagnosed TCC/PCA dogs and those undergoing treatment ($P = 1.0000$), but the uCalR was significantly lower in dogs diagnosed with a UTI compared to all other disease groups of dogs: treatment-naïve TCC/PCA dogs ($P = 0.0014$) (Fig. 3), TCC/PCA dogs undergoing treatment ($P < 0.0001$), non-neoplastic urinary tract diseases ($P = 0.0049$), and neoplastic disease not involving the urinary tract ($P = 0.0364$).

$S100A8/A9_{Prot}$ and $S100A12_{Prot}$ were significantly higher in dogs with TCC/PCA than those with non-neoplastic urinary tract diseases ($P = 0.0079$ and 0.0485, respectively) or other neoplasms ($P < 0.0001$ and 0.0056, respectively) but were comparable to those in dogs with a UTI (both $P = 1.0000$) and healthy controls (both $P = 1.0000$).

Comparing urinary canine S100/calgranulin concentrations amongst the same groups of dogs after exclusion of all dogs <6 years of age yielded similar results, with the exception that the difference did not reach significance for $S100A12_{USG}$ in treatment-naïve TCC/PCA dogs compared to dogs with non-neoplastic urinary tract disease ($P = 0.0574$) and healthy control dogs ($P = 0.0566$), for $S100A12_{Cre}$ between treatment-naïve TCC/PCA dogs and those dogs with TCC/PCA under treatment ($P= 0.1526$), and for $S100A12_{Prot}$ between treatment-naïve TCC/PCA dogs and dogs with non-neoplastic urinary tract disease ($P = 0.2245$).

Within group comparisons

In patients with TCC/PCA, $S100A8/A9_{USG}$, $S100A8/A9_{Cre}$, $S100A8/A9_{Prot}$, $S100A12_{USG}$, $S100A12_{Cre}$, $S100A12_{Prot}$, and uCalR did not differ between dogs with a single tumor site (bladder, urethra, or prostate; $n = 53$) and dogs with more than one of those sites affected ($n = 9$; all $P > 0.05$). This finding was no different in treatment-naïve TCC/PCA dogs (all $P > 0.05$) and those dogs receiving antitumor therapy at the time of sample collection (all $P > 0.05$).

$S100A8/A9_{Prot}$ and $S100A12_{Prot}$ were significantly higher in treatment-naïve TCC/PCA dogs with a positive urine culture ($n = 5$; median [IQR]: 604.8 [392.9–10,353.6] and 39.8 [13.4–870.0], respectively) than dogs without a concurrent UTI ($n = 7$; median [IQR]: 44.5 [32.4–181.2] and 2.5 [1.1–6.1], respectively; both $P = 0.0230$), whereas no differences in $S100A8/A9_{USG}$, $S100A8/A9_{Cre}$,

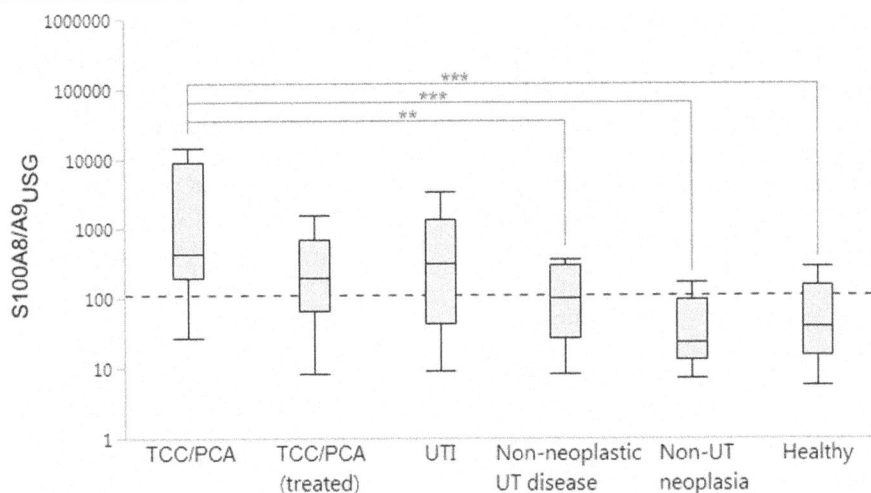

Fig. 2 Urinary concentrations of S100A8/A9 normalized against urine specific gravity ($S100A8/A9_{USG}$) were significantly higher in newly diagnosed TCC/PCA dogs compared to dogs with non-neoplastic urinary tract (UT) diseases ($P = 0.0088$), dogs with neoplastic diseases not involving the urinary tract ($P < 0.0001$), and healthy control dogs ($P < 0.0001$); but did not differ from $S100A8/A9_{USG}$ measured in dogs with TCC/PCA undergoing cancer therapy ($P = 0.2587$) or dogs with a bacterial urinary tract infection (UTI; $P = 0.1763$). Boxes: interquartile range (IQR); vertical lines within boxes: medians; whiskers: determined by the outermost data points or values computed as (25th quartile − 1.5 × IQR) or (75th quartile +1.5 × IQR); dashed line: optimum cut-off concentration (≥109.9) to distinguish dogs with TCC/PCA from those of other groups; **significant difference at $P < 0.01$; ***significant difference at $P < 0.001$

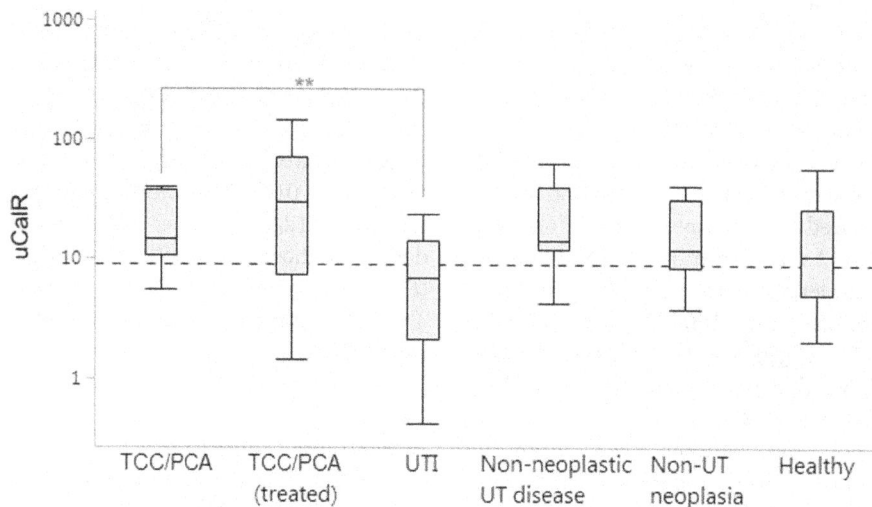

Fig. 3 Urinary S100A8/A9-to-S100A12 ratios (uCalR) were significantly lower in dogs diagnosed with a urinary tract infection (UTI) compared to treatment-naïve TCC/PCA dogs (P = 0.0014), but did not differ between newly diagnosed TCC/PCA dogs and all other disease groups (all P = 1.0000) or healthy control dogs (P = 0.3030). *Boxes*: interquartile range (IQR); vertical lines within boxes: medians; whiskers: determined by the outermost data points or values computed as (25th quartile – 1.5 × IQR) or (75th quartile +1.5 × IQR); *dashed line*: optimum cut-off concentration (≥9.1) to distinguish dogs with TCC/PCA from dogs with a UTI; **significant difference at P < 0.01

$S100A12_{USG}$, $S100A12_{Cre}$, or uCalR were seen between both groups of dogs (all $P > 0.05$).

$S100A8/A9_{USG}$, $S100A8/A9_{Cre}$, $S100A8/A9_{Prot}$, $S100A12_{USG}$, $S100A12_{Cre}$, $S100A12_{Prot}$, and uCalR did not differ among the three different primary tumor sites in newly diagnosed TCC/PCA dogs (all global $P > 0.05$), whereas $S100A8/A9_{USG}$, $S100A12_{USG}$, $S100A12_{Cre}$, and $S100A12_{Prot}$ were significantly lower with primary involvement of the urinary bladder ($n = 31$; median [IQR]: 161.4 [67.3–361.5], 3.3 [2.3–13.5], 6.6 [3.6–32.9], and 2.0 [0.7–9.5], respectively) than the prostate ($n = 7$; median [IQR]: 1849.6 [563.1–5641.2], 239.6 [10.3–1274.4], 254.0 [18.9–2196.2], and 58.1 [9.2–119.0], respectively) in dogs undergoing treatment ($P = 0.0274$, 0.0020, 0.0128, and 0.0165, respectively). Also, $S100A8/A9_{USG}$, $S100A8/A9_{Cre}$, $S100A8/A9_{Prot}$, $S100A12_{USG}$, $S100A12_{Cre}$, $S100A12_{Prot}$, and uCalR did not differ between dogs treated with a single agent ($n = 30$) compared to combination protocols ($n = 10$; all $P > 0.05$) nor those treated with an NSAID ($n = 37$) compared to dogs not receiving an NSAID ($n = 3$; all $P > 0.05$).

In patients diagnosed with a UTI, $S100A8/A9_{USG}$, $S100A8/A9_{Cre}$, $S100A8/A9_{Prot}$, $S100A12_{USG}$, $S100A12_{Cre}$, $S100A12_{Prot}$, and uCalR did not differ in dogs with a single bacterial isolate ($n = 43$) from those with a polymicrobial UTI ($n = 7$; all $P > 0.05$); and there were no differences seen in dogs where only *Enterococcus* sp. ($n = 5$) and/or other isolates ($n = 45$) were cultured from urine samples (all $P > 0.05$).

Diagnostic accuracy

The area under the ROC curve (AUROC), optimum cut-off concentrations (and cut-off concentrations for at least a 90% sensitivity and a 90% specificity, respectively), sensitivities, and specificities are summarized in Table 2.

Using a uCalR of ≥9.3 or a $S100A8/A9_{USG}$ of ≥109.9 to screen middle-aged to older dogs (≥ 6 years of age) for TCC/PCA (0.7% estimated prevalence of TCC/PCA) yielded an NPV of 100% (1.000 for both) and a PPV between 1 and 2% (0.011 and 0.019, respectively). If a UTI has been excluded in the same population of dogs (estimated prevalence of TCC/PCA: 1%), a $S100A8/A9_{USG} ≥ 109.9$ resulted in a NPV of ~100% (1.000) and a PPV of ~4% (0.038). In dogs ≥6 years of age, a uCalR of ≥5.2 [or ≥9.1] or a $S100A8/A9_{USG}$ of ≥96.3 differentiated patients with TCC/PCA from those with non-neoplastic causes of similar presenting signs (estimated prevalence of TCC/PCA in this population: 20%) with a NPV of 96–100% (1.000 [0.956] and 0.975, respectively) and a PPV of 29–31% (0.294 [0.308] and 0.301, respectively).

Use of a uCalR of ≥9.1 combined with a $S100A8/A9_{USG}$ of ≥109.9 to screen middle-aged to older dogs (≥ 6 years of age) for TCC/PCA (estimated prevalence: 0.7%) yielded a sensitivity of 86% (95% CI: 67–95%) and a specificity of 80% (95% CI: 72–87%; OR: 25.6, 95% CI: 7.3–88.5) (Fig. 4), with a NPV of ~100% (0.999; 95% CI: 0.997–1.000) and a PPV of 3% (0.030; 95% CI: 0.020–0.044).

Table 2 Sensitivities and specificities at the optimal cut-off values (and cut-offs for resulting in a sensitivity and specificity of at least 90% each), and area under the receiver operating characteristic curve (AUROC) for urinary S100/calgranulins and the S100A8/A9-to-S100A12 ratio (uCalR) to distinguish treatment-naïve dogs with transitional cell carcinoma (TCC)/prostatic carcinoma (PCA) from other groups of dogs (all dogs ≥6 years of age [n = 141])

Parameter	AUROC[†]	Cut-off	Sensitivity	Specificity
Treatment-naïve TCC/PCA (n = 22) vs. UTI (n = 35)				
S100A8/A9$_{USG}$	**0.671**	≥96.3	96%	43%
		≥8180.7	32%	94%
S100A8/A9$_{Cre}$	0.612	≥160.0	96%	35%
S100A12$_{USG}$	0.516	≤3.2	91%	29%
S100A12$_{Cre}$	0.521	≤117.9	68%	62%
uCalR	**0.751**	≥9.1	91%	60%
		≥5.2	100%	49%
		≥72.2	18%	94%
Treatment-naïve TCC/PCA vs. other diseases causing lower urinary tract signs (n = 45)				
S100A8/A9$_{USG}$	**0.684**	≥96.3	96%	44%
		≥8230.7	32%	96%
S100A8/A9$_{Cre}$	0.631	≥167.8	96%	39%
S100A12$_{USG}$	0.548	≥7.0	82%	42%
S100A12$_{Cre}$	0.517	≥8.7	96%	34%
uCalR	**0.698**	≥5.2	100%	40%
		≥9.1	91%	49%
		≥72.2	18%	96%
Treatment-naïve TCC/PCA vs. other disease groups (n = 86)[a]				
S100A8/A9$_{USG}$	**0.807**	≥109.9	96%	64%
		≥2274.8	36%	92%
S100A8/A9$_{Cre}$	0.763	≥188.9	96%	55%
		≥8603.1	27%	91%
S100A12$_{USG}$	0.712	≥4.0	91%	57%
		≥776.1	23%	93%
S100A12$_{Cre}$	0.697	≥8.7	96%	78%
		≥2538.9	18%	95%
uCalR	**0.664**	≥9.3	91%	42%
		≥83.4	18%	96%
Treatment-naïve TCC/PCA vs. all other groups (n = 119)[a]				
S100A8/A9$_{USG}$	**0.824**	≥109.9	96%	66%
		≥2274.8	36%	93%
S100A8/A9$_{Cre}$	0.787	≥188.9	96%	59%
		≥5783.2	36%	92%
S100A12$_{USG}$	0.740	≥7.0	82%	66%
		≥221.0	27%	90%
S100A12$_{Cre}$	0.722	≥8.7	96%	57%
		≥833.8	23%	90%

Table 2 Sensitivities and specificities at the optimal cut-off values (and cut-offs for resulting in a sensitivity and specificity of at least 90% each), and area under the receiver operating characteristic curve (AUROC) for urinary S100/calgranulins and the S100A8/A9-to-S100A12 ratio (uCalR) to distinguish treatment-naïve dogs with transitional cell carcinoma (TCC)/prostatic carcinoma (PCA) from other groups of dogs (all dogs ≥6 years of age [n = 141]) *(Continued)*

Parameter	AUROC[†]	Cut-off	Sensitivity	Specificity
uCalR	**0.657**	≥9.3	91%	41%
		≥83.4	18%	96%
Treatment-naïve TCC/PCA vs. all other groups, excl. Urinary tract infections (n = 84)				
S100A8/A9$_{USG}$	**0.896**	≥109.9	96%	75%
		≥374.9	59%	95%
S100A8/A9$_{Cre}$	**0.875**	≥188.9	96%	70%
		≥792.7	55%	91%
S100A12$_{USG}$	**0.850**	≥8.6	77%	86%
		≥4.0	91%	71%
S100A12$_{Cre}$	**0.838**	≥10.7	91%	76%
		≥92.3	32%	91%
uCalR	0.612	≥9.3	91%	33%

[a]excluding TCC/PCA dogs undergoing anticancer therapy
[†]values in boldface are significant at P < 0.05

Discussion

This study evaluated the diagnostic utility of measuring urine concentrations of S100A8/A9 and S100A12 as well as the uCalR in dogs with TCC/PCA (treatment-naïve or undergoing antineoplastic therapy). Measurement of these biomarkers in urine specimens has the advantage of yielding information from the urinary tract. However, the results may be skewed by prerenal factors (e.g., increased amino acid turnover with neoplastic diseases causing glomerular

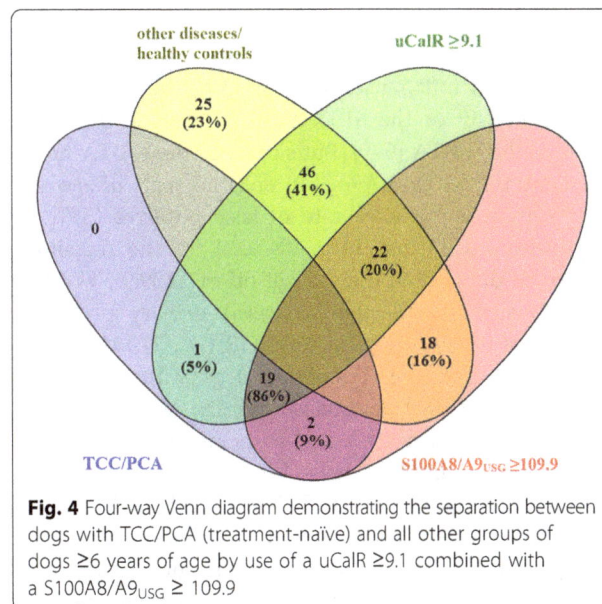

Fig. 4 Four-way Venn diagram demonstrating the separation between dogs with TCC/PCA (treatment-naïve) and all other groups of dogs ≥6 years of age by use of a uCalR ≥9.1 combined with a S100A8/A9$_{USG}$ ≥ 109.9

hyperfiltration [35]), renal diseases (e.g., chronic kidney disease), and/or other diseases of the lower urinary tract (e.g., bacterial cystitis or urolithiasis). Thus, dogs with other non-neoplastic diseases of the urinary tract and dogs with neoplastic conditions not involving the urinary tract were included as disease control groups of dogs.

Diagnostic accuracy of the urinary canine S100/calgranulins was evaluated in dogs ≥6 years of age to mimic the situation of using these biomarkers in the clinical setting to screen for or diagnose dogs with TCC/PCA. The results of this study showed that urine S100A8/A9 and the uCalR may have limited diagnostic utility in dogs with TCC/PCA. Concentrations of urine S100A8/A9 as well as the parameters of diagnostic accuracy (AUROC, sensitivity, and specificity) and the optimum cut-offs for the separation of dogs diagnosed with TCC/PCA from the other groups of dogs were comparable to those in one study evaluating urine S100A8/A9 concentrations in humans with bladder cancer [30]. The study by Ebbing et al. also showed higher urine concentrations of S100A8/A9 in people with higher grade urothelial carcinomas [30]. However, the possibility of a correlation between urinary concentrations of the S100/calgranulins and the results of complete cancer staging and/or grading, response to treatment, and the individual patient outcome were not investigated as part of our study, and this will need to be further explored. Further research is also needed to determine when changes in S100A8/A9 and S100A12 could possibly occur along the spectrum of tumor development and whether these tests can detect pre-cancerous pathology or early cancer.

The components of diagnostic accuracy for the urinary S100/calgranulins in this study were higher than the sensitivity and specificity reported for urine sediment analysis, where neoplastic cells are detectable in approximately 30% of patients with TCC but neoplastic cells can be difficult to distinguish from reactive epithelial cells associated with inflammation [3, 5]. Also, both sensitivity and specificity of the S100A8/A9$_{USG}$ were higher than those of the V-BTA [6–9]. But similar to the V-BTA measurement, the S100A8/A9$_{USG}$ in dogs ≥6 years of age also suffers from a moderate rate of false positives (59% for dogs with a UTI and 24% [18–33%] for the remaining groups of dogs when using a cut-off of ≥109.9), which is also consistent with the increased urinary proteome fraction of S100A8/A9 and S100A12 (i.e., S100A8/A9$_{Prot}$ and S100A12$_{Prot}$) in TCC/PCA dogs with concurrent UTI. An additional advantage over the V-BTA test [8], S100A8/A9$_{USG}$ is not affected by hematuria and offers a quantitative result [34].

The high sensitivity and NPV of S100A8/A9$_{USG}$ observed in this study suggest that measuring S100A8/A9$_{USG}$ could be a good screening test for TCC/PCA in dogs, especially patients where a UTI has been ruled out

as a cause of clinical signs of lower urinary tract disease, and that a negative test result (i.e., a S100A8/A9$_{USG}$ of <109.9) essentially excludes a diagnosis of TCC/PCA in dogs. The uCalR, on the other hand, appears to be a better marker to distinguish patients with a UTI from those with TCC/PCA. However, the false negative rate of the uCalR in dogs ≥6 years old with a UTI was still moderate (54% and 43% when using ≥5.2 and ≥9.1 as the cut-off concentration, respectively), but a combination of S100A8/A9$_{USG}$ and the uCalR improved the diagnostic accuracy (i.e., specificity) for the detection of TCC/PCA in dogs. Similar to the V-BTA test [8], the PPV of the uCalR and S100A8/A9$_{USG}$ increased to about 30% if used in a population of dogs with a higher index of suspicion for lower urinary tract disease. Further prospective studies are warranted in a larger cohort of dogs to validate our findings and to directly compare the diagnostic performance of the urinary S100/calgranulins with the V-BTA test.

Dog breeds reported to have a higher risk of developing TCC (Scottish Terrier, West Highland White Terrier, Shetland Sheepdog, Beagle, and Dachshund) [1–3, 36] were overrepresented (36%) in our study. The female:male ratio (1.4:1) as well as the urinary bladder trigone being the most common tumor site were similar to previous reports [1, 3, 4, 8]. Detection of a concurrent UTI in 42% of the dogs with TCC/PCA (both treatment-naïve dogs and dogs undergoing anticancer therapy) and the spectrum of organisms isolated are also in line with the results of others [37].

An interesting finding of the current study is that, compared to dogs with TCC/PCA that received anticancer treatment at the time of urine sample collection, treatment-naïve dogs with TCC/PCA had 2.1- to 2.5-fold higher urinary S100A8/A9 concentrations and 2.5- to 2.9-fold higher urinary S100A12 concentrations (albeit statistical significance was reached only for S100A12$_{Cre}$). While the cause of urinary S100/calgranulins being lower in dogs with TCC/PCA under treatment cannot be evaluated through this study, potential explanations include a decreased expression of these proteins by tumor cells or reduction of tumor-associated inflammation (particularly tumor-associated or even metastasis-associated macrophages) in response to treatment [38]. However, with the source and treatment-induced change of S100A8/A9 and S100A12 expression in canine TCC/PCA being unknown and the relatively large variation in the uCalR seen in the group of TCC/PCA dogs receiving anticancer treatment, it remains to be determined whether the S100/calgranulins are part of a pro-tumorigenic [39] or anti-tumorigenic [40] signature in canine TCC/PCA [38], or if they may even have a dual role. This distinction is particularly important as the synergism and convergence in the signaling pathways of inflammation and cancer – especially the release of damage-associated molecular pattern molecules (such as S100A8/A9 and S100A12), downstream activation of nuclear factor-κB, and expression of inflammatory cytokines and chemokines – can lead to positive feedback loops perpetuating chronic inflammation and thus a pro-tumorigenic microenvironment [13, 38].

From a clinical perspective, these aspects lend themselves to research of novel molecular-based therapeutic strategies aimed at targeting tumor-associated inflammation, which can drive tumor progression and metastasis [38, 41]. From a comparative oncology standpoint, study of the S100/calgranulins in canine TCC/PCA is of very high interest because here the spontaneous disease in dogs serves as a better model for human urothelial carcinoma than murine models (rodents lack S100A12 and S100A8 appears to functionally resemble S100A12 [42–44]).

Another interesting finding in TCC/PCA dogs receiving anticancer therapy is that urinary S100A8/A9 and S100A12 concentrations were lower with primary involvement of the urinary bladder than that of the prostate. Whether this reflects a higher degree of tumor-associated inflammation with prostatic involvement, the response (increased antitumor immunity or treatment-induced inflammation) or even lack of response to treatment [38] requires further study. In view of this finding, the lack of a difference in urinary S100/calgranulin concentrations between TCC/PCA dogs given an NSAID (either alone or as part of a combination protocol) and those receiving other forms of antineoplastic therapy was unexpected as metronomic NSAIDs predominantly affect the tumor-promoting inflammation [1, 38] and the expression of S100A8 and S100A9 has been indirectly linked to the cyclooxygenase (COX)-2/cAMP pathway [45, 46].

We acknowledge the limitation of the study that healthy control dogs did not undergo the same diagnostic evaluation as patients with TCC/PCA or other urinary tract or non-urinary tract diseases. Thus, the possibility of an occult urinary tract disease (including TCC/PCA) cannot be excluded with certainty in this group of dogs.

Conclusions

The results of this study show that urine S100A8/A9 and the uCalR have utility as an exclusionary tool in dogs with suspected TCC/PCA. Despite a limited diagnostic value (i.e., as a confirmatory test), the high sensitivity and NPV of S100A8/A9$_{USG}$ suggests that S100A8/A9 could be a good screening test for TCC/PCA in dogs and that the uCalR can help differentiate dogs with a UTI. Further studies are warranted to validate our findings in a larger cohort of dogs, to evaluate the source of S100A8/A9 and S100A12 expression in canine TCC/PCA patients, and to determine whether S100A8/A9 and/or S100A12 expression correlates with tumor grade and/or

complete tumor stage, response to treatment, progression of cancer, and/or survival time.

Endnotes

[1]Clinical refractometer, Atago USA Inc., Bellevue, WA, USA.
[2]Sirrus Creatinine LiquiColor, Stanbio Laboratory, Boerne, TX, USA.
[3]Coomassie protein Bradford assay, Thermo Fisher Scientific Inc., Rockford, IL, USA.
[4]Analyse-it® v4.20.1 Method validation edition, Analyse-it Software, Leeds, West Yorkshire, UK.
[5]JMP® v12.0, SAS Institute Inc., Cary, NC, USA.

Abbreviations
AUROC: Area under the ROC curve; CI: Confidence interval; NPV: Negative predictive value; PCA: Prostatic carcinoma; PPV: Positive predictive value; ROC: Receiver operating characteristic curve; S100A12: S100A12 protein; S100A8/A9: S100A8/A9 (calprotectin) protein complex; TCC: Transitional cell carcinoma; uCalR: Urine S100A8/A9-to-S100A12 ratio; USG: Urine specific gravity; UTI: Urinary tract infection

Acknowledgements
The authors acknowledge the help of Dr. Mary Nabity, Dr. Stephanie Smith, Dr. Tomomi Minamoto, Ms. Kelly Salgado, and Ms. Katja Weber with the collection and processing of urine samples.
Part of the data were presented at the 34rd Annual Meeting of the American College of Veterinary Internal Medicine (ACVIM), Denver, CO, USA (8–11 June, 2016).

Funding
This study was not supported by a grant or otherwise.

Authors' contributions
RMH, EAM, NG, DJL, and JMS designed the study and enrolled patients into the study. RMH, NG, and DJL analysed the specimens from dogs enrolled in the study. RMH, EAM, NG, DJL, and JSS analysed and interpreted the patient and biomarker data. All authors read and approved the final manuscript.

Competing interests
The authors declare that they have no competing interests.

Consent for publication
Not applicable.

Author details
[1]College of Veterinary Medicine, University of Leipzig, An den Tierkliniken 23, DE-04103 Leipzig, Germany. [2]Gastrointestinal Laboratory, Texas A&M University, TAMU 4474, College Station, TX 77843-4474, USA. [3]Cummings School of Veterinary Medicine, Tufts University, 200 Westboro Rd, North Grafton, MA 01536, USA. [4]College of Veterinary Medicine, Michigan State University, 784 Wilson Rd, East Lansing, MI 48824, USA. [5]Farm Animal Clinic,

Vetsuisse Faculty, University of Bern, Bremgartenstrasse 109a, CH-3012 Bern, BE, Switzerland.

References

1. Mutsaers AJ, Widmer WR, Knapp DW. Canine transitional cell carcinoma. J Vet Intern Med. 2003;17(2):136–44.

2. Knapp DW, Ramos-Vara JA, Moore GE, et al. Urinary bladder cancer in dogs, a naturally occurring model for cancer biology and drug development. ILAR J. 2014;55(1):100–18.

3. Fulkerson CM, Knapp DW. Management of transitional cell carcinoma of the urinary bladder in dogs: a review. Vet J. 2015;205(2):217–25.

4. Knapp DW, Glickman NW, Denicola DB, et al. Naturally-occurring canine transitional cell carcinoma of the urinary bladder. A relevant model of human invasive bladder cancer. Urol Oncol. 2000;5(2):47–59.

5. Norris AM, Laing EJ, Valli VE, et al. Canine bladder and urethral tumors: a retrospective study of 115 cases (1980-1985). J Vet Intern Med. 1992;6(3):145–53.

6. Borjesson DL, Christopher MM, Ling GV. Detection of canine transitional cell carcinoma using a bladder tumor antigen urine dipstick test. Vet Clin Pathol. 1999;28(1):33–8.

7. Billet JP, Moore AH, Holt PE. Evaluation of a bladder tumor antigen test for the diagnosis of lower urinary tract malignancies in dogs. Am J Vet Res. 2002;63(3):370–3.

8. Henry CJ, Tyler JW, McEntee MC, et al. Evaluation of a bladder tumor antigen test as a screening test for transitional cell carcinoma of the lower urinary tract in dogs. Am J Vet Res. 2003;64(8):1017–20.

9. Sotirakopoulos AJ, Armstrong PJ, Heath L, et al. Evaluation of microsatellite instability in urine for the diagnosis of transitional cell carcinoma of the lower urinary tract in dogs. J Vet Intern Med. 2010;24(6):1445–51.

10. Allen DK, Waters DJ, Knapp DW, Kuczek T. High urine concentrations of basic fibroblast growth factor in dogs with bladder cancer. J Vet Intern Med. 1996;10(4):231–4.

11. Zhang J, Wei S, Liu L, et al. NMR-based metabolomics study of canine bladder cancer. Biochim Biophys Acta. 2012;1822(11):1807–14.

12. Bracha S, McNamara M, Hilgart I, et al. A multiplex biomarker approach for the diagnosis of transitional cell carcinoma from canine urine. Anal Biochem. 2014;455:41–7.

13. Foell D, Wittkowski H, Roth J. Mechanisms of disease: a 'DAMP' view of inflammatory arthritis. Nat Clin Pract Rheumatol. 2007;3(7):382–90.

14. Manolakis AC, Kapsoritakis AN, Tiaka EK, Potamianos SP. Calprotectin, calgranulin C, and other members of the S100 protein family in inflammatory bowel disease. Dig Dis Sci. 2011;56(6):1601–11.

15. Yao R, Lopez-Beltran A, Maclennan GT, et al. Expression of S100 protein family members in the pathogenesis of bladder tumors. Anticancer Res. 2007;27(5A):3051–8.

16. Duan L, Wu R, Ye L, et al. S100A8 and S100A9 are associated with colorectal carcinoma progression and contribute to colorectal carcinoma cell survival and migration via Wnt/β-catenin pathway. PLoS One. 2013;8(4):e62092.

17. De Ponti A, Wiechert L, Schneller D, et al. A pro-tumorigenic function of S100A8/A9 in carcinogen-induced hepatocellular carcinoma. Cancer Lett. 2015;369(2):396–404.

18. Zhang L, Jiang H, Xu G, et al. Proteins S100A8 and S100A9 are potential biomarkers for renal cell carcinoma in the early stages: results from a proteomic study integrated with bioinformatics analysis. Mol Med Rep. 2015;11(6):4093–100.

19. Hermani A, De Servi B, Medunjanin S, et al. S100A8 and S100A9 activate MAP kinase and NF-kB signaling pathways and trigger translocation of RAGE in human prostate cancer cells. Exp Cell Res. 2006;312(2):184–97.

20. Hiratsuka S, Watanabe A, Aburatani H, Maru Y. Tumour-mediated upregulation of chemoattractants and recruitment of myeloid cells predetermines lung metastasis. Nat Cell Biol. 2006;8(12):1369–75.

21. Rafii S, Lyden D. S100 chemokines mediate bookmarking of premetastatic niches. Nat Cell Biol. 2006;8(12):1321–3.

22. Rehman I, Azzouzi AR, Catto JW, et al. Proteomic analysis of voided urine after prostatic massage from patients with prostate cancer: a pilot study. Urology. 2004;64(6):1238–43.

23. Hermani A, Hess J, De Servi B, et al. Calcium-binding proteins S100A8 and S100A9 as novel diagnostic markers in human prostate cancer. Clin Cancer Res. 2005;11(14):5146–52.

24. Tolson JP, Flad T, Gnau V, et al. Differential detection of S100A8 in transitional cell carcinoma of the bladder by pair wise tissue proteomic and immunohistochemical analysis. Proteomics. 2006;6(2):697–708.

25. Müller H, Haug U, Rothenbacher D, et al. Evaluation of serum and urinary myeloid related protein-14 as a marker for early detection of prostate cancer. J Urol. 2008;180(4):1309–12.

26. Ha YS, Kim MJ, Yoon HY, et al. mRNA expression of S100A8 as a prognostic marker for progression of non-muscle-invasive bladder cancer. Korean J Urol. 2010;51(1):15–20.

27. Kim SK, Kim EJ, Leem SH, et al. Identification of S100A8-correlated genes for prediction of disease progression in non-muscle invasive bladder cancer. BMC Cancer. 2010;10:21.

28. Kim WJ, Kim SK, Jeong P, et al. A four-gene signature predicts disease progression in muscle invasive bladder cancer. Mol Med. 2011;17(5–6):478–85.

29. Kim WT, Kim J, Yan C, et al. S100A9 and EGFR gene signatures predict disease progression in muscle invasive bladder cancer patients after chemotherapy. Ann Oncol. 2014;25(5):974–9.

30. Ebbing J, Mathia S, Seibert FS, et al. Urinary calprotectin: a new diagnostic marker in urothelial carcinoma of the bladder. World J Urol. 2014;32(6):1485–92.

31. Hsieh HL, Schäfer BW, Sasaki N, Heizmann CW. Expression analysis of S100 proteins and RAGE in human tumors using tissue microarrays. Biochem Biophys Res Commun. 2003;307(2):375–81.

32. Khorramdelazad H, Bagheri V, Hassanshahi G, et al. S100A12 and RAGE expression in human bladder transitional cell carcinoma: a role for the ligand/RAGE axis in tumor progression? Asian Pac J Cancer Prev. 2015;16(7):2725–9.

33. Shapiro SG, Raghunath S, Williams C, et al. Canine urothelial carcinoma: genomically aberrant and comparatively relevant. Chromosom Res. 2015;23(2):311–31.

34. Heilmann RM, Wright ZM, Lanerie DJ, et al. Measurement of urinary canine S100A8/A9 and S100A12 concentrations as candidate biomarkers of lower urinary tract neoplasia in dogs. J Vet Diagn Investig. 2014;26(1):104–12.

35. Hjorth L, Wiebe T, Karpman D. Hyperfiltration evaluated by glomerular filtration rate at diagnosis in children with cancer. Pediatr Blood Cancer. 2011;56(5):762–6.

36. Davis BW, Ostrander EA. Domestic dogs and cancer research: a breed-based genomics approach. ILAR J. 2014;55(1):59–68.

37. Budreckis DM, Byrne BA, Pollard RE, et al. Bacterial urinary tract infections associated with transitional cell carcinoma in dogs. J Vet Intern Med. 2015;29(3):828–33.

38. Raposo TP, Beirão BC, Pang LY, et al. Inflammation and cancer: till death tears them apart. Vet J. 2015;205(2):161–74.

39. Turovskaya O, Foell D, Sinha P, et al. RAGE, carboxylated glycans and S100A8/A9 play essential roles in colitis-associated carcinogenesis. Carcinogenesis. 2008;29(10):2035–43.

40. Ehrchen JM, Sunderkötter C, Foell D, et al. The endogenous toll-like receptor 4 agonist S100A8/A9 (calprotectin) as innate amplifier of infection, autoimmunity, and cancer. J Leukoc Biol. 2009;86(3):557–66.

41. Hanada T, Nakagawa M, Emoto A, et al. Prognostic value of tumor-associated macrophage count in human bladder cancer. Int J Urol. 2000;7(7):263–9.

42. Foell D, Frosch M, Sorg C, Roth J. Phagocyte-specific calcium-binding S100 proteins as clinical laboratory markers of inflammation. Clin Chim Acta. 2004;344(1–2):37–51.

43. Fuellen G, Nacken W, Sorg C, Kerkhoff C. Computational searches for missing orthologs: the case of S100A12 in mice. OMICS. 2004;8(4):334–40.

44. Hsu K, Champaiboon C, Guenther BD, et al. Anti-infective protective properties of S100 calgranulins. Antiinflamm Antiallergy Agents Med Chem. 2009;8(4):290–305.

45. Hsu K, Passey RJ, Endoh Y, et al. Regulation of S100A8 by glucocorticoids. J Immunol. 2005;174(4):2318–26.

46. Xu K, Yen T, Geczy CL. IL-10 up-regulates macrophage expression of the S100 protein S100A8. J Immunol. 2001;166(10):6358–66.

5

Vertical transmission of avian leukosis virus subgroup J (ALV-J) from hens infected through artificial insemination with ALV-J infected semen

Yang Li[1,2†], Shuai Cui[1†], Weihua Li[2], Yixin Wang[1], Zhizhong Cui[1*], Peng Zhao[1*] and Shuang Chang[1*]

Abstract

Background: Avian leukosis virus (ALV) is one of the main causes of tumour development within the poultry industry in China. The subgroup J avian leukosis viruses (ALV-J), which induce erythroblastosis and myelocytomatosis, have the greatest pathogenicity and transmission ability within this class of viruses. ALV can be transmitted both horizontally and vertically; however, the effects of ALV infection in chickens—especially roosters—during the propagation, on future generations is not clear. Knowing the role of the cock in the transmission of ALV from generation to generation might contribute to the eradication programs for ALV.

Results: The results showed that two hens inseminated with ALV-J-positive semen developed temporary antibody responses to ALV-J at 4–5 weeks post insemination. The p27 antigen was detected in cloacal swabs of six hens, and in 3 of 26 egg albumens at 1–6 weeks after insemination. Moreover, no viremia was detected at 6 weeks after insemination even when virus isolation had been conducted six times at weekly intervals for each of the 12 females. However, ALV-J was isolated from 1 of their 34 progeny chicks at 1 week of age, and its *gp85* had 98.4%–99.2% sequence identity with the *gp85* of ALV-J isolated from semen samples of the six cocks.

Conclusions: Our findings indicated that females that were late horizontally infected with ALV-J by artificial insemination might transmit the virus to progeny through eggs, which amounts to vertical transmission.

Keywords: Avian leukosis virus subgroup J, Semen, Vertical transmission, Specific pathogen free, Artificial insemination, Progeny chicks

Background

Avian leukosis virus (ALV) is one of the major causes of disease in poultry, and commonly produces tumours in those infected. This virus is recognized by host cell specificity and is susceptible to the virus neutralization reaction, which is mainly associated with the envelope protein, *gp85*. ALVs belong to the genus *Alpharetrovirus* of the family Retroviridae [1], and are divided into 10 subgroups, A to J, according to their host range, cross-neutralization, and viral interference [2]. The subgroup J avian leukosis viruses (ALV-J), which induce erythroblastosis and myelocytomatosis, have a greater pathogenicity and transmission ability than the other subgroups.

ALV-J was first isolated in 1988 from meat-type chickens in Great Britain and it mainly induced myelocytomatosis and nephromas [3]. During the last 10 years, ALV-J has been reported in many areas of the world [4–9]. Some previous studies have demonstrated that this tumorigenic virus can cause immune suppression [5], growth retardation, and tissue tumours in infected fowl [10, 11], which can cause substantial damage to the poultry industry [12, 13].

ALV can be transmitted horizontally and vertically [14–16]; however, the effects of ALV infection in chickens, especially roosters, during reproduction are not clear [17, 18]. In the cock reproductive organs, the virus budding phenomenon

* Correspondence: zzcui@sdau.edu.cn; zhaopeng@sdau.edu.cn; changshuang81@126.com
†Equal contributors
[1]College of Veterinary Medicine, Shandong Agricultural University, Tai'an 271018, China
Full list of author information is available at the end of the article

has been observed through electron microscopy in all structures except germ cells [17]. This indicates that the virus cannot proliferate in the germ cells. Therefore, the rooster may infect other chickens through contact or mating and will act only as a carrier of the virus [19–21]. It is not clear whether hens, after mating or other contact with infected semen, can produce viremia, especially for further vertical transmission to future generations [3].

In this study, each embryonated chicken egg was intravenously infected with ALV-J, and semen was collected from cocks with persistent viremia and used to inseminate specific pathogen free (SPF) hens. This research explores the possibility that hens infected with ALV-J through cock semen transmitted this virus to their offspring, and further clarifies the role of the cock on the infection and spread of ALV-J in chicken flocks.

Results

Isolation and identification of ALV-J in semen

Seminal fluid was collected from six cocks with persistent viremia and inoculated separately into DF-1 cells for ALV-J isolation. All supernatants inoculated with semen samples were positive for the p27 antigen using an ELISA, and IFA detection was positive using the ALV-J-specific monoclonal antibody JE9. At the same time, all negative semen from ALV-J negative control cocks was inoculated into DF-1 cells for p27 and IFA. The results indicated that all six cocks with persistent viremia could release ALV-J into their semen.

Comparison of hens artificially inseminated with the ALV-J-positive or -negative semen for their viremia, antibody responses, and p27 shedding

The results showed that no viremia was detected in any of the hens at 1–6 weeks after insemination with ALV-J-positive semen. The ALV-J antibody response was negative at 1–4 weeks after insemination for all 12 hens. The ALV-J antibody response was positive at 5–6 weeks after insemination in 2 hens, while the other 10 hens were negative for ALV-J. The results of the p27 antigen detection experiments from the cloaca swabs showed a different percentage of p27 positive hens until the end of the experiment at 6 weeks. Viremia was not detected in hens during this experiment; however, 6

of the 12 hens were p27-positive when samples were taken from cloacal swabs at 4, 5, and 6 weeks. Therefore, the control group was inseminated with semen that was negative for ALV-J; all samples were negative for virus viremia, an ALV-J antibody response, and the p27 antigen at 1–6 weeks after insemination. These results indicated that some hens were infected horizontally through artificial insemination.

Comparison of hens artificially inseminated with the ALV-J-positive or -negative semen for p27 antigens in their egg albumens

Eggs were collected from hens that were artificially inseminated with ALV-J-positive or -negative semen, and at one week post insemination, we attempted to detect p27 in the egg albumen. The results indicated that p27 was detected in the albumen of 3 of 26 eggs (11.54%) collected from hens inseminated with ALV-J positive semen, and the S/P values were 0.256, 0.322, and 0.565, which were significantly higher than the 0.2 baseline (S:P ratios that are greater than 0.2 were considered positive for ALV). In contrast, all 26 eggs of the control group were negative for p27, and their ELISA S/P values were less than 0.04. This indicated that some hens shed virus antigens into their egg albumen.

Vertical transmission was confirmed in SPF hens artificially inseminated with ALV-J-positive semen

SPF hens were artificially inseminated, and after one week, eggs were collected for hatching. Hatched progeny chicks were tested for viremia and the presence of p27 by cloacal swabs. As indicated in Table 1, p27 was detected in cloacal swabs of approximately 20–30% of chicks from group 1 hens at 1 d, 1–3 weeks of age, whereas all samples were negative for p27 at 3 weeks of age for control group 2, indicating the possibility of vertical transmission for hens inseminated with ALV-J-positive semen. Importantly, ALV-J was isolated from 1 of 34 chicks at 1 week of age from hens inseminated with ALV-J-positive semen (Table 1). This was subsequently confirmed by IFA with the ALV-J-specific monoclonal antibody JE9 (Fig. 1) and gp85 sequence analysis (see below). This is direct experimental evidence that hens artificially inseminated with ALV-J-positive semen may induce vertical transmission of the disease.

Table 1 The results of viremia and cloacal swab testing of progeny chicks after artificial insemination using the ALV-J positive and negative semen

	1d		1w		2w		3w	
	experimental	Control	experimental	Control	experimental	Control	experimental	Control
viremia	0/34	0/31	1/30[a] (3.3%)	0/30	0/25	0/30	0/22	0/28
cloacal swabs	7/34 (20.6%)	0/31	9/30[b] (30%)	0/30	5/25 (20%)	0/30	4/22 (18.2%)	0/28

[a]The chicken were dead at 10-days-old
[b]Three chickens were dead between 7 to 14 days of age in these nine chickens

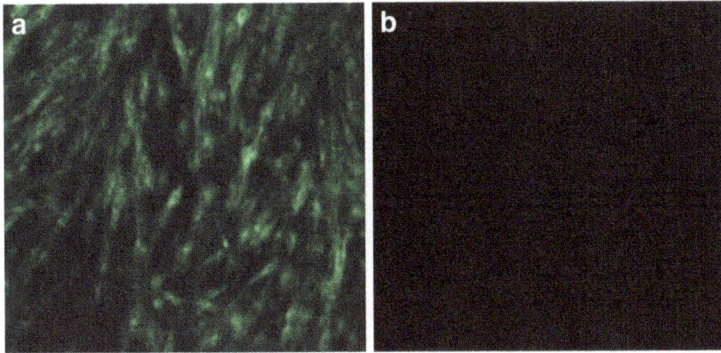

Fig. 1 IFA detection for ALV-J of DF-1 cells of the progeny chicks. **a** Fluorescence from one of the progeny chicks' plasma as detected by IFA using monoclonal antibodies JE9. **b** negative control

gp85 sequence comparisons between ALV-J isolated from progeny, semen, and original challenge virus

The length of the *gp85* gene from ALV-J isolates is 921 bp. Sequence analysis demonstrated that *gp85* from ALV-J isolated from the progeny chick had a very high sequence identity of 98.4–99.2% when compared to viruses isolated from six semen plasma samples from cocks in group 1. Moreover, the sequence identity of ALV-J isolated from chicks was 98.1–99.0% when compared to the original ALV-J strain, 733, which was the original challenging virus for cocks. Furthermore, the ALV-J from six semen plasma samples had a *gp85* sequence identity of 97.6–98.8% when compared to the original strain (Table 2). This was strong evidence that the ALV-J isolated from the progeny chick came from the semen used to inseminate SPF hens.

Discussion

ALV can be transmitted horizontally and vertically, but congenital transmission through eggs is more important to leukosis outbreaks because most tumour cases occur in vertically transmitted or early horizontally infected chickens [22]. The critical roles of infected hens in transmission of ALV from generation to generation in chicken farms have been described and emphasized previously, especially for ALV-J eradication programs [3, 22], as Payne and Nair (2012) described that myelomatosis leukosis (ML) could occur in both congenital and early infected chickens.

Table 2 Sequence comparisons of gp85 of ALV-J isolated from the progeny, the semen, and original challenge virus

	733[a]	seminal fluid	progeny chicks
733[a]	-	97.6%–98.8%	98.1%–99.0%
seminal fluid	97.6%–98.8%	-	98.4%–99.2%
progeny chicks	98.1%–99.0%	98.4%–99.2%	-

[a]733 = original challenge virus

However, the role of cocks in ALV transmission is still not fully understood, and was described as "The role of males in the transmission of ALV is at best equivocal. Infection of the cock apparently does not influence the rate of congenital infection of progeny" and "The cock, therefore, is likely to act only as a virus carrier and source of contact of venereal infection to other birds." Such conclusions were mainly based on early studies [15, 17, 19–21]. Even a more recent schematic description of ALV-J transmission failed to mention the role of infected cocks [3], as venereal infections are able to cause only late infections in females and unable to induce congenital infections in progeny.

The widespread outbreaks of ALV-J were reported in layers and in some Chinese indigenous breeds in recent years in China [23–25]. Studies of this epidemic indicated that the ALV-J infection of cocks might be responsible for the congenital infection of progeny. It was found that ALV was isolated from male chickens, but not female birds, in a large breeding farm, and their progeny developed tumours. In some indigenous chicken breed flocks, a high percentage of progeny were positive for ALV-J viremia when v + (i.e. viremia positive) rates were high in male breeders (e.g. >10%), but very low (e.g. <1%) in their female breeders (unpublished data). Such epidemic phenomena encouraged us to further elucidate the role of the cock in transmission of ALV from generation to generation, especially given that numerous breeding companies are interested in eradication programs for ALV.

In this study, six cocks maintained persistent viremia and shed the virus into their semen (they were termed 'shedders' and designated v + s+). The results indicated that the v + s + cocks might enable female breeders to transmit the virus to their progeny through their eggs. As Table 1 demonstrates, viremia was proven in 1 of 30 chicks hatched from eggs of 12 SPF hens artificially inseminated with v + semen, although all 12 hens remained viremia negative 6 weeks after insemination (Table 3). At

Table 3 The results of viremia, antibody response, and cloacal swab testing of hens after artificial insemination using the ALV-J positive and negative semen

week	group	viremia	ALV-J antibody response	cloacal swabs
1w	experimental	0/12	0/12	2/12
	Control	0/12	0/12	0/12
2w	experimental	0/12	0/12	5/12
	Control	0/12	0/12	0/12
3w	experimental	0/12	0/12	6/12
	Control	0/12	0/12	0/12
4w	experimental	0/12	0/12	6/12
	Control	0/12	0/12	0/12
5w	experimental	0/12	2/12[a]	6/12
	Control	0/12	0/12	0/12
6w	experimental	0/12	2/12[a]	6/12
	Control	0/12	0/12	0/12

[a]Hens are the same in two different times to produce antibody response

the same time, p27 was detected in cloacal swabs from 20 to 30% of the chicks in the experimental group in the first 3 weeks, whereas none of the chicks from the control group was positive for p27. Sequence comparisons indicated that *gp85* of ALV-J isolated from the progeny chick and the semen had very high homology, with a sequence identity of 98.1–99.7% (Table 2), suggesting that ALV-J isolated from the one week old chick originated from the semen used for artificial insemination.

This is the first report to demonstrate that females infected late with ALV-J by artificial insemination may transmit the virus to their progeny through their eggs. It was reported that ALV does not multiply in germ cells of cocks [17], but ALV-J in the semen caused the venereal infection in hens, which further caused a congenital infection in progeny in this experiment. It was recognized that the genetics of different hosts and strains of ALV influence shedding and congenital transmission potentials after horizontal infection [18]. As such, further studies are needed to understand if the phenomena demonstrated in this manuscript would occur when different ALV-J strains and chicken breeds were involved. This study suggests that tests for male virus carriers would be as important as those for female breeders in eradication programs for ALV.

Conclusions

Our findings indicated that females that were late horizontally infected with ALV-J by artificial insemination might transmit the virus to their progeny through their eggs, which amounts to vertical transmission of the virus.

Methods

Virus strains

ALV-J strain 733 was isolated from commercial layer hens and stored after replication in DF-1 cells (American Type Culture Collection, Manassas, VA) in our lab in China in 2012 [26]. The strain shows the typical myelocytomatosis, but no contamination of reticuloendotheliosis virus (REV), infectious bursal disease virus (IBDV), avian reovirus (ARV), chicken infectious anemia virus (CIAV), and Marek's disease virus (MDV) by indirect immunofluorescence assay (IFA), reverse transcription polymerase chain reaction (RT-PCR), and dot-blot hybridization. There were 10^4 $TCID_{50}$ in each 0.1 mL of DF-1 cellular supernatant, which was diluted with PBS 1:10 before inoculating chick embryos.

The infection experiment of ALV-J in cocks

SPF chicken embryos were obtained from the SPAFAS Co. (Jinan, China; a joint venture with Charles River Laboratory, Wilmington, MA, USA) and SPF chickens were normally hatched in our lab. Approximately 100 SPF chicken embryos were divided into 2 groups. All 11-day old chick embryos were intravenously inoculated with ALV-J of 1000 $TCID_{50}$ (50 chicken embryos, group 1). The chicken embryos from the control group were inoculated with PBS (50 chicken embryos, group 2). For group 1, all hens were weeded out after eggs hatched and cocks were kept in a separate isolator. For group 2, all chickens were raised in another separate isolator. Blood samples were aseptically collected from all chickens in heparinized tubes at the age of 4, 8, 16, 20, and 24 weeks. For ALV viremia detection, DF-1 cells were inoculated with plasma samples from the chickens.

Isolation and identification of the ALV-J in seminal fluid

Six cocks, which showed positive persistent viremia and negative viremia, were chosen for the collection of seminal fluid from group 1 after being raised to 24 weeks of age in isolators. The resulting seminal fluid was diluted 1:10 with Gibco Dulbecco Modified Eagle medium (DMEM, Life Technologies, Carlsbad, CA). The samples were then centrifuged at 10,000 g for 15 min at 4 °C. The supernatant was removed and filtered through a 0.22 μm filter (EMD Millipore, Billerica, MA), which was used to inoculate the DF-1 cells. The cells were cultured for 2 h at 37 °C, and the supernatant was replaced with fresh medium containing 1% foetal bovine serum [27]. The cells were incubated for an additional 7 d, and blind passages were performed for 2 generations over a total period of 21 d.

A 100 μL aliquot of cell culture supernatant was analysed for the presence of p27 from ALV using the Avian Leukosis Virus Antigen Test Kit (IDEXX Laboratories,

Westbrook, ME). The ALV-positive supernatant samples were stored at −80 °C. The ALV-positive cells were fixed in an acetone-ethanol (3:2) bath for 5 min, and analysed using IFA with the JE9 anti-ALV-J monoclonal antibody [28] and an ALV-A/B antiserum [9], as previously described. Primary antibody reactivity was detected using a fluorescein isothiocyanate-labelled anti-mouse IgG antibody (Sigma-Aldrich, Saint Louis, MO). A drop of 50% glycerol was added to the coverslip, and the cells were observed using a fluorescence microscope.

Detection of ALV-J infection in hens inseminated with the ALV-J infected semen

Semen samples were collected from six cocks with persistent viremia and mixed for artificial insemination of 12 SPF hens as the experimental group after the hens started producing eggs. Another 12 SPF hens were artificially inseminated with the semen collected from four cocks with no ALV-J infection as the control group. All hens of the two groups were bled once a week for 6 weeks after insemination. Plasma and serum were prepared for each individual hen for virus isolation in cell cultures or ALV-J antibody tests with ELISA antibody detection kits (IDEXX Laboratories, Westbrook, ME). At the same time, cloaca swabs were collected for each hen for p27 antigen detection with the Avian Leukosis Virus Antigen Test Kit (IDEXX Laboratories, Westbrook, ME). The eggs were collected to detect the presence of the p27 antigen from the egg albumen. Eggs were collected 1–3 weeks after insemination and hatched.

Determination of ALV-J infection in progeny chicks

Anticoagulated blood samples from each chicken were collected at the age of 1 d. Subsequently, it took 1–3 weeks to inoculate DF-1 cells in order to conduct virus isolation tests as previously described. The cloacal swabs and meconium were analysed for the presence of the p27 antigen using the Avian Leukosis Virus Antigen Test Kit (IDEXX Laboratories), according to the manufacturer's instructions. All samples collected were analysed in duplicate.

Amplification and sequence analysis of viral RNA

The viral RNAs were extracted from the ALV strain 733, semen plasma samples, and ALV-J isolated from the progeny chicks using the Viral RNA Kit (Omega Bio-Tek, Doraville, CA). The purified RNAs were used for ALV detection by RT-PCR. The primers used for the amplification of the gp85 cDNA from the ALV isolate were designed based on previous studies of representative ALV strains. The primers were as follows: F: 5′-GAT-GAGGCGAGCCCTCTCTTTG-3′; R: 5′-TGTTGGGA GGTAAAATGGCGT-3′. The PCR products were separated by electrophoresis on a 1% agarose gel. The gp85 cDNA bands were purified from the gel using the EZNA Gel Extraction Kit (Omega), and ligated into the PMD-18 T plasmid (Takara Bio, Shiga, Japan). The vector was used to transform competent DH5α *Escherichia coli*. The sequence of the gp85 cDNA was determined by a commercial service (Invitrogen, Shanghai, China). At least three independent RT-PCR experiments were performed for each sample to ensure the accuracy of the results. The sequence alignment was performed using with the Clustal application in the MegAlign program of DNAStar, version 7.01, software suite (DNAStar, Madison, WI, USA).

Abbreviations

ALV: Avian leukosis virus; ALV-J: Avian leukosis virus subgroup J; ARV: Avian reovirus; CIAV: Chicken infectious anemia virus; DMEM: Dulbecco Modified Eagle medium; IBDV: Infectious bursal disease virus; IFA: Indirect immunofluorescence assay; MDV: Marek's disease virus; ML: Myelomatosis leukosis; REV: Reticuloendotheliosis virus; RT-PCR: Reverse transcription polymerase chain reaction; SPF: Specific-pathogen-free

Acknowledgements

The authors would like to thank Enago (www.enago.cn) for critical modification of this manuscript.

Funding

This work was supported by the National Key Research and Development Program of China (2016YFD0501606).

Authors' contributions

YL and SC conducted the experiments, analyzed the data, and drafted the manuscript. WL contributed in experiment design and manuscript revision. YW coordinated supported the challenge experiments. ZC conceived the idea, and revised the manuscript. PZ and SCh conceived and designed the challenge experiments, supervised the project, edited and finalized the manuscript. All authors provide input in interpretation and presentation of the results, and approved the final manuscript.

Consent for publication

Not applicable.

Competing interests

The authors declare that they have no competing interests.

Author details

¹College of Veterinary Medicine, Shandong Agricultural University, Tai'an 271018, China. ²China Animal Health and Epidemiology Center, Qingdao 266032, China.

References

1. Payne LN, Brown SR, Bumstead N, Howes K, Frazier JA, et al. A novel subgroup of exogenous avian leukosis virus in chickens. J Gen Virol. 1991;72:801–7.
2. Chesters PM, Howes K, Petherbridge L, Evans S, Payne LN, et al. The viral envelope is a major determinant for the induction of lymphoid and myeloid tumours by avian leukosis virus subgroups a and J, respectively. J Gen Virol. 2002;83:2553–61.
3. Payne LN, Nair V. The long view: 40 years of avian leukosis research. Avian Pathol. 2012;41:11–9.
4. Cui Z, Du Y, Zhang Z, Silva R. Comparison of Chinese field strains of avian leukosis subgroup J viruses with prototype strain HPRS-103 and United States strains. Avian Dis. 2003;47:1321–30.

5.   Cui Z, Sun S, Wang J. Reduced serologic response to Newcastle disease virus in broiler chickens exposed to a Chinese field strain of subgroup J avian leukosis virus. Avian Dis. 2006;50:191–5.

6.   Malkinson M, Banet-noach C, Davidson I, Fadly AM, Witter RL. Comparison of serological and virological findings from subgroup J avian leukosis virus-infected neoplastic and non-neoplastic flocks in Israel. Avian Pathol. 2004;33:281–7.

7.   Thapa B, Omar A, Arshad S, Hair-Bejo M. Detection of avian leukosis virus subgroup J in chicken flocks from Malaysia and their molecular characterization. Avian Pathol. 2004;33:359–63.

8.   Lai H, Zhang H, Ning Z, Chen R, Zhang W, Qing A, et al. Isolation and characterization of emerging subgroup J avian leukosis virus associated with hemangioma in egg-type chickens. Vet Microbiol. 2011;151:275–83.

9.   Li Y, Liu X, Liu H, Xu C, Liao Y, Wu X, et al. Isolation, identification, and phylogenetic analysis of two avian leukosis virus subgroup J strains associated with hemangioma and myeloid leukosis. Vet Microbiol. 2013;166:356–64.

10. Zavala G. An overview of myeloid leukosis in meat-type chickens. Technical News, Special Technical Bulletin, 1998; January: S1–S4.

11. Stedman NL, Brown TP. Body weight suppression in broilers naturally infected with avian leukosis virus subgroup. J Avian Dis. 1999;43:604–10.

12. Cheng Z, Liu J, Cui Z, Zhang L. Tumors associated with avian leukosis virus subgroup J in layer hens during 2007 to 2009 in China. Journal of Veterinary Medical Sci. 2010;72:1027–33.

13. Gao YL, Qin LT, Pan W, Wang YQ, Qi XL, Gao HL, et al. Avian leukosis virus subgroup J in layer chickens. China Emerg Infect Dis. 2010;16:1637–8.

14. Cottral GE, Burmester BR, Waters NF. Egg transmission of avian lymphomatosis. Poult Sci. 1954;33:1174–84.

15. Rubin H, Cornelius A, Fanshier L. The pattern of congenital transmission of an avian leukosis virus. Proc Natl Acad Sci. 1961;47:1058.

16. Rubin H, Fanshier L, Cornelius A, Hughes WF. Tolerance and immunity in chickens after congenital and contact infection with an avian leukosis virus. Virol. 1962;17:143–56.

17. Di Stefano HS, Dougherty RM. Multiplication of avian leukosis virus in the reproductive system of the rooster. J Natl Cancer Inst. 1968;41:451–64.

18. Crittenden LB, Smith EJ, Fadly AM. Influence of endogenous viral (ev)gene expression and strain of exogenous avian leukosis virus (ALV) on mortality and ALV infection and shedding in chickens. Avian Dis. 1984:1037–56.

19. Spencer JL, Gavora JS, Gowe RS. Lymphoid leukosis virus: natural transmission and nonneoplastic effects. Viruses in Naturally Occurring Cancers (Book A). 1980; 533.

20. Segura JC, Gavora JS, Spencer JL, Fairfull RW, Gowe RS, Buckland RB. Semen traits and fertility of white leghorn males shown to be positive or negative for lymphoid leukosis virus in semen and feather pulp. British Poultry Sci. 1988;29:545–53.

21. Smith EJ, Fadly AM. Male-mediated venereal transmission of endogenous avian leukosis virus. Poultry Sci. 1994;73:488–94.

22. Nair V, Fadly AM. Leukosis/sarcoma group. Diseases of Poultry. Ames, IA: Wiley-Blackwell. 2013; 553–592.

23. Cui Z, Sun S, Zhang Z, Meng S. Simultaneous endemic infections with subgroup J avian leukosis virus and reticuloendotheliosis virus in commercial and local breeds of chickens. Avian Pathol. 2009;38:443–8.

24. Mao Y, Li W, Dong X, Liu J, Zhao P. Different quasispecies with great mutations hide in the same subgroup J field strain of avian leukosis virus. Sci ChinaLife Sci. 2013;56:414–20.

25. Dong X, Zhao P, Li W, Chang S, Li J, Li Y, et al. Diagnosis and sequence analysis of avian leukosis virus subgroup J isolated from Chinese partridge shank chickens. Poultry Sci. 2015;94:668–72.

26. Bian X, Li D, Zhao P, Cui Z. Continuous observation of subgroup J avian leukosis for three groups of commercial layer chicken. Sci Agric Sin. 2013;46:409–16.

27. Qin L, Gao Y, Ni W, Sun M, Wang Y, Yin C, et al. Development and application of real-time PCR for detection of subgroup J avian leukosis virus. J Clin Microbiol. 2013;51:149–54.

28. Qin A, Lee LF, Fadly A, Hunt H, Cui Z. Development and characterization of monoclonal antibodies to subgroup J avian leukosis virus. Avian Dis. 2001; 45:938–45.

6

Antiproliferative effects of masitinib and imatinib against canine oral fibrosarcoma *in vitro*

Milan Milovancev[1*], Stuart C. Helfand[1], Kevin Marley[1], Cheri P. Goodall[1], Christiane V. Löhr[2] and Shay Bracha[1]

Abstract

Background: Canine oral fibrosarcoma (COF) is one of the most common oral tumors in dogs and carries a guarded prognosis due to a lack of effective systemic therapeutic options. Mastinib and imatinib are two commonly used tyrosine kinase inhibitors (TKIs) in veterinary oncology but their potential efficacy against COF is uncharacterized. To begin investigating the rationale for use of these TKIs against COF, the present study tested for the presence TKI targets PDGFR-α, PDGFR-β, Kit, and VEGFR-2 and examined the *in vitro* effects on cell viability after TKI treatment alone or with doxorubicin.

Immunohistochemistry for PDGFR-α, PDGFR-β, Kit, and VEGFR-2 was performed in 6 COF tumor biopsies. Presence of these same receptors within 2 COF cell lines was probed by reverse transcription-polymerase chain reaction and, for those with mRNA detected, confirmed via western blot. Effects on cell viability were assessed using an MTS assay after masitinib or imatinib treatment alone (0-100 μM), or in combination with doxorubicin (0-3000 nM doxorubicin). Anti-*PDGFRB* siRNA knockdown was performed and the effect on cell viability quantified.

Results: Expression of the TKI targets evaluated was similar between the 2 COF cell lines and the 6 COF tumor biopsies: PDGFR-α and PDGFR-β were detected in neoplastic cells from most COF tumor biopsies (5/6 and 6/6, respectively) and were present in both COF cell lines; *KIT* and *KDR* were not detected in any sample. Masitinib and imatinib IC50 values ranged from 7.9–33.4 μM, depending on the specific TKI and cell line tested. The addition of doxorubicin resulted in synergistic cytotoxicity with both TKIs. Anti-*PDGFRB* siRNA transfection reduced PDGFR-β protein expression by 77 % and 67 % and reduced cell viability by 24 % ($p < 0.0001$) and 28 % ($0 = 0.0003$) in the two cell lines, respectively.

Conclusions: These results provide rationale for further investigation into the use of TKIs, possibly in combination with doxorubicin, as treatment options for COF.

Keywords: Dog, Oral fibrosarcoma, Masitinib, Imatinib, Platelet-derived growth factor receptor

Background

Canine oral fibrosarcoma (COF) is one of the three most common oral neoplasms in dogs [1]. Compared to other anatomic locations, COF exhibits a biologically aggressive behavior with recurrence rates following resection of 24–59 %, metastasis in up to 30 % of cases, and reported median survival times of 7–24 months [2–9]. The most recent of these studies included 65 dogs and found significant predictors of median survival time to include tumor location (maxillary location better than mandibular), size (smaller tumors better), type of surgery (aggressive surgery better than conservative), histologic margin status, and grade (low grade better). This study included 14 dogs that received adjuvant systemic therapy (4 received doxorubicin and 10 received metronomic chemotherapy) but because of this low sample size and the fact that therapy was often initiated after relapse of disease, no conclusions could be drawn regarding the potential efficacy of this treatment strategy [8]. Currently, the prognosis for this disease remains guarded due to a lack of effective systemic therapeutic options to address potential metastasis as well as local recurrence [1–9].

* Correspondence: milan.milovancev@oregonstate.edu
[1]Department of Clinical Sciences, College of Veterinary Medicine, Oregon State University, Corvallis, OR 97331, USA
Full list of author information is available at the end of the article

The use of receptor tyrosine kinase inhibitors (TKIs) for targeted therapy in veterinary oncology is increasing as indicated by the growing number of clinical reports [10–15]. Although some reports describe use of TKIs alone, others have reported on observed clinical efficacy when combined with traditional cytotoxic chemotherapeutic agents and/or piroxicam [10, 11, 13, 15, 16]. Proposed mechanisms behind combination therapy include chemosensitization as well as immunomodulatory effects such as suppression of regulatory T cells and restoration of T cell-mediated immune responses [16]. Masitinib is conditionally approved by the United States Food and Drug Administration and the European Medicines Agency for use against canine mast cell tumors. Masitinib targets PDGFR-α and -β, Kit, Lyn, and to a lesser degree, the FGFR3 and FAK pathways [16]. Masitinib may also affect VEGFR-2 levels [14]. Imatinib is another TKI that targets some of the same kinases as masitinib, including PDGFR-α, PDGFR-β, and Kit [16, 17]. Although not approved by the United States Food and Drug Administration for use in veterinary patients, off-label veterinary use of imatinib has been reported with favorable results in canine and feline cancer patients [18–21].

To our knowledge, there are no reports that have profiled expression of tyrosine kinases in COF, nor the potential for targeting by masitinib or imatinib. The purpose of this study was to (1) evaluate the expression of PDGFR-α, PDGFR-β, Kit, and VEGFR-2 in archived COF biopsies and immortalized cell lines and (2) assess the effects on cell viability of two TKIs (masitinib and imatinib), either alone or in combination with doxorubicin, against the cell lines *in vitro*. The results presented herein begin to shed light on this strategy as a potential future therapy for COF.

Results
Archived canine oral fibrosarcoma tumors express PDGFR-α and –β protein

Immunohistochemistry (IHC) for PDGFR-α, PDGFR-β, Kit, and VEGFR-2 demonstrated differential expression of each protein amongst the six archived tumor specimens with good agreement between subjective observer-derived assessments and semi-quantitative software-derived results (Table 1). Representative photomicrographs for each of the proteins evaluated are shown in Fig. 1. A representative software threshold-processed image of tumor cell immunoreactivity for PDGFR-β is shown in Fig. 2. Higher percentages represent more immunoreactivity (i.e. pixels above the user-defined threshold for IHC stain). Mitotic counts in five of six sarcomas were low, ranging from 1 to 4 in ten 400x high power fields. Case 3 had a much higher mitotic count (*n* = 15). This tumor also had the largest nuclei, poorest overall

Table 1 Immunohistochemistry reactivity scores

Protein	Dog #	% Cells	Location	Intensity	% Area
PDGFR-α	1	75	C, N	+	29.4
	2	80	C, N	+	26.2
	3	100	C, N	++	21.6
	4	90	C, N	++	43.9
	5	0	–	–	0
	6	90	C, N	+	11.6
PDGFR-β	1	90	C, M	+++	34.8
	2	70	C, M	++	40.8
	3	100	C	+++	38.1
	4	60	C	+++	23.8
	5	90	C	+	19.6
	6	80	C	++	21.8
Kit	1	0	–	–	0
	2	0	–	–	0
	3	0	–	–	0
	4	0	–	–	0
	5	0	–	–	0
	6	0	–	–	0
VEGFR-2	1	0	–	–	0
	2	0	–	–	0
	3	0	–	–	0
	4	0	–	–	0
	5	0	–	–	0
	6	0	–	–	0

Subjective scoring of immunoreactivity of 6 archived canine oral fibrosarcoma cases for VEGFR-2, PDGFR-α, PDGFR-β, and Kit. The estimated percentage of tumor cells displaying immunoreactivity, the predominant location(s) of staining (C = cytoplasmic, M = membranous, or N = nuclear), and the subjective intensity of staining (+, ++, or +++) are displayed along with semi-quantitative measurement of immunoreactivity using computer image analysis software and threshold-processed photomicrographs

organization, and most intense IHC staining for both PDGFRs.

Staining for PDGFR-α was detected in the cytoplasm and nuclei of 75–100 % of neoplastic cells in five of the six tumor samples, with a relatively uniform staining intensity among samples. In all sections, PDGFR-α staining was also present in the cytoplasm and nuclei of endothelial cells including neoplastic endothelial cells of a canine metastatic hemangiosarcoma control sample. Similarly, PDGFR-β was detected in the cytoplasm of 60–100 % of neoplastic cells in all six tumor samples. There was relatively uniform intensity and subcellular location of immunostaining of neoplastic cells in five of the biopsy samples with a similar distribution but weaker staining intensity in the remaining sample. Two samples also showed cell membrane associated PDGFR-β staining. PDGFR-β stained the cytoplasm of endothelial cells in all sections including neoplastic endothelial

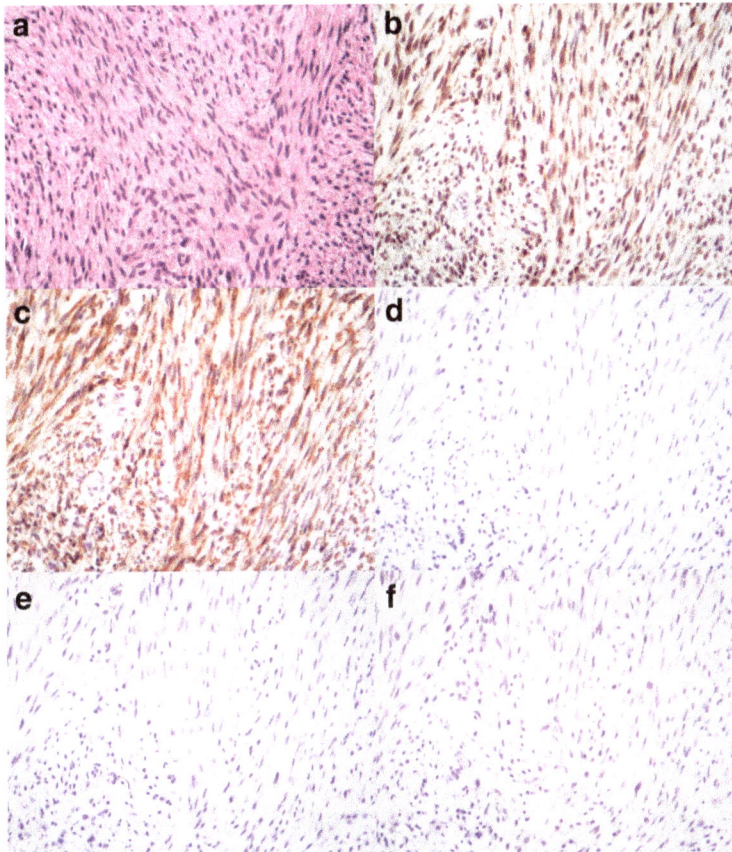

Fig. 1 Immunohistochemistry of archived canine oral fibrosarcoma tumor biopsies. Representative photomicrographs of an archived canine oral fibrosarcoma tumor specimen (dog #4) stained with (**a**) hematoxylin and eosin, **b** PDGFR-α immunohistochemistry, **c** PDGFR-β immunohistochemistry, **d** Kit immunohistochemistry, **e** VEGFR-2 immunohistochemistry, and **f** rabbit negative control; 400×. Immunoreactivity for PDGFR-α (both cytoplasmic and nuclear locations) and PDGFR-β (predominantly cytoplasmic location) is visible. No staining is seen for VEGFR-2, Kit, or in the rabbit negative control

cells in the hemangiosarcoma control sample. VEGFR-2 and Kit staining were uniformly negative in neoplastic cells of all six COF tumor samples. Endothelial cells around but not within the tumors had cytoplasmic staining for VEGFR-2, whereas neoplastic cells of a metastatic hemangiosarcoma did not stain. Most sections had interstitial mast cells that displayed a largely membrane-associated staining pattern for Kit. In the mast cell tumor control sample, most neoplastic cells had cytoplasmic, perinuclear, punctate staining for Kit (pattern 2); less than 5 % showed diffuse cytoplasmic staining (pattern 3) [22].

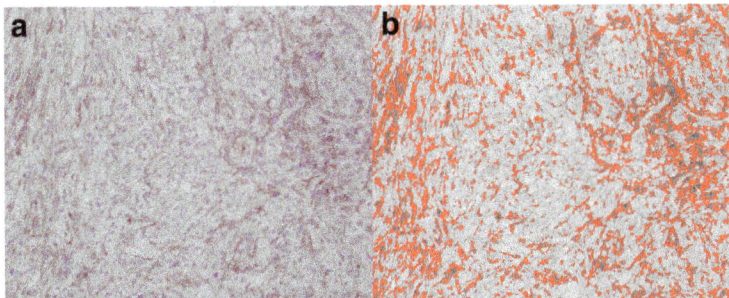

Fig. 2 Semi-quantitative assessment of immunoreactivity via image threshold-processing. Representative photomicrograph of PDGFR-β immunohistochemical staining of an archived canine oral fibrosarcoma tumor specimen (dog #6) before (**a**) and after (**b**) threshold-processing for semi-quantitative assessment of immunoreactivity; 400×. Red pixels are reported as percentage of total image pixels to provide a semi-quantified measure of immunoreactivity

Canine oral fibrosarcoma cell lines express PDGFR-α and –β at both mRNA and protein levels

PDGFRA and *PDGFRB* mRNA was reverse transcribed and amplified from exponentially growing MBSa1 and CoFSA cells by reverse transcription-polymerase chain reaction (RT-PCR; Fig. 3a). Amplicons were of the predicted size and sequencing reaction results matching the published sequence with 100 % homology. Transcripts for *KIT* and *KDR* were not detected (Fig. 3a) despite using two different canine-specific primer sets.

Western blots showed strong expression of both PDGFR-α and –β in cell lysates from CoFSA, with weaker expression in MBSa1 (Fig. 3b). These data coincide with the apparent mRNA signals shown in these two cell lines (Fig. 3a).

Masitinib or imatinib alone, or in combination with doxorubicin, inhibit canine oral fibrosarcoma cell viability

Masitinib treated cells displayed decreased viability relative to the vehicle-treated control at concentrations of 10, 30, and 100 μM for both MBSa1 and CoFSA cell lines ($p < 0.0001$; Fig. 4a). The calculated IC50 of masitinib for MBSa1 and CoFSA is 9.1 and 12.0 μM,

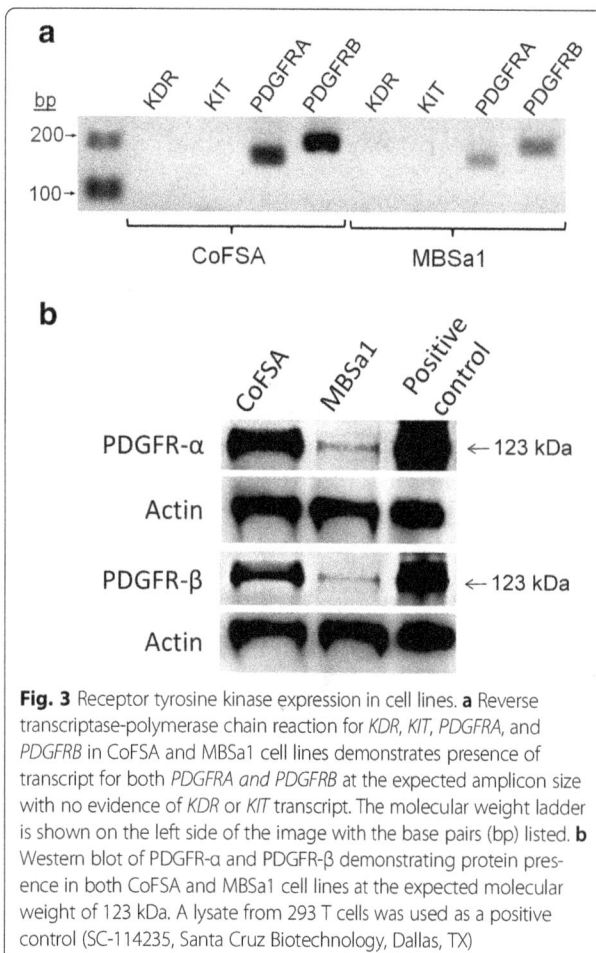

Fig. 3 Receptor tyrosine kinase expression in cell lines. **a** Reverse transcriptase-polymerase chain reaction for *KDR, KIT, PDGFRA*, and *PDGFRB* in CoFSA and MBSa1 cell lines demonstrates presence of transcript for both *PDGFRA and PDGFRB* at the expected amplicon size with no evidence of *KDR* or *KIT* transcript. The molecular weight ladder is shown on the left side of the image with the base pairs (bp) listed. **b** Western blot of PDGFR-α and PDGFR-β demonstrating protein presence in both CoFSA and MBSa1 cell lines at the expected molecular weight of 123 kDa. A lysate from 293 T cells was used as a positive control (SC-114235, Santa Cruz Biotechnology, Dallas, TX)

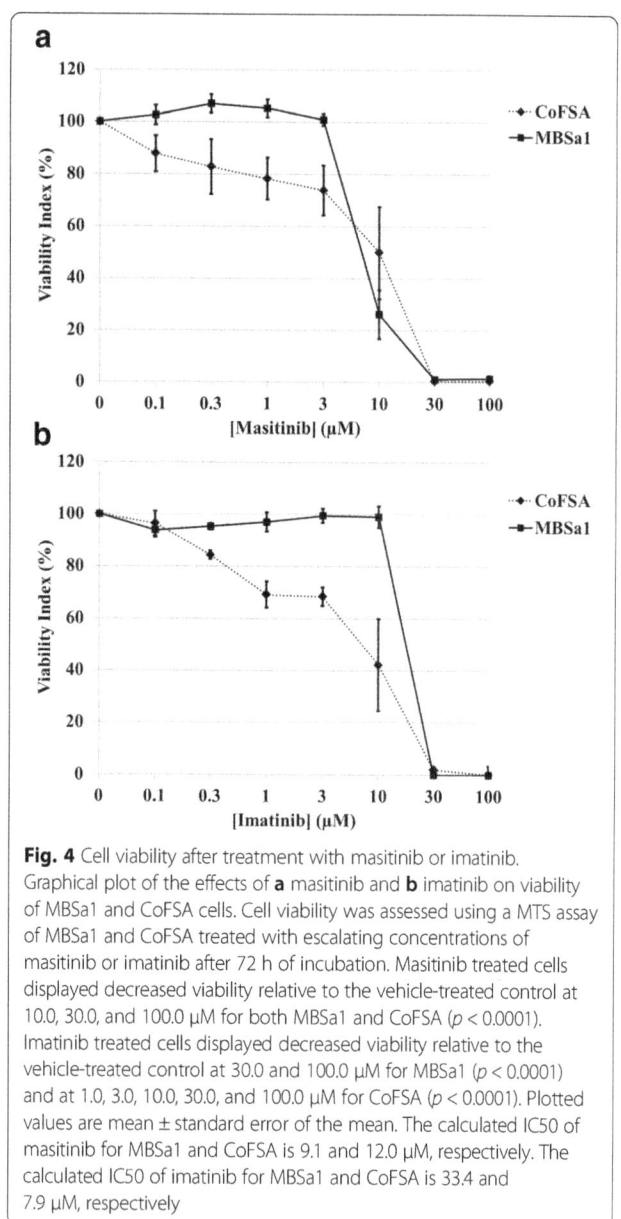

Fig. 4 Cell viability after treatment with masitinib or imatinib. Graphical plot of the effects of **a** masitinib and **b** imatinib on viability of MBSa1 and CoFSA cells. Cell viability was assessed using a MTS assay of MBSa1 and CoFSA treated with escalating concentrations of masitinib or imatinib after 72 h of incubation. Masitinib treated cells displayed decreased viability relative to the vehicle-treated control at 10.0, 30.0, and 100.0 μM for both MBSa1 and CoFSA ($p < 0.0001$). Imatinib treated cells displayed decreased viability relative to the vehicle-treated control at 30.0 and 100.0 μM for MBSa1 ($p < 0.0001$) and at 1.0, 3.0, 10.0, 30.0, and 100.0 μM for CoFSA ($p < 0.0001$). Plotted values are mean ± standard error of the mean. The calculated IC50 of masitinib for MBSa1 and CoFSA is 9.1 and 12.0 μM, respectively. The calculated IC50 of imatinib for MBSa1 and CoFSA is 33.4 and 7.9 μM, respectively

respectively. Imatinib treated cells displayed decreased viability relative to the vehicle-treated control at 30.0 and 100.0 μM for MBSa1 ($p < 0.0001$) and at 1.0, 3.0, 10.0, 30.0, and 100.0 μM for CoFSA ($p < 0.0001$; Fig. 4b). The calculated IC50 of imatinib for MBSa1 and CoFSA is 33.4 and 7.9 μM, respectively.

The combination of either 1.0 μM masitinib or imatinib with doxorubicin yielded synergistic reductions in cell viability for both cell lines (Fig. 5). Combination treatment demonstrated synergism in MBSa1 cells at all doxorubicin concentrations for masitinib and at 1, 3, 10, 30, and 100 nM doxorubicin concentrations for imatinib (Fig. 5a). Due to the greater reduction in cell viability seen with 1.0 μM of either TKI alone in CoFSA cells, synergism was shown only at the highest doxorubicin

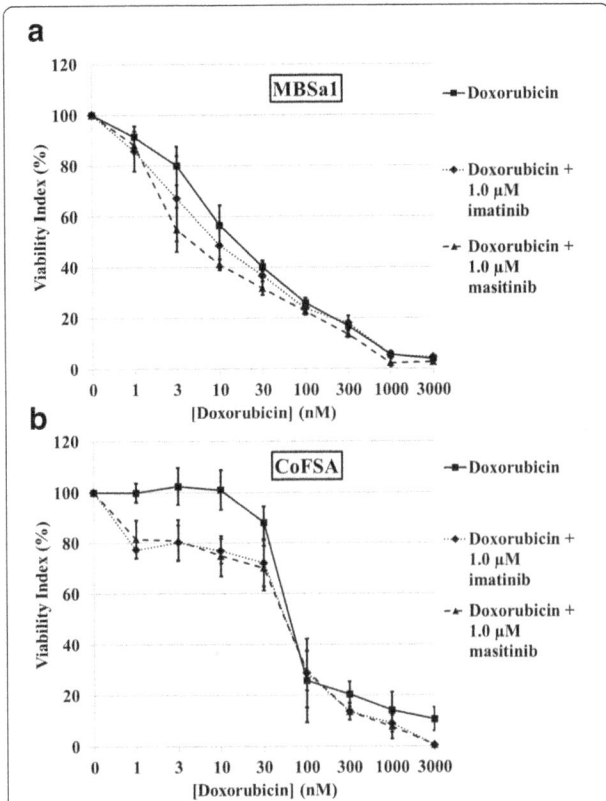

Fig. 5 Cell viability following doxorubicin treatment alone or combined with 1.0 μM of either masitinib or imatinib. Graphical plot of the effects of treatment with escalating concentrations of doxorubicin alone or combined with 1.0 μM of either masitinib or imatinib on viability of (**a**) MBSa1 and (**b**) CoFSA cells. Cell viability was assessed using a MTS assay following treatment with the above drug concentrations after 72 h of incubation. Masitinib showed a synergistic interaction with doxorubicin at all concentrations for MBSa1 and at 10, 300, 1000, and 3000 nM for CoFSA. Imatinib showed a synergistic interaction with doxorubicin at 1, 3, 10, 30, and 100 nM for MBSa1 and at 300, 1000, and 3000 nM for CoFSA. Plotted values are mean ± standard error of the mean. Synergism was defined as being present when the surviving fraction of cells exposed to the combination of doxorubicin and either tyrosine kinase inhibitor was lower than the product of the surviving fraction of cells exposed to the tyrosine kinase inhibitor alone multiplied by the surviving fraction of cells exposed to doxorubicin alone. See Materials and Methods section for detailed synergism calculation methods

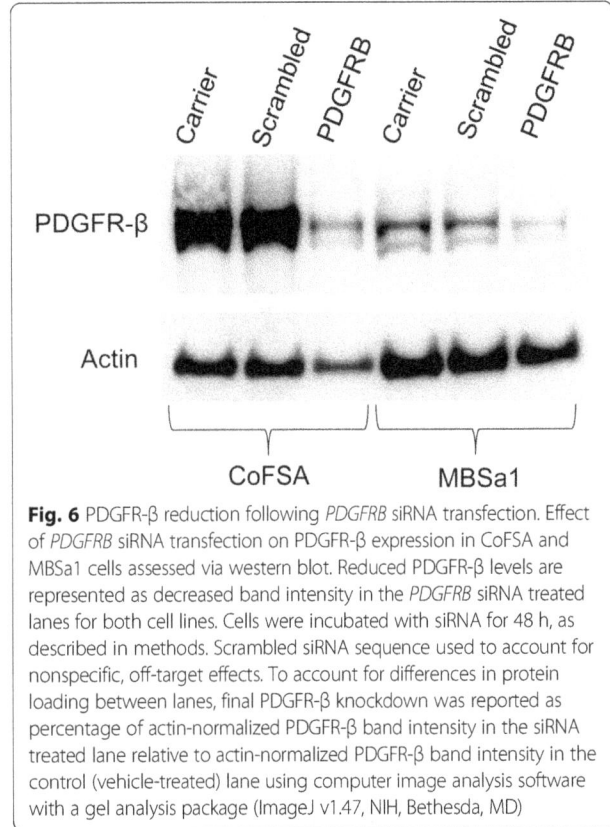

Fig. 6 PDGFR-β reduction following *PDGFRB* siRNA transfection. Effect of *PDGFRB* siRNA transfection on PDGFR-β expression in CoFSA and MBSa1 cells assessed via western blot. Reduced PDGFR-β levels are represented as decreased band intensity in the *PDGFRB* siRNA treated lanes for both cell lines. Cells were incubated with siRNA for 48 h, as described in methods. Scrambled siRNA sequence used to account for nonspecific, off-target effects. To account for differences in protein loading between lanes, final PDGFR-β knockdown was reported as percentage of actin-normalized PDGFR-β band intensity in the siRNA treated lane relative to actin-normalized PDGFR-β band intensity in the control (vehicle-treated) lane using computer image analysis software with a gel analysis package (ImageJ v1.47, NIH, Bethesda, MD)

concentrations tested: 10, 300, 1000, and 3000 nM for masitinib and 300, 1000, and 3000 nM for imatinib (Fig. 5b).

PDGFRB siRNA knocks down PDGFR-β protein expression and reduces oral fibrosarcoma cell line viability

Western blot analysis demonstrated that PDGFR-β is expressed in both MBSa1 and CoFSA cell lines, with a marked reduction in PDGFR-β expression evident in both cell lines after *PDGFRB* siRNA transfection (Fig. 6). Densitometry measurements of actin-normalized PDGFR-β band intensity (expressed as a percentage of the vehicle-only treated control cells) revealed a reduction of PDGFR-β

protein in MBSa1 and CoFSA cells of 77.4 % and 67.4 %, respectively.

Cell viability after *PDGFRB* siRNA transfection was significantly reduced in both MBSa1 (mean reduction of 24.0 %; $p < 0.0001$) and CoFSA (mean reduction of 27.6 %; $p = 0.0003$) cell lines compared to vehicle-treated control cells (Fig. 7). Visual comparison of siRNA-transfected cells to control cells revealed a greater negative effect on cell viability than was reflected by the MTS assay results (Fig. 7).

Effect of masitinib and imatinib, alone or combined with doxorubicin, on oral fibrosarcoma cell line caspase activity

MBSa1 cells did not demonstrate significant changes in caspase-3/7 activity at any drug concentration tested (Fig. 8a and c). In contrast, CoFSA cells did display significantly increased caspase activity at 1.0 μM masitinib alone (Fig. 8b) and at 300 nM doxorubicin combined with either 1.0 μM masitinib or imatinib (Fig. 8d); CoFSA cells showed significantly reduced caspase activity following treatment with 30 μM masitinib alone (Fig. 8b).

Discussion

This study begins to explore the potential rationale for using two commonly prescribed TKIs (masitinib and imatinib) as adjunctive treatment in COF. The stimulus

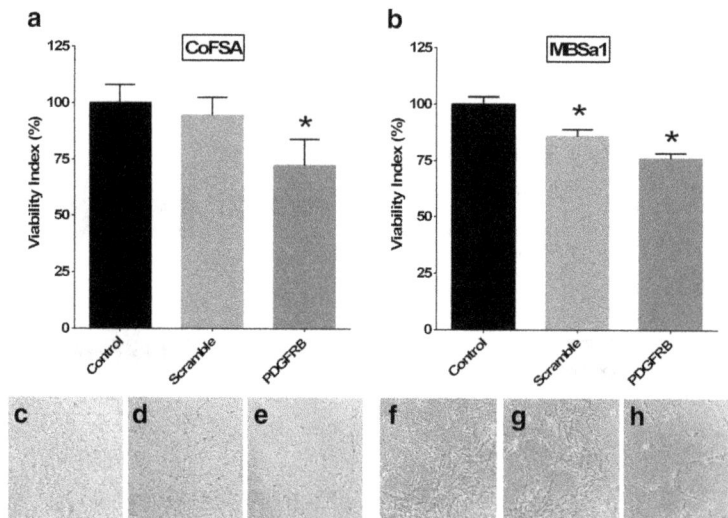

Fig. 7 Cell viability following *PDGFRB* siRNA transfection. Effect of *PDGFRB* siRNA transfection on (**a**) CoFSA and (**b**) MBSa1 cell viability assessed via an MTS assay after 72 h of incubation, with representative photomicrographs of cells under each condition (CoFSA cells treated with (**c**) vehicle alone, **d** scrambled siRNA sequence, and **e** *PDGFRB* siRNA; MBSa1 cells **f** treated with vehicle alone, **g** scrambled siRNA sequence, and **h** *PDGFRB* siRNA). Scrambled siRNA sequence used to account for nonspecific, off-target effects. "*" indicates statistically significant ($p < 0.05$) differences in cell viability compared to vehicle-treated controls. Because siRNA transfection was performed during two independent experiments, statistical analysis for these data was performed using the 6 replicates within one representative siRNA experiment. Visual assessment of cellular appearance in *PDGFRB* siRNA treated samples (**e** and **h**) display apoptotic bodies and marked cellular morphologic deterioration

for this investigation is based on the premise that targeted small molecule therapy may provide an adjuvant therapeutic strategy for control of COF following surgery, given the challenge of obtaining complete surgical tumor excision and the reluctance of many pet owners to pursue adjuvant radiotherapy. We began by testing for the presence of targets of these two TKIs, including PDGFR-α, PDGFR-β, VEGFR-2, and Kit, in six archived COF tumors and two immortalized COF cell lines. Our results demonstrate a similar expression profile between the immortalized cell lines and the archived tumor samples, leading into the second aim of the study: assessing the effects of the two TKIs on cell viability, either alone or in combination with doxorubicin. Our data show both cell lines were relatively resistant to single-agent TKI treatment, with substantial reductions in cell viability and an increase in apoptotic activity being seen only at relatively high concentrations in most experiments. Both TKIs met the criteria for synergistic *in vitro* cytotoxicity when combined with doxorubicin, although the magnitude of this effect was relatively small. Cumulatively, the present study provides insight into the potential validity of future *in vivo* investigations exploring the use of TKIs, possibly in combination with traditional cytotoxic chemotherapeutic agents, as adjuvant treatment options in COF.

Of the four potential TKI targets evaluated via IHC, PDGFR-β was the most consistently expressed (6/6 of archived tumors) and showed the strongest immunoreactivity

across tumor samples. Furthermore, PDGFR-β was detected within both cell lines at the mRNA and protein levels. PDGFR-α was also frequently detected with 5/6 archived tumor samples showing immunoreactivity, but with lower subjective staining intensity and scoring lower on our semi-quantitative immunoreactivity measurements. Both cell lines also expressed PDGFR-α at both mRNA and protein levels. The COF tumor sample with the highest mitotic count and least degree of differentiation was among the tumors with the most intense IHC staining for PDGFR-β and PDGFR-α, consistent with the positive effect of PDGF on cell proliferation. Neither Kit nor VEGFR-2 were detected at the protein level within tumor samples or at mRNA levels within the cell lines. These data indicate that at least two targets of the TKIs used in this study are present within COF tumors and provided a rationale for proceeding with the evaluation of cell viability following TKI treatment.

The *in vitro* effect of the tested TKIs on CoFSA and MBSa1 cell viability was observed to be relatively similar between the two drugs. These observations are consistent with the shared targets between the two TKIs [15, 16]. MBSa1 cells were consistently resistant to either TKI, with significant cytotoxic effects seen only at high concentrations and no significant changes in apoptosis elicited by any drug concentration tested. By comparison, CoFSA cells were similarly resistant to masitinib but slightly more sensitive to imatinib, with a modest but statistically significant reduction in cell viability at ≥ 1 μM concentrations. CoFSA cells also demonstrated significant increases in apoptosis at

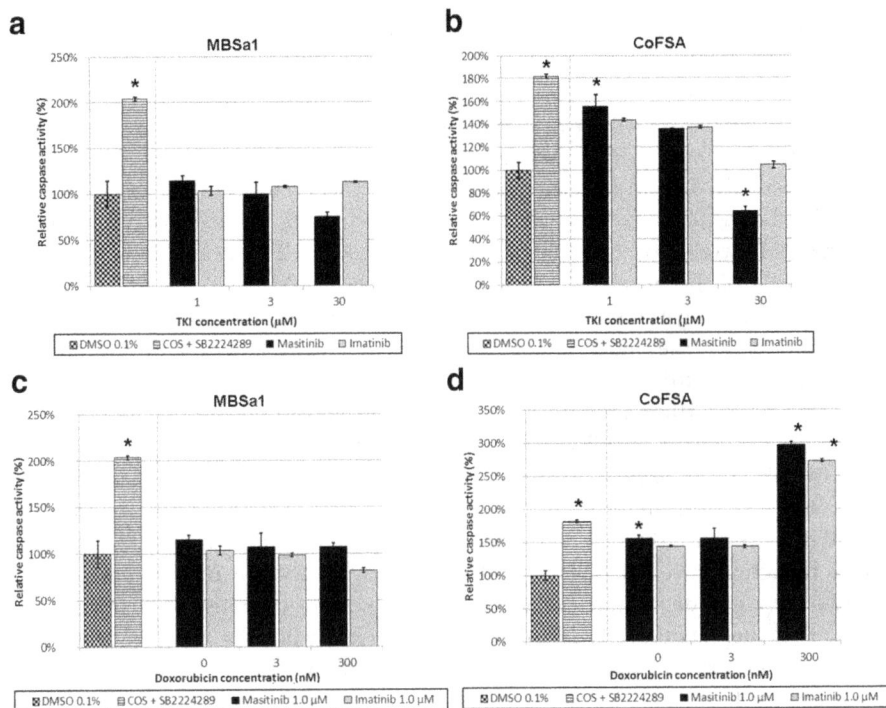

Fig. 8 Cell apoptosis following treatment with imatinib and masitinib, alone or combined with doxorubicin. Graphical plot of relative caspase activity following treatment with escalating concentrations of masitinib and imatinib alone (**a** and **b**) and doxorubicin combined with 1.0 μM of either masitinib or imatinib (**c** and **d**) on MBSa1 and CoFSA cells, respectively. Caspase activity was assessed using a luminogenic caspase-3/7 substrate assay following treatment with the above drug concentrations after 72 h of incubation and expressed as a percentage of caspase activity within vehicle-treated (DMSO 0.1 %) control cells. COS cells treated with SB2224269 represent a positive control. Plotted values are mean ± standard error of the mean. "*" indicates statistically significant ($p < 0.001$) difference compared to the vehicle-treated controls indicated by a one-way ANOVA with Dunnett's correction

select drug concentrations, consistent with their increased sensitivity to the treatments evaluated in this study. CoFSA cells also showed a significant decrease in relative caspase activity at 30 μM masitinib, which may reflect a paucity of cells with caspase activity due to the extremely low cell viability at this TKI concentration, as supported by our MTS assay results. These relatively minor differences in TKI sensitivity between cell lines may reflect a combination of differences in drug targets between the two TKIs tested along with differences in the cell lines used [14, 16]. To the authors' knowledge, no studies have characterized specific receptor tyrosine kinase pathway dependence in either MBSa1 or CoFSA cell lines. Several other *in vitro* veterinary studies have reported similarly high masitinib or imatinib IC50 concentrations in canine hemangiosarcoma and feline injection site sarcoma cell lines [12, 14, 23]. In contrast, the cell-based IC50s for masitinib against PDGFR-α, PDGFR-β, and Kit have been reported as 0.3, 0.05, and 0.15 μM, respectively, in an IL3-dependent hematopoietic cell line [24]. These values are markedly lower than the IC50 values seen in the present and prior *in vitro* veterinary studies, raising the possibility that the observed reductions in cell viability may be due to off-target effects. This is also compatible

with the calculated IC50 values from another veterinary study evaluating *in vitro* masitinib effects on a variety of immortalized canine cancer cell lines [25]. The reason for this relative resistance to single-agent TKI treatment in the cell lines in the present report, as well as in the those cell lines used in the referenced studies, is not fully understood but likely reflects the cell lines' lack of dependence on the targeted pathways for survival [12, 14, 23, 25]. However, as pointed out in previous reports, findings such as described in the current study do not preclude a potential clinical benefit of masitinib therapy either as a single agent targeting tumor-related angiogenesis, or perhaps more importantly, as a potential chemosensitizer [25].

To begin to investigate the potential role of either masitinib or imatinib as chemosensitizers in COF, we performed MTS assays using a range of doxorubicin concentrations, with or without 1.0 μM of either TKI. This concentration of TKI was chosen because pharmacokinetic studies in healthy Beagle dogs have shown that a clinically-relevant oral dose of 10 mg/kg of masitinib results in a serum maximum concentration of 1.3–1.5 μM [26]. Our data support an *in vitro* synergistic effect of either TKI with doxorubicin in both cell lines, although the effect was modest. The potential for myelo-suppression, or other side-effects, may be increased when TKIs are combined with traditional cytotoxic chemotherapeutic agents *in vivo*, as shown in a study evaluating the safety of toceranib combined with vinblastine in dogs with mast cell tumors [16]. Maximal sensitization factors, potential alterations in drug pharmacokinetics, and alternative methods for determining pharmacologic synergism were not considered as they extend beyond the scope of the present study, but may form the basis for future investigations.

As PDGFR-β was found to be the most uniformly expressed receptor tyrosine kinase for TKI targeting in the present study, we chose to further investigate the contribution of PDGFR-β signaling to viability of COF cell lines. Knockdown of PDGFR-β protein expression via siRNA transfection was successful in both cell lines. The effect of this PDGFR-β protein reduction was associated with a significant reduction in cell viability in both cell lines as well as visibly apparent degenerative changes in cellular morphology. This suggests that PDGFR-β signaling plays a partial role in maintaining viability of COF cells, but the overall significance of this single signaling pathway to COF cell survival requires further investigation.

Although a thorough discussion of the mechanism of action of imatinib and masitinib is beyond the scope of this report, a few select points are worth highlighting. Both TKIs are considered small molecule inhibitors that selectively interfere with specific receptor tyrosine kinase activity (PDGFR-α, -β, and Kit; masitinib also targets Lyn, the FGFR3 and FAK pathways and possibly VEGFR-2 levels) [14, 16, 27]. Through occupying the receptor's active site, thereby blocking receptor tyrosine kinase phosphorylation, TKIs prevent subsequent activation of downstream pathways. Depending on the cell's dependence on the targeted pathways, this may result in cell death [16]. Some TKIs, such as masitinib, have shown an anticancer action that extends beyond inhibition of its primary targets, and may include disruption of additional signaling pathways associated with tumor progression, metastasis, and chemoresistance [25, 26, 28, 29]. The *in vivo* tumor microenvironment is characterized by varying levels of hypoxia and acidity, which influence tumor cell behavior and drug sensitivity, potentially rendering them more or less sensitive to TKI treatment [30]. PDGFR is emerging as a key regulator of mesenchymal cells within the tumor microenvironment of many common human malignancies [31]. Blockade of PDGFR signaling has been shown to reduce metastasis in *in vivo* murine models of colorectal and prostate cancers [32–34]. These points serve to illustrate some of the impetus behind this study's investigations into the use of TKIs as a potential treatment strategy, although their

applicability to imatinib and/or masitinib treatment of COF remain unknown at this time.

The primary limitations of the present study center on its *in vitro* nature and the limited experimental methods used. This study tested for receptor tyrosine kinase expression but did not evaluate receptor phosphorylation status (i.e. activation), receptor over- or under-expression, or effect of ligand stimulation on the receptors present. The presence of TKI targets does not necessarily imply their requirement for cell survival or a gain-of-function structural aberration conferring malignant behavior. This study evaluated effects of TKI treatment on COF cell line viability using an MTS assay, supplemented with an apoptosis assay for select drug concentrations, representing only a partial evaluation of potential TKI effects. Examples of additional treatment effects that could be examined in future studies include COF cell migration and/or metastasis. Finally, it is difficult to extrapolate *in vitro* results of TKI treatment to the far more complex *in vivo* scenario that includes interactions with the tumor microenvironment and the host immune system.

Conclusions

In conclusion, this study identified expression of PDGFR-α and –β in COF tumor biopsies and cell lines. Treatment with masitinib or imatinib yielded *in vitro* reductions in cell viability which was enhanced synergistically by the addition of doxorubicin. Furthermore, the tested COF cell lines exhibited partial PDGFR-β dependency for survival. Taken together, these data support further investigation into the potential use of TKIs, potentially in combination with doxorubicin, to augment existing treatment options for COF.

Methods
Immunohistochemistry of archived canine oral fibrosarcomas

Medical records from dogs seen at the Oregon State University Lois Bates Acheson Veterinary Teaching Hospital between 2007 and 2011 were searched to identify histologically confirmed COF tumor biopsies. All tumors were comprised of elongate to spindle cells arranged in streams or bundles and whorls that produced variable amounts of collagenous matrix. Four of the tumors had small heterochromatic nuclei, case 1 had medium-sized and case 3 had large euchromatic nuclei. The diagnosis of COF was confirmed by examination of a representative hematoxylin and eosin stained section from each biopsy by a single board-certified veterinary anatomic pathologist (CVL). Serial sections 4–5 μm thick from paraffin-embedded formalin-fixed tumor biopsies were mounted on positively charged slides for IHC analysis of PDGFR-α, PDGFR-β, Kit, and VEGFR-2 expression using anti-human receptor-specific polyclonal rabbit antibodies (detailed in Table 2) [35–37].

High temperature antigen retrieval was performed with a microwave pressure cooker using Dako Target Retrieval solution (pH 6, 10 mins) according to the manufacturer's recommendations[a]. IHC staining was performed on a Dako Autostainer (Dako North America, Carpinteria, CA) at room temperature (21 °C) after blocking for 10 mins with 3 % H_2O_2 (Sigma Laboratories, Santa Fe, NM) in TBST (Biocare Medical, Concord, CA) followed by Dako serum-free protein block (Dako North America, Carpinteria, CA) for 10 mins. The primary antibodies were diluted in Dako antibody diluent (Dako North America, Carpinteria, CA) and applied for 30 mins. Conditions and manufacturer information are detailed in Table 2. Specific antibody binding was detected using MaxPoly-One polymer HRP rabbit (ImmunoBioScienceIH-8064-custom-OrSU, ImmunoBioScience, Mukilteo, WA) for 10 mins followed by Nova Red (SK-4800, Vector Laboratories, Burlingame, CA) for 5 mins. Hematoxylin (Dako North America, Carpinteria, CA) diluted 1:3 in distilled water for 5 mins was used as a counter stain. Washes between steps were performed using TBST (Biocare Medical, Concord, CA), except no wash was performed for the protein block. Dako Universal Negative Control-Rabbit (Dako North America, Carpinteria, CA) was used as the negative control. Peritumoral non-neoplastic tissues were used as internal positive (endothelium or mast cells) and negative (epidermis) controls, a canine cutaneous mast cell tumor submitted as biopsy served as positive control for Kit staining, and a canine metastatic hemangiosarcoma (liver, kidney, testis, spleen) collected during necropsy was used as a positive control [37–39]. Evaluation of IHC staining for specificity was performed by a board-certified veterinary anatomic pathologist (CVL).

Immunohistochemistry scoring

Immunoreactivity for PDGFR-α, PDGFR-β, Kit, and VEGFR-2 were scored by three of the investigators (CVL, MM, and SB) with the results representing a consensus agreement between the observers. The criteria evaluated included: percentage of tumor cells displaying immunoreactivity (assessed from a representative 40× field, after examining the slide in its entirety), the predominant location of staining (cytoplasmic, membranous, or nuclear), and relative visual intensity of staining (+, ++, or +++).

In addition, semi-quantitative measurement of immunoreactivity for the same proteins (using a photomicrograph of the same IHC field as described above) was carried out using a computer image analysis software package (ImageJ v1.47, NIH, Bethesda, MD) as previously described [40]. Output data recorded was the percentage of image pixels above the user-defined threshold to capture immunoreactivity.

Cell lines and reagents

Two immortalized COF cell lines were tested: MBSa1 (provided by Dr. Marlene Hauck, North Carolina State University, Raleigh, NC, USA) and CoFSA (provided by Dr. Melanie Wergin, University of Zurich, Zurich, Switzerland). Both cell lines were derived from biopsies acquired from clinically affected dogs presented for spontaneously arising COF [41, 42]. Cells were cultured in RPMI-1640 medium supplemented with 10 % fetal bovine serum, 2 mM glutamine, 2 mM sodium pyruvate, 2 mM HEPES, and 1 % pen-strep in a humidified 5 % CO_2 atmosphere at 37 °C.

Masitinib powder (provided by AB Science, Paris, France) was suspended in DMSO and stored at -80 °C until use. Imatinib was purchased from a commercial supplier (LC Labs, Woburn, MA), suspended in DMSO and stored at -80 °C until use. Doxorubicin HCl (2 mg/ ml) in isotonic solution was purchased from a commercial supplier (Amneal-Agila, Glasgow, KY). Dimethyl sulofoxide concentrations in all experiments never exceeded 0.3 %.

Reverse transcription-polymerase chain reaction

Expression of transcripts for *PDGFRA*, *PDGFRB*, *KIT*, and *KDR* was assessed in MBSa1 and CoFSA cells using RT-PCR. Cells were seeded into six-well plates (3×10^5/ well) suspended in 2.0 mL supplemented medium and allowed to adhere overnight. The cells were rinsed in PBS and RNA was isolated (RNeasy, Qiagen, Valencia, CA) and reverse transcribed to cDNA (High Capacity Reverse Transcription, Applied Biosystems, Foster City, CA) according to the manufacturers' instructions. Targets were amplified from cDNA using the specific

Table 2 Antibodies and conditions used for immunohistochemical staining of archived canine oral fibrosarcoma tumor specimens

Target	Manufacturer	Antibody	Dilution	Species	HTAR
VEGFR-2	Novus Biologicals, Littleton, CO	NBP1-74001	1:100	Rabbit	+
PDGFR-α	Santa Cruz Biotechnology, Dallas, TX	SC-338	1:200	Rabbit	+
PDGFR-β	BioGenex Laboratories, San Ramon, CA	N463-UC	1:200	Rabbit	+
Kit	Dako North America, Carpinteria, CA	A4502	1:500	Rabbit	+

HTAR High temperature antigen retrieval at pH 6

primers (Invitrogen, Carlsbad, CA) listed in Table 3 with the following accession numbers: [*PDGFRA* GenBank: XM532374.5; *PDGFRB* GenBank: NM001003382.1; *KIT* GenBank: XM005627969.2; and *KDR* GenBank: NM001048024.1]. Reverse transcription-polymerase chain reaction was performed according to standard methods [43] using Taq DNA polymerase (Invitrogen, Carlsbad, CA), with an annealing temperature of 58 °C, melting temperature of 94 °C, and run for 34 cycles on a thermocycler (Bio-rad Laboratories, Hercules, CA). Products were separated by agarose gel electrophoresis and visualized under ultra-violet light with propidium iodide and recorded using an Image Quant LAS4000 digital image capture system (GE Healthcare, Pittsburg, PA). Amplicons were purified using magnetic beads (Invitrogen, Carlsbad, CA) and sequenced on an ABI Prism 3730 Genetic Analyzer (Applied Biosystems, Grand Island, NY) using the Sanger method (BigDye Terminator v. 3.1 Cycle Sequencing Kit, Life Technologies, Grand Island, NY). Results reported are representative of three independent experiments, with each cell line tested in triplicate during each experiment.

Western blot

Western blots were performed against proteins for which mRNA transcripts were detected via RT-PCR in MBSa1 and CoFSA cells. Cells were seeded in 6-well plates (3×10^6/well) and allowed to adhere overnight as described above. The cells were detached using a cell scraper, transferred to a micro-centrifuge tube, and centrifuged in a tabletop centrifuge (3 min, $1200 \times g$). Cell pellets were rinsed by re-suspending twice in 3 mL ice cold PBS and extracted in 50 μL ice cold RIPA buffer with protease and phosphatase inhibitor cocktail (Sigma Laboratories, Santa Fe, NM). Extracts were sonicated four times (1 s each) using a Model 150 T ultrasonic dismembrator (Fisher Scientific, Pittsburg, PA) and pelleted at $10,000 \times g$ to remove cellular debris. Protein concentration was measured using a Bradford assay (Bio-rad Laboratories, Hercules, CA) according to the manufacturer's instructions. Proteins (20 μg/lane) were separated on 4–12 % SDS polyacrylamide gels (Bio-rad Laboratories, Hercules, CA) and transferred to PVDF membranes. The membranes were blocked in 1.5 % bovine serum albumin and probed with either anti-PDGFR-β antibody (BioGenex, Fremont, CA) or anti-PDGFR-α antibody

(antibody #SC-388, Santa Cruz Biotechnology, Dallas, TX) diluted 1:1000 and incubated overnight at 4 °C. The membranes were washed, probed with horseradish peroxidase-linked secondary antibody (SC-2005, Santa Cruz Biotechnology, Dallas, TX) diluted 1:20000, and exposed to substrate (ECL Select, GE Healthcare, Pittsburg, PA). A lysate from 293 T cells was used as a positive control (SC-114235, Santa Cruz Biotechnology, Dallas, TX). Bands were visualized and recorded using an Image Quant LAS4000 digital image capture system. Western blot results reported are representative of two independent experiments.

Cell viability assay

An MTS colorimetric assay (CellTiter 96 Aqueous One Solution Cell Proliferation Assay, Promega, Madison, WI) was used according to the manufacturer's instructions to assess the effects of masitinib and imatinib on viability of COF cell lines. Briefly, growing cells were seeded into 96-well plates at 2,500 cells/well suspended in 100 μL of supplemented medium and incubated overnight prior to adding drugs to allow adherence. Frozen aliquots of each TKI were thawed and diluted to twice the desired concentrations in supplemented medium prior to adding 100 μL to wells containing cells. The final TKI concentrations included the following: 0, 0.1, 0.3, 1.0, 3.0, 10.0, 30.0, and 100.0 μM. Cultures were maintained for 72 h following addition of the drugs, after which 150 μL of the media was removed and replaced with 20 μL MTS reagent premixed with 50 μL supplemented media. Cells were incubated in the presence of the MTS reagent for 2–4 h. Two cell-free, media-only wells were included in each experiment to generate assay background values, which were subtracted from the absorbance of each well prior to calculating viability indices. Results from TKI treated cells were compared against controls comprised of cells cultured under identical conditions with 0.3 % DMSO, but without added TKI. There was no difference in viability between cell lines treated with DMSO only (data not shown).

To assess the potential for a chemosensitizing effect of the tested TKIs with doxorubicin, MTS cell viability experiments were performed as described above with doxorubicin either alone or combined with 1.0 μM of either masitinib or imatinib. This concentration of TKI was

Table 3 Primers used for reverse transcriptase-polymerase chain reaction of immortalized canine oral fibrosarcoma cell lines

Target	Forward primer sequence (5'-3')	Reverse primer sequence (5'-3')	Spanned mRNA sequence	Product size (bp)
PDGFRA	CCTCGATCCTTCCAAATGAA	GGTCACAAAAAGGCCACTGT	357-523	167
PDGFRB	GTGGTATGGGAACGGTTGTC	GTGGGATCTGGCACAAAGAT	228-421	194
KIT	CCCATTTAACCGAACGAGAA	TCTCCGTGATCTTCCTGCTT	2016-2226	211
KDR	GATCGGTGAGAAATCCCTGA	CTGGAAGTCATCCACGTTT	1266-1473	208

chosen because pharmacokinetic studies in healthy Beagle dogs show that a clinically-relevant oral dose of 10 mg/kg of masitinib results in a serum maximum concentration of 1.3–1.5 µM [26]. Doxoribucin concentrations tested included 0, 1, 3, 10, 30, 100, 300, 1000, and 3000 nM. Results from drug-treated cells were compared to controls of cells cultured under identical conditions with 0.3 % DMSO and without added doxorubicin or TKI.

Three MTS experiments were performed independently and each condition was run in triplicate within each experiment.

The type of interaction between each TKI and doxorubicin was determined using the following equations [44]:

$$\text{Synergistic} = SF_{t+y} < SF_t \times SF_y$$
$$\text{Additive} = SF_{t+y} = SF_t \times SF_y$$
$$\text{Sub-additive} = SF_t \times SF_y < SF_{t+y} < SF_t \text{ and } SF_y$$
$$\text{Antagonistic} = SF_{t+y} > SF_t \text{ or } SF_y$$

SF_{t+y} = surviving fraction of cells exposed to the combination of either TKI and doxorubicin, SF_t = surviving fraction of cells exposed to either TKI alone, SF_y = surviving fraction of cells exposed to doxorubicin alone. These equations are appropriate provided the drug effect is reduced cell viability [45], a condition that was met at all drug concentrations except at 3 and 10 nM doxorubicin in CoFSA where the mean cell viability values for doxorubicin treatment alone were slightly increased. In these exceptions, the SF of the control group (i.e. cells, but no doxorubicin or TKI) was substituted in the equation for the SF of doxorubicin, as it was the more stringent condition for evaluating drug interaction.

All MTS testing was performed during three independent experiments, with each condition run in triplicate during each experiment.

Inhibition of PDGFR-β expression by siRNA
PDGFR-β knockdown was used to assess the role of PDGFR-β in sustaining viability of COF cell lines MBSa1 and CoFSA. Cells were seeded into 96-well plates (5 × 10^3 cells/well) and allowed to adhere overnight before transfection with a combination of four commercially purchased target-specific siRNAs (Life Technologies, Carlsbad, CA; 3 pmol per reaction) against canine *PDGFRB* (Dharmacon, Lafayette, CO) or a scrambled sequence (Mission siRNA Universal Negative Control #1, Sigma Laboratories, Santa Fe, NM) using Lipofectamine RNAiMAX (Invitrogen, Carlsbad, CA) according to the manufacturer's directions. Cell viability was measured in 96-well plate format 72 h after siRNA transfection using the MTS colorimetric assay (CellTiter 96 Aqueous One Solution Cell Proliferation Assay, Promega, Madison, WI) as described above.

The *PDGFRB* siRNAs used were (5′–3′):

Sequence #1: CCUUCAAGGUGGUGGUGAUUTT
Sequence #2: CCAUGAACGAACAGUUCUAUTT
Sequence #3: GAAAUGAGGUGGUUAACUUTT
Sequence #4: GAAUGACCAUCGAGAUGAATT

All siRNA data were normalized to the readouts taken from control cells treated with the transfection reagent alone, and included scrambled sequence controls to assess for nonspecific, off-target effects. Results from siRNA knockdown reported are representative of two independent experiments, with each condition run in sextuplicate during each experiment.

Western blot was repeated after siRNA treatment, as described above, using only the anti-PDGFR-β antibody (BioGenex, Fremont, CA). Quantification of siRNA PDGFR-β protein knockdown was performed using computer image analysis software with a gel analysis package (ImageJ v1.47, NIH, Bethesda, MD). PDGFR-β signal intensities in each lane were expressed as percentage of the total protein control (actin) loaded into respective lanes. Final PDGFR-β protein knockdown was reported as percentage of actin-normalized PDGFR-β band intensity in the siRNA treated lane relative to actin-normalized PDGFR-β band intensity in the control (vehicle-treated) lane.

Apoptosis
A luminogenic caspase-3/7 substrate assay (Caspase-Glo 3/7, Promega, Madison, WI) was used to determine relative caspase activity in COF cell lines after TKI treatment, either alone or with doxorubicin. The drug concentrations tested were selected based on MTS results in order to represent the range of observed effects on cell viability. Cells were seeded in 96-well culture plates at a density of 2,500 cells/well and challenged with the following drugs (concentrations): masitinib (0, 1, 3, and 30 µM), imatinib (0, 1, 3, and 30 µM), masitinib 1.0 µM + doxorubicin (3 and 300 nM), and imatinib 1.0 µM + doxorubicin (3 and 300 nM). For an apoptosis positive control, COS cells were incubated with 6.25 µM SB2224289 (Tocris, Bristol, UK) [46]. For a vehicle control, cells were incubated with 0.1 % DMSO in media. Drugs were dissolved in DMSO, with cells exposed to a final vehicle concentration of 0.1 %. Cells were challenged for 72 h, after which the caspase-3/7 activity was quantified. The caspase activity assay was performed according to the manufacturer's protocol. Cumulative luminescence over 1 s was measured using a luminometer (GloMax 96 Microplate Luminometer, Promega, Madison, WI). Relative caspase activity was calculated using the formula: relative caspase activity = (mean luminescence of treated cells)/(mean luminescence of vehicle control) × 100.

As this experiment was intended to act as a supplement to the MTS assay observations, only a single independent experiment (with each drug treatment condition in triplicate) was performed.

Statistical analysis

Mean cell viability (as described above) was compared to vehicle-treated control cells using a one-way ANOVA with Dunnett's multiple comparisons post-test. Except for siRNA experiments, all statistical analyses were performed using means from each independent experiment with standard deviations representing differences between the means. Because siRNA transfection was performed during two independent experiments, statistical analysis for these data were performed using the 6 replicates within one representative siRNA experiment. The 50 % inhibitor concentration (IC50) of masitinib and imatinib for CoFSA and MBSa1 were calculated using non-linear regression of the log of the inhibitor versus a variable slope response equation, with constraints set at 100 % for the top and 0 % for baseline. Relative caspase activities within the various drug treatment conditions were compared to vehicle-treated control cells with a one-way ANOVA with Dunnett's correction using the technical replicate data from the apoptosis experiment. Significance was set at $p < 0.05$ and all statistical testing was performed using a commercially available computer software program (Graphpad Prism v6.02 for Windows, Graphpad Software, San Diego, CA).

Abbreviations
COF, canine oral fibrosarcoma; TKIs, tyrosine kinase inhibitors; IHC, immunohistochemistry; RT-PCR, reverse transcription-polymerase chain reaction.

Acknowledgements
The authors wish to thank Alain Moussy of AB Science (Paris, France) for providing masitinib, Novartis (Basel, Switzerland) for the donation of imatinib, Dr. Marlene Hauck (North Carolina State University, Raleigh, NC, USA) and Dr. Melanie Wergin (University of Zurich, Zurich, Switzerland) for their generous provision of the MBSa1 and CoFSA cell lines, respectively, Dr. Gerd Bobe for his assistance with the data analysis, and Mrs. Kay Fischer for her technical expertise in performing the IHC preparations for this project.

Funding
This study was supported by intramural funding through Oregon State University's College of Veterinary Medicine Department of Clinical Sciences by provision of laboratory space and equipment to perform the study experiments.

Authors' contributions
All authors (MM, SCH, KM, CPG, CVL, and SB) participated in conceptual study design, analyzing and interpreting the data, and provided revisions to the manuscript. Additional individual author contributions are as follows: KM and CPG performed the *in vitro* experiments including cell cultures; CVL, SB, and MM performed the immunohistochemistry analysis; MM primarily authored the manuscript text. All authors have read and approve of the final version of the manuscript.

Competing interests
The authors declare that they have no competing interests.

Consent for publication
Not applicable.

Author details
[1]Department of Clinical Sciences, College of Veterinary Medicine, Oregon State University, Corvallis, OR 97331, USA. [2]Department of Biomedical Sciences, College of Veterinary Medicine, Oregon State University, Corvallis, OR 97331, USA.

References
1. Liptak JM, Withrow SJ. Cancer of the gastrointestinal tract. In: Withrow SJ, Vail DM, Page RL, editors. Withrow & MacEwen's Small Animal Clinical Oncology. 5th ed. St. Louis, MO: Saunders Elsevier; 2013. p. 381–431.
2. Todoroff RJ, Brodey RS. Oral and pharyngeal neoplasia in the dog: a retrospective survey of 361 cases. J Am Vet Med Assoc. 1979;175:567–71.
3. Kosovsky JK, Matthiesen DT, Marretta SM, Patnaik AK. Results of partial mandibulectomy for the treatment of oral tumors in 142 dogs. Vet Surg. 1991;20:397–401.
4. Wallace J, Matthiesen DT, Patnaik AK. Hemimaxillectomy for the treatment of oral tumors in 69 dogs. Vet Surg. 1992;21:337–41.
5. Schwarz PD, Withrow SJ, Curtis CR, Powers BE, Straw RC. Mandibular resection as a treatment for oral cancer in 81 dogs. J Am Anim Hosp Assoc. 1991;27:601–10.
6. Schwarz PD, Withrow SJ, Curtis CR, Powers BE, Straw RC. Partial maxillary resection as a treatment for oral cancer in 61 dogs. J Am Anim Hosp Assoc. 1991;27:617–24.
7. Ciekot PA, Powers BE, Withrow SJ, Straw RC, Ogilvie GK, LaRue SM. Histologically low-grade, yet biologically high-grade, fibrosarcomas of the mandible and maxilla in dogs: 25 cases (1982-1991). J Am Vet Med Assoc. 1994;204:610–5.
8. Gardner H, Fidel J, Haldorson G, Dernell W, Wheeler B. Canine oral fibrosarcomas: a retrospective analysis of 65 cases (1998-2010). Vet Comp Oncol. 2015;13:40–7.
9. Frazier SA, Johns SM, Ortega J, Zwingenberger AL, Kent MS, Hammond GM, et al. Outcome in dogs with surgically resected oral fibrosarcoma (1997-2008). Vet Comp Oncol. 2011;10:33–43.
10. Chon E, McCartan L, Kubicek LN, Vail DM. Safety evaluation of combination toceranib phosphate (Palladia®) and piroxicam in tumour-bearing dogs (excluding mast cell tumours): a phase I dose-finding study. Vet Comp Oncol. 2012;10:184–93.
11. de Vos J, Ramos Vega S, Noorman E, de Vos P. Primary frontal sinus squamous cell carcinoma in three dogs treated with piroxicam combined with carboplatin or toceranib. Vet Comp Oncol. 2012;10:206–13.
12. Lawrence J, Saba C, Gogal Jr R, Lamberth O, Vandenplas ML, Hurley DJ, et al. Masitinib demonstrates anti-proliferative and pro-apoptotic activity in primary and metastatic feline injection-site sarcoma cells. Vet Comp Oncol. 2012;10:143–54.
13. London C, Mathie T, Stingle N, Clifford C, Haney S, Klein MK, et al. Preliminary evidence for biologic activity of toceranib phosphate (Palladia®) in solid tumours. Vet Comp Oncol. 2012;10:194–205.
14. Lyles SE, Milner RJ, Kow K, Salute ME. In vitro effects of the tyrosine kinase inhibitor, masitinib mesylate, on canine hemangiosarcoma cell lines. Vet Comp Oncol. 2012;10:223–35.
15. Robat C, London C, Bunting L, McCartan L, Stingle N, Selting K, et al. Safety evaluation of combination vinblastine and toceranib phosphate (Palladia®) in dogs: a phase I dose-finding study. Vet Comp Oncol. 2012;10:174–83.
16. Bavcar S, Argyle DJ. Receptor tyrosine kinase inhibitors: molecularly targeted drugs for veterinary cancer therapy. Vet Comp Oncol. 2012;10:163–73.
17. Pardanani A, Tefferi A. Imatinib targets other than bcr/abl and their clinical relevance in myeloid disorders. Blood. 2004;104:1931–9.
18. Kobayashi M, Kuroki S, Ito K, Yasuda A, Sawada H, Ono K, et al. Imatinib-associated tumour response in a dog with a non-resectable gastrointestinal stromal tumour harbouring a c-kit exon 11 deletion mutation. Vet J. 2013; 198:271–4.

19. Yamada O, Kobayashi M, Sugisaki O, Ishii N, Ito K, Kuroki S, et al. Imatinib elicited a favorable response in a dog with a mast cell tumor carrying a c-kit c.1523A>T mutation via suppression of constitutive KIT activation. Vet Immunol Immunopathol. 2011;142:101–6.

20. Isotani M, Tamura K, Yagihara H, Hikosaka M, Ono K, Washizu T, et al. Identification of a c-kit exon 8 internal tandem duplication in a feline mast cell tumor case and its favorable response to the tyrosine kinase inhibitor imatinib mesylate. Vet Immunol Immunopathol. 2006;114:168–72.

21. Katayama R, Huelsmeyer MK, Marr AK, Kurzman ID, Thamm DH, Vail DM. Imatinib mesylate inhibits platelet-derived growth factor activity and increases chemosensitivity in feline vaccine-associated sarcoma. Cancer Chemother Pharmacol. 2004;54:25–33.

22. Kiupel M, Webster JD, Kaneene JB, Miller R, Yuzbasiyan-Gurkan V. The use of KIT and tryptase expression patterns as prognostic tools for canine cutaneous mast cell tumors. Vet Pathol. 2004;41:371–7.

23. Dickerson EB, Marley K, Edris W, Tyner JW, Schalk V, Macdonald V, et al. Imatinib and dasatinib inhibit hemangiosarcoma and implicate PDGFR-beta and Src in tumor growth. Trans Oncol. 2013;6:158–68.

24. Dubreuil P, Letard S, Ciufolini M, Gros L, Humbert M, Casteran N, et al. Masitinib (AB1010), a potent and selective tyrosine kinase inhibitor targeting KIT. PLoS One. 2009;4:e7258.

25. Thamm DH, Rose B, Kow K, Humbert M, Mansfield CD, Moussy A, et al. Masitinib as a chemosensitizer of canine tumor cell lines: a proof of concept study. Vet J. 2012;191:131–4.

26. Hahn KA, Oglivie G, Rusk T, Devauchelle P, Leblanc A, Legendre A, et al. Masitinib is safe and effective for the treatment of canine mast cell tumors. J Vet Int Med. 2008;22:1301–9.

27. Roskoski R. A historical overview of protein kinases and their targeted small molecule inhibitors. Pharmacol Res. 2015;100:1–23.

28. Humbert M, Casteran N, Letard S, Hanssens K, Iovanna J, Finetti P, et al. Masitinib combined with standard gemcitabine chemotherapy: in vitro and in vivo studies in human pancreatic tumour cell lines and ectopic mouse model. PLoS One. 2010;5:e9430.

29. Mitry E, Hammel P, Deplanque G, Mornex F, Levy P, Seitz JF, et al. Safety and activity of masitinib in combination with gemcitabine in patients with advanced pancreatic cancer. Cancer Chemother Pharmacol. 2010;66:395–403.

30. Filippi I, Naldini A, Carraro F. Role of the hypoxic microenvironment in the antitumor activity of tyrosine kinase inhibitors. Curr Med Chem. 2011;18:2885–92.

31. Paulsson J, Ehnman M, Ostman A. PDGF receptors in tumor biology: prognostic and predictive potential. Future Oncol. 2014;10:1695–708.

32. Uehara H, Kim SJ, Karashima T, Shepherd DL, Fan D, Tsan R, et al. Effects of blocking platelet-derived growth factor-receptor signaling in a mouse model of experimental prostate cancer bone metastases. J Natl Cancer Inst. 2003;95(6):458–70.

33. Najy AJ, Jung YS, Won JJ, Conley-LaComb MK, Saliganan A, Kim CJ, et al. Cediranib inhibits both the intraosseous growth of PDGF D-positive prostate cancer cells and the associated bone reaction. Prostate. 2012;72:1328–38.

34. Shinagawa K, Kitadai Y, Tanaka M, Sumida T, Onoyama M, Ohnishi M, et al. Stroma-directed imatinib therapy impairs the tumor-promoting effect of bone marrow-derived mesenchymal stem cells in an orthotopic transplantation model of colon cancer. Int J Cancer. 2013;132:813–23.

35. Urie BK, Russell DS, Kisseberth WC, London CA. Evaluation of expression and function of vascular endothelial growth factor receptor 2, platelet derived growth factor receptors-alpha and -beta, KIT, and RET in canine apocrine gland anal sac adenocarcinoma and thyroid carcinoma. BMC Vet Res. 2012;8:67–75.

36. Webster JD, Yuzbasiyan-Gurkan V, Miller RA, Kaneene JB, Kiupel M. Cellular proliferation in canine cutaneous mast cell tumors: associations with c-KIT and its role in prognostication. Vet Pathol. 2007;44:298–308.

37. Yonemaru K, Sakai H, Murakami M, Yanai T, Masegi T. Expression of vascular endothelial growth factor, basic fibroblast growth factor, and their receptors (flt-1, flk-1, and flg-1) in canine vascular tumors. Vet Pathol. 2006;43:971–80.

38. Asa SA, Murai A, Murakami M, Hoshino Y, Mori T, Maruo K, et al. Expression of platelet-derived growth factor and its receptors in spontaneous canine hemangiosarcoma and cutaneous hemangioma. Histol Histopathol. 2012;27:601–7.

39. Sabattini S, Bettini G. An immunohistochemical analysis of canine haemangioma and haemangiosarcoma. J Comp Pathol. 2009;140:158–68.

40. Jensen EC. Quantitative analysis of histological staining and fluorescence using ImageJ. Anat Rec. 2013;296:378–81.

41. Wergin MC. Effect of ionizing radiation molecular parameters in spontaneous canine tumors and canine tumor cell lines. Zurich: University of Zurich Press; 2007.

42. Snyder SA, Linder K, Hedan B, Hauck ML. Establishment and characterization of a canine soft tissue sarcoma cell line. Vet Pathol. 2011;48:482–5.

43. Marley K, Helfand SC, Edris WA, Mata JE, Gitelman AI, Medlock J, et al. The effects of taurolidine alone and in combination with doxorubicin or carboplatin in canine osteosarcoma in vitro. BMC Vet Res. 2013;9:15.

44. Aapro MS, Alberts DS, Salmon SE. Interactions of human leukocyte interferon with vinca alkaloids and other chemotherapeutic agents against human tumors in clonogenic assay. Cancer Chemother Pharmacol. 1983;10:161–6.

45. Wolfesberger B, Hoelzl C, Walter I, Reider GA, Fertl G, Thalhammer JG, et al. In vitro effects of meloxicam with or without doxorubicin on canine osteosarcoma cells. J Vet Pharmacol Ther. 2006;29:15–23.

46. Viall AK, Goodall CP, Stand B, Marley K, Chappell PE, Bracha S. Antagonism of serotonin receptor 1B decreases viability and promotes apoptosis in the COS canine osteosarcoma cell line. Vet Comp Oncol. 2014. doi:10.1111/vco.12103.

7

Reference gene validation for gene expression normalization in canine osteosarcoma: a geNorm algorithm approach

Gayathri Thevi Selvarajah[1,2*], Floor A. S. Bonestroo[1], Elpetra P. M. Timmermans Sprang[1], Jolle Kirpensteijn[1] and Jan A. Mol[1]

Abstract

Background: Quantitative PCR (qPCR) is a common method for quantifying mRNA expression. Given the heterogeneity present in tumor tissues, it is crucial to normalize target mRNA expression data using appropriate reference genes that are stably expressed under a variety of pathological and experimental conditions. No studies have validated specific reference genes in canine osteosarcoma (OS). Previous gene expression studies involving canine OS have used one or two reference genes to normalize gene expression. This study aimed to validate a panel of reference genes commonly used for normalization of canine OS gene expression data using the geNorm algorithm. qPCR analysis of nine canine reference genes was performed on 40 snap-frozen primary OS tumors and seven cell lines.

Results: Tumors with a variety of clinical and pathological characteristics were selected. Gene expression stability and the optimal number of reference genes for gene expression normalization were calculated. RPS5 and HNRNPH were highly stable among OS cell lines, while RPS5 and RPS19 were the best combination for primary tumors. Pairwise variation analysis recommended four and two reference genes for optimal normalization of the expression data of canine OS tumors and cell lines, respectively.

Conclusions: Appropriate combinations of reference genes are recommended to normalize mRNA levels in canine OS tumors and cell lines to facilitate standardized and reliable quantification of target gene expression, which is essential for investigating key genes involved in canine OS metastasis and for comparative biomarker discovery.

Keywords: Quantitative real-time PCR, Osteosarcoma, Bone tumor, Dog, Reference genes

Background

Osteosarcoma (OS) is the primary malignant bone tumor in dogs. Apart from having complex metastatic characteristics, OS has been observed to have a complex histopathology that develops due to predominantly osteoblastic cell differentiation as well as a mixture of fibroblastic and chondroblastic cell differentiation, with varying degrees of necrosis and tumor matrix present within a tumor [1, 2]. Gene expression studies in canine OS are valuable, as dogs develop OS spontaneously and have many common clinical and molecular characteristics that are invaluable resources for biomarker discovery and offer translational opportunities [3, 4]. Furthermore, publication of the canine genome along with the advent of quantitative real-time PCR (qPCR) and other high-throughput technologies have enabled studies of key genes involved in OS metastasis and disease progression.

qPCR is a sensitive method for quantifying mRNA gene transcripts; the two most popular real-time assays use SYBR® green fluorescent dye and the Taqman® probe. Many reports have demonstrated the importance of studying gene expression at the mRNA transcription level using snap-frozen tissues, micro-dissected tumors

* Correspondence: gayathri@upm.edu.my
[1]Department of Clinical Sciences of Companion Animals, Faculty of Veterinary Medicine, University of Utrecht, Yalelaan 104, 3584, CM, Utrecht, The Netherlands
[2]Department of Veterinary Clinical Studies, Faculty of Veterinary Medicine, University Putra Malaysia, UPM, 43400 Serdang, Malaysia

from paraffin-embedded blocks [5], cellular content from fine needle aspirates of primary tumors, and various cell culture models. The quantification of gene expression using the qPCR method requires appropriate standardization from initial tissue sampling, RNA extraction protocols, cDNA synthesis, assay characteristics, and reference gene validation [6, 7]. Furthermore, it is important to incorporate internal standards such as reference genes to normalize mRNA expression levels between different samples to precisely compare mRNA transcription levels. Ideally, a reference gene should be stably expressed in tissues or cells regardless of the histology, pathological condition, or cellular physiological-metabolic state.

Reference gene expression validation studies have been conducted in several types of normal, diseased, and tumor canine tissues [8, 9]. These studies suggested that stably expressed genes can differ according to the tissue origin and disease condition, particularly in cancer. Most gene expression studies examining canine OS have included one or two reference genes as the internal control for data normalization [4, 10–14]. Given the biological and pathological diversity of OS tumors, it is crucial to determine the stability of reference genes and their suitability for normalization to accurately quantify gene expression data. Thus, in the present study, the mRNA expression of nine commonly used canine reference genes was quantified using the SYBR® green fluorescent dye qPCR assay with canine OS snap-frozen tissues and cell lines. The geNorm algorithm approach was utilized to determine the reference gene(s) showing stable expression for normalization of canine OS mRNA expression data.

Methods

All procedures were approved by the University of Utrecht, Netherlands ethical committee, as required under Dutch legislation. Naturally developed bone tumors were obtained from privately owned euthanized animals or obtained through a routine medical treatment for cancer (surgical resection of tumors) at the Department of Clinical Sciences of Companion Animals (University Clinic for Companion Animals) in Utrecht, The Netherlands. No experimental animals were used for the sole purpose of this study.

Tissue specimens and clinical-pathological data

Of the dogs with OS clinically diagnosed at the University Clinic for Companion Animals in Utrecht, The Netherlands, 40 with histologically confirmed primary tumors were selected for this study. Tissues from these samples were harvested under sterile conditions during surgery (amputation/marginal resection/total resection), snap-frozen in liquid nitrogen, and stored at −70 °C. Histopathology diagnosis and grading [2] were performed by a certified veterinary pathologist. These 40 tumors were selected after screening from 60 OS tumors randomly selected from the snap-frozen tumor archive at the Department of Clinical Sciences of Companion Animals, University of Utrecht; first based on RNA quantity (minimum 100 ng/μL in 30 μL) and followed by RNA quality (RIN > 6.5). The samples that didn't qualify these two stages of screening were not included in this study. The medical records of the selected 40 tumors were reviewed retrospectively.

Cell lines and culture conditions

Seven well-characterized canine OS cell lines were used in this study. The cell lines COS31 [15], HMPOS [16], and POS [17] were obtained through a collaboration with the University of Florida, USA; KOS-001, KOS-002, KOS-003 and KOS-004 were kindly gifted by the National Cancer Institute, NIH, Bethesda, MD, USA. All cell lines tested negative for mycoplasma using a myco-sensor qPCR assay kit according to the manufacturer's protocol (Agilent Technologies, CA, USA). Cells were maintained in a sub-confluent monolayer in DMEM supplemented with 10% fetal bovine serum (Invitrogen, CA, USA) at 37 °C in a humidified atmosphere with 5% CO_2.

RNA isolation and cDNA synthesis

RNA in snap-frozen OS tumor materials was isolated as described previously [3, 18]. Briefly, frozen bone tumor materials were ground to form bone powder, which was subjected to RNA isolation protocols. For cells grown in culture, 1 mL of RLT lysis buffer (Qiagen, Germany) was used to lyse 75–90% confluent cells grown in 75 mL flasks, following a single wash of the cells with Hank's Balance Salt Solution (PAA Laboratories, GmbH, UK). These three samples were collected from three independent passages in culture. RNA was isolated and cDNA synthesis done independently for the three samples and not pooled together. The three samples were considered as three independent biological replicates from each cell line. In addition to that, for qPCR assay, each of these biological replicate was assessed for gene expression in duplicate (technical replicate) using qPCR assays. RNA isolation and purification was performed using the RNeasy mini kit according to the manufacturer's protocol (Qiagen). The RNA samples were treated with the Qiagen RNase-free DNase kit (DNase-I) and eluted in purified water. Total RNA was quantified using the Nanodrop ND-1000 spectrophotometer (Isogen Lifesciences, The Netherlands). RNA quality was evaluated using the Agilent 2100 Bioanalyzer (Agilent Technologies). The cDNA was synthesized using 0.5 μg total RNA into a total reaction volume of 20 μL from each sample using the iScript kit cDNA Synthesis Kit according to the manufacturer's protocol (Bio-Rad, CA, USA).

Quantitative real-time PCR

Primers were designed and qPCR products were sequenced for specificity as previously described [19, 20]. cDNA samples from both cell lines and tumors were diluted by two-fold, pooled, and diluted with purified water in a four-fold serial dilution to assess the amplification efficiency of each gene. The remaining cDNA samples were diluted by two-fold and 2 μL was used as a template to measure the gene expression in technical duplicates. qPCR was conducted on separate plates for the OS cell lines from the primary tumors using the SYBR® green fluorescent dye method. Initial screening for genomic DNA contamination was performed on all samples using a non-reversed-transcribed RNA template. qPCR was performed on a MyiQ™ quantitative real-time PCR machine (Bio-Rad). Reactions were conducted in duplicate, involving two-step reaction protocols, except for HPRT which involved a three-step reaction protocol, for up to 40 qPCR cycles [19, 20].

Data analysis

Individual reaction data were corrected for qPCR efficiencies and analyzed using IQ5 software (Bio-Rad). A box-plot was generated from the absolute qPCR cycle threshold (Cq) values [6] referring to the RNA transcription of the tested reference genes in OS tissues and cell lines using the statistical software SPSS version 16.0 (SPSS, Inc., Chicago, IL, USA). Cases with values between 1.5 and 3.0 box length, from the upper or lower edges of the box, are presented as outliers and indicated by a dark dot. The expression stability of each reference gene in tumors and cell lines was calculated independently, and their average values were recalculated using step-wise exclusion and pairwise variation analyses, all of which were analyzed using geNorm (version 3.5) software [21]. GeNorm calculates the stability of expression (M) of one gene based on the average pairwise variation between all studied reference genes. The pairwise variation (V) value illustrates the variation generated by incorporating various numbers of reference genes for normalization based on individual absolute (M) values. A lower V value indicates lower variation between the selected combinations of reference genes. Stepwise elimination of the least stable gene reveals the two most stable genes.

Results

Canine OS samples and reference gene selection

Clinical and pathological data of 40 primary canine OS tissues from differently sized (medium to large) breeds used in this study are summarized in Table 1. The tissues were obtained upon amputation or tumor resection prior to the initiation of chemotherapy. These tumors consisted of mixed histopathology characteristics. Seven canine OS cell lines with varying characteristics, including

Table 1 Characteristics of canine OS tissues (n = 40) used for this study

Parameter	n	%
Histological subtype[a]		
OB + FB	12	30
OB + TL	5	12.5
OB + CB + FB	7	17.5
OB + FB + TL	2	5
OB	14	35
Histological grade		
High	28	70
Medium-low	12	30
Necrosis		
< 50% (low)	12	30
> 50% (high)	28	70
Sex		
Female	14	35
Male	26	65
Neuter status		
Intact	22	55
Neutered	18	45
Location of primary tumor		
Extraskeletal	1	2.5
Femur	1	2.5
Humerus	8	20
Mandible/maxilla	3	7.5
Radius/ulna	14	35
Rib	2	5
Scapula	3	7.5
Tibia/fibula/metatarsus	8	20

[a]CB chondroblastic, FB fibroblastic, OB osteoblastic, TL telangiectic

morphology, cell proliferation, colony-forming abilities, migration, and apoptotic rates, were selected. Sub-confluent cells from 3 independent passages were lysed for RNA isolation, as representatives for biological replicates from each cell line. The reference genes selected for this study were previously described (e.g. RPS19, HPRT, GAPDH) [3, 18] and several putative reference genes that have not been used in OS studies, but were expressed in other canine tissues (e.g. SRPR, HNRNPH, GUSB, RPL8, RPS5, B2M) [19, 20]. These genes represent different functional groups, thus avoiding having a cluster of genes co-regulated in a specific cellular mechanism (Table 2).

Pre-qPCR quality control measures and qPCR efficiencies

RNA quantity in tumors ranged from 173.0 to 2399.3 ng/μL, while the RNA quality of all samples was acceptable with a 260/280 ratio of 1.97–2.11. RNA integrity number

Table 2 Reference genes for canine OS and their cellular function(s)

Gene symbol	Name	Function
RPS5	Ribosomal protein S5	Ribosomal protein that is a component of the 40S subunit, belongs to the S7P family of ribosomal proteins
RPS19	Ribosomal protein S19	Ribosomal protein that is a component of the 40S subunit, belongs to the S19E family of ribosomal proteins
HPRT	Hypoxanthine guanine phosphoribosyl transferase	Purine metabolism, salvage of purines from degraded RNA
HNRNPH	Heterogeneous nuclear ribonucleoprotein H	RNA-binding protein that forms a complex with heterogeneous nuclear RNA (hnRNA). These proteins are associated with pre-mRNAs in the nucleus and appear to influence pre-mRNA processing and other aspects of mRNA metabolism and transport
RPL8	Ribosomal protein L8	Ribosomal protein that is a component of the 60S subunit which catalyzes protein synthesis
GAPDH	Glyceraldehyde-3-phosphate dehydrogenase	Enzyme in glycolysis and gluconeogenesis pathway
B2M	β-2-Microglobulin	Beta chain of MHC class I molecules
SRPR	Signal recognition particle receptor	Ensures, in conjunction with the signal recognition particle, the correct targeting of the nascent secretory proteins to the endoplasmic reticulum membrane system
GUSB	β-glucuronidase	Role in degradation of dermatan and keratin sulphates

(RIN) values were 9.5–10.0 for the cell lines and above 6.5 for the snap-frozen tumors. Primer sequences, product size, and optimal annealing temperature for each reference gene were previously verified [19, 20] and are summarized in Table 3. qPCR was performed in duplicate for each sample in which separate assays for cell lines and tumors were performed. Both the non-reverse transcribed template control samples were below the detection limits in every qPCR. qPCR efficiencies were between 91.1% and 103.1% for the cell lines and between 94.9% and 104.1% for the tumors. All qPCRs exhibited a single melting curve representing a specific product.

Reference gene expression variation in OS tumors and cell lines

Reference genes that were highly expressed in both OS tumors and cell lines, based on average Cq values, were GAPDH, followed by the ribosomal RNA genes RPS19, RPS5, and RPL8. SRPR showed the lowest expression. Although the absolute Cq range differed slightly between the tumor and cell line assays, a coherent expression pattern was observed. The expression range and average Cq values for each reference gene in OS tumors and cell lines are shown in Fig. 1.

Expression stability of reference genes in canine OS tumors and cell lines

The average reference gene expression stability (M value) upon step-wise exclusion and pairwise variation (V value) were calculated using the geNorm algorithm approach for the tumors and cell lines individually. A higher absolute M value indicates lower expression stability and vice versa (Table 4). Among the reference genes tested for the canine OS cell lines, HNRNPH was the most stable gene with an M value of 0.420, while SRPR appeared to be the least stably expressed gene with an M value of 0.588, although all reference genes had acceptable M values. For OS tumors, absolute M values ranged from 0.790 for RPS19 (most stable) to 1.210 for B2M (least stable) compared to the other reference genes. The average expression stabilities

Table 3 Details of primers and qPCR conditions for the putative reference genes assessed in this study

Reference gene	Accession number	Forward primer 5′ to 3′	Reverse primer 5′ to 3′	Product length (bp)	T_a (°C)
RPS5	XM_533568	TCACTGGTGAGAACCCCCT	CCTGATTCACACGGCGTAG	141	62.5
RPS19	XM_533657	CCTTCCTCAAAAAGTCTGGG	GTTCTCATCGTAGGGAGCAAG	95	61
HPRT	AY_283372	AGCTTGCTGGTGAAAAGGAC	TTATAGTCAAGGGCATATCC	114	56
HNRNPH	XM_53857	CTCACTATGATCCACCACG	TAGCCTCCATAACCTCCAC	151	61.2
RPL8	XM_532360	CCATGAATCCTGTGGAGC	GTAGAGGGTTTGCCGATG	64	55
GAPDH	NM_001003142	TGTCCCCACCCCCAATGTATC	CTCCGATGCCTGCTTCACTACCTT	100	58
B2M	XM_535458	TCCTCATCCTCCTCGCT	TTCTCTGCTGGGTGTCG	85	61.2
SRPR	XM_03184	GCTTCAGGATCTGGACTGC	GTTCCCTTGGTAGCACTGG	81	61.2
GUSB	NM_001003191	AGACGTTCCAAGTACCCC	AGGTGTGGTGTAGAGGAGCAC	103	62

T_a annealing temperature, *bp* base pair

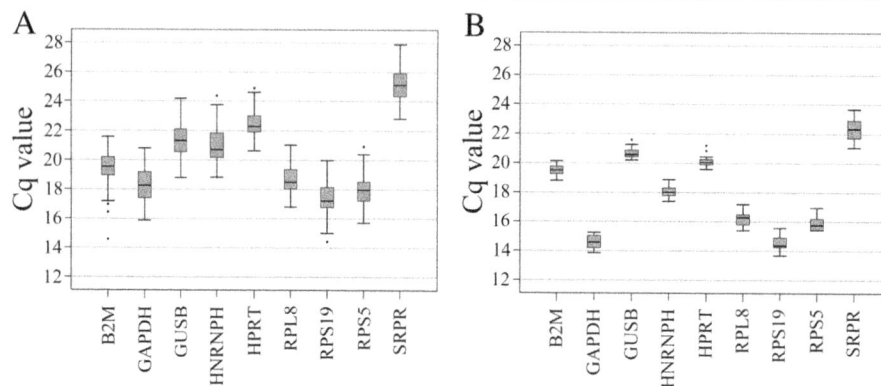

Fig. 1 Box-plots demonstrating the absolute Cq values, 25%/75% percentiles, and outliers (indicated by dark dots) for mRNA transcription quantified for the putative reference genes in: **a** canine OS snap-frozen primary tumors and **b** for canine OS cell lines

of the 9 tested reference genes among cell lines and tumors upon the stepwise exclusion algorithm are depicted in Fig. 2. *HNRNPH* and *RPS5* expression, together, showed the lowest variability for the cell lines, while *RPS19* and *RPS5* were the best combination for the tumors.

Pairwise variation (V value), which reflects the optimal number of reference genes for normalization in tumors and cell lines, was also calculated. A lower the V value indicates lower variation between the selected combinations of reference genes. Normalization of gene expression data among 40 OS tumors required a minimum combination of 3 (V value is 0.15) and optimally 4 reference genes (V value <0.15), while a combination of 2 reference genes was sufficient for the OS cell lines (Fig. 3). These values were determined according to a cut-off V value of 0.15 as per published recommendations [21].

Discussion

Selection of suitable reference genes is crucial for accurate interpretation of gene expression data [21, 22]. Many quality control measures, from initial sample collection

Table 4 Reference genes ranked based on their expression stability, M, in canine osteosarcoma primary tumors and cell lines

Primary tumors (tissues)		Cell lines	
Gene	M value	Gene	M value
RPS19	0.790	HNRNPH	0.420
RPS5	0.796	RPS5	0.423
HNRNPH	0.803	B2M	0.475
HPRT	0.808	RPS19	0.494
GUSB	0.816	GUSB	0.508
GAPDH	0.835	HPRT	0.510
RPL8	0.842	GAPDH	0.510
SRPR	0.921	RPL8	0.579
B2M	1.210	SRPR	0.588

The lower the M value for a gene, the more stable expression is across the samples

to data analysis, should be evaluated critically prior to analysis of gene expression data [23, 24]. Reference genes, previously known as 'housekeeping genes,' are essential not only for normalizing the mRNA expression of target genes, but also for correcting variations in initial RNA sample input, extraction methods, and reaction efficiencies [25]. Failure to normalize gene expression data may result in inaccurate interpretation and promote false perception of target gene expression.

Numerous studies have been conducted to validate panels of reference genes in different tissues from different animals [26–29], including dogs. Previous studies on reference gene analysis using the GeNorm approach was done on soft tissues from dogs including skin, prostate, kidney, mammary gland, heart and liver tissues [19, 20]. Bone tissues are of mesenchymal origin and certainly have a set of genes expressed differentially compared to soft tissues. It is not known if the optimal reference genes would be the same as other soft tissues, hence this study was necessary. Besides that, there are only two other studies on reference genes on tumor specimens using the GeNorm analysis which are on canine soft tissue sarcoma ($n = 6$ tumors) [30] and canine mammary gland tumors ($n = 22$ tumors) [9]. Reference genes stably expressed in canine soft tissue sarcoma are β-Glucuronidase (GUSB) and proteasome subunit, beta type, 6 (PSMB6); while in canine mammary gland tumors were a combination of hypoxanthine-phosphoribosyl transferase, ATP-synthase subunit 5B, ribosomal protein L32 and ubiquitin. These two studies suggest different set of reference gene which are stably expressed as compared to the current study on canine osteosarcoma.

This study investigated the reliability of several reference genes expression in snap-frozen tumors and in cell lines of canine OS origin. The present study validated a panel of nine reference genes commonly used for qPCR investigations on dog tissues. Although this is not the first study to demonstrate the need for reference gene

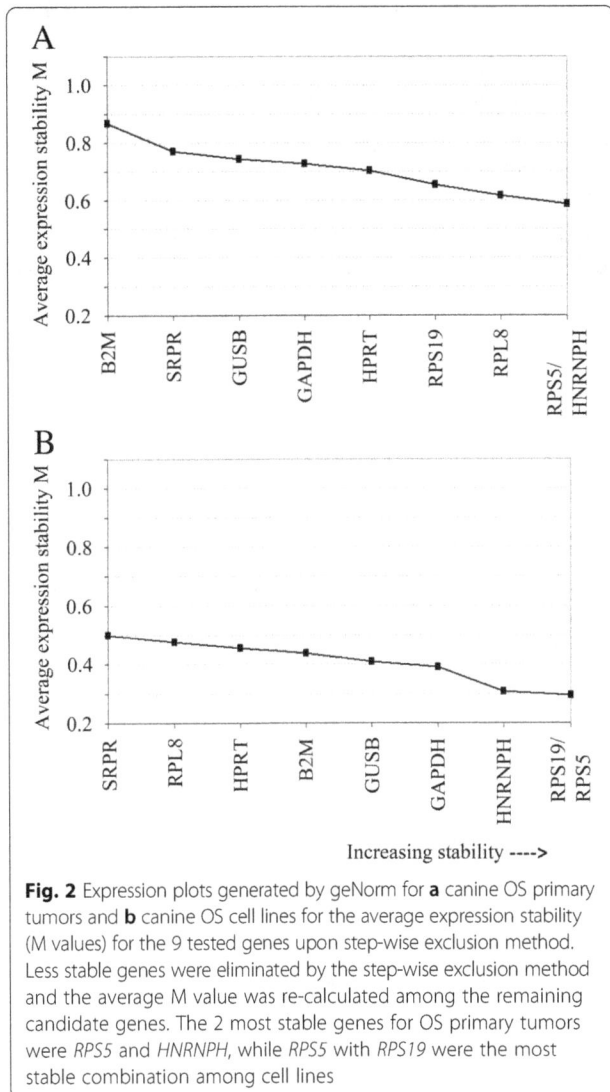

Fig. 2 Expression plots generated by geNorm for **a** canine OS primary tumors and **b** canine OS cell lines for the average expression stability (M values) for the 9 tested genes upon step-wise exclusion method. Less stable genes were eliminated by the step-wise exclusion method and the average M value was re-calculated among the remaining candidate genes. The 2 most stable genes for OS primary tumors were *RPS5* and *HNRNPH*, while *RPS5* with *RPS19* were the most stable combination among cell lines

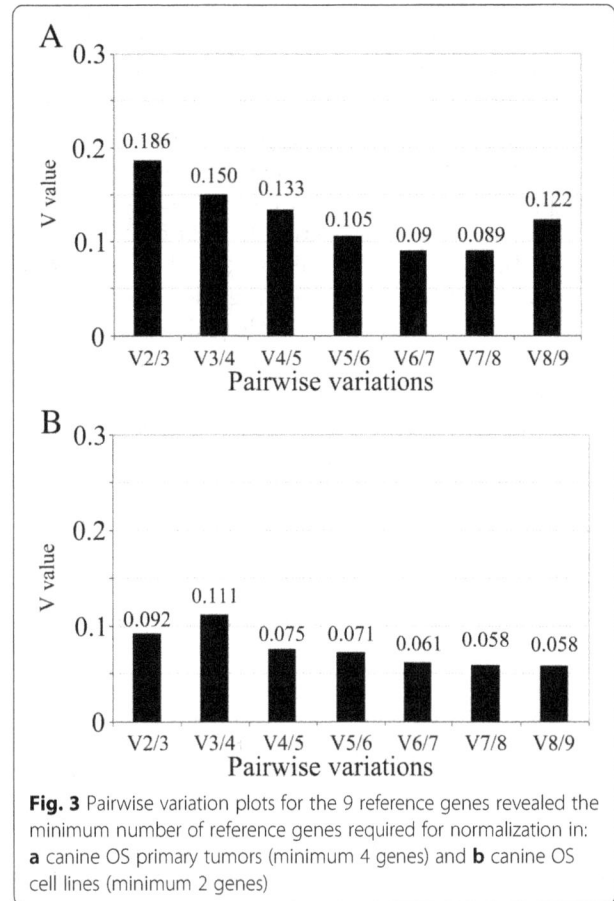

Fig. 3 Pairwise variation plots for the 9 reference genes revealed the minimum number of reference genes required for normalization in: **a** canine OS primary tumors (minimum 4 genes) and **b** canine OS cell lines (minimum 2 genes)

validation in tumor tissues from dogs, this is the first study to use OS tissues and to incorporate the largest number of snap-frozen canine tumor tissues and cell lines in a single canine reference gene validation study. The popular and established statistical tool geNorm (version 3.5) was used to calculate reference gene expression stability. For technical considerations, most 'essential' criteria outlined in the MIQE (Minimum Information for Publication of Quantitative Real-Time PCR Experiments) standards were employed in the current investigation in canine OS tissues [6]. The present study was unable to examine gene expression for biological replicates of OS tumors as recommended in the MIQE guidelines and power analysis was not conducted prior to the experiment to determine the number of samples necessary for valid conclusions, as the samples were obtained from naturally developed tumors in dogs and not from an experimental laboratory setting where the

sample size can be controlled. The sample size in this study was based on sample availability, and with good quality RNA and sufficient RNA (quantity).

All nine reference genes tested in both canine OS snap-frozen tumors and cell lines showed acceptable expression stability with M values below 1.5. Overall, reference genes were much more stably expressed in cell lines (M values of 0.420–0.588) compared to those in tumor tissues (M values of 0.790–1.210), clearly indicating homogeneity among cell populations in cultured systems. In contrast, tumor tissues contain more heterogeneous cell populations.

Ribosomal protein genes (components of both 40S and 60S subunits) are highly expressed in various tissues and are preferred references for normalization in various models [8, 19, 20, 29], including in the present study of canine OS. Although there were slight differences in the ranking of genes (according to absolute M values) between those tested for the cell lines and tumors, *RPS5* was the most stable gene in both model systems. *RPS5* in combination with *RPS19* (for tumor tissues) or *HNRNPH* (for cell lines) showed the highest expression stability compared to other genes such as *B2M* and *GAPDH*, which are the most commonly used reference genes in many human and canine OS studies to date [10, 18, 31]. *GAPDH* expression did not appear to differ remarkably between OS samples, but its expression stability was much lower than the other reference genes investigated in the present study, which agrees with several previous reports [32, 33]. GAPDH is an enzyme involved in several metabolic pathways that are essential for cell growth and proliferation, and its expression has shown to differ in different tissue types and environment conditions [22, 34]. In an investigation of canine articular connective tissue, *GAPDH* and *B2M* were found to be highly stable [35], while in canine mammary tumors, *GAPDH* was less stable [9]. Furthermore, GAPDH protein expression in cultured cells may change depending upon cell density [34], and it was also found to be differentially expressed between tumors of epithelial origin and their normal counterparts [22]. Among canine OS tumors, *B2M* showed the lowest expression stability compared to the other eight candidate genes investigated in this study. Therefore, it is not recommended to rely on *B2M* nor *GAPDH* as a sole reference gene to normalize gene expression data.

Pairwise analysis of a combination of genes that can be used for normalization revealed that four reference genes for canine OS tumors and two for the cell lines were essential based on a recommended cut-off point. A lower V indicated smaller variation, suggesting that adding an additional gene did not significantly improve normalization. A cut-off value of 0.15 for pairwise variation is commonly used, indicating that the use of a set of reference genes with a pairwise variation results in valid normalization. As more genes are incorporated for normalization, the V value decreases to an optimal seven reference genes, which can be considered during normalization, given the expression data across canine OS tumors. When sample availability and RNA yield is limited, particularly from OS tumor materials, a minimum of three reference genes is acceptable, and four reference genes are optimal for normalization. OS typically shows a complex heterogeneous phenotype, and thus we recommend including multiple reference genes for the normalization of mRNA gene expression data.

The current study incorporated canine OS tumors, which are chemo-naive, and thus we cannot exclude the possibility of changes in reference gene stability in tumors induced by the various therapeutic modalities employed in clinical and experimental settings. If gene expression quantification comparing the effects of a given therapy is required, screening of a panel of reference genes may be essential prior to data normalization. Additionally, based on the assumption that RNA isolated from a specific tissue section represents the overall pooled expression in the tumor, RNA transcription in canine OS tumor tissues was quantified from a single tissue section from an individual OS tumor. Several other studies have recommended incorporating different parts of the same tumor to include separate biological replicates to more accurately quantify gene expression. However, this is often not feasible because of limited tissue availability. Further studies are necessary to test other potential or novel reference genes identified by global gene expression profiling methods and subsequently validated using other statistical algorithms. Because canine spontaneous OS is a clinically and biologically relevant model for human OS [36], we propose that multiple reference genes should be included in future normalization of gene expression data for both species to improve the accuracy and reliability of gene expression quantification.

Conclusions

In conclusion, this study agreed with the consensus opinion that no single reference gene can accurately normalize given expression data. A combination of reference genes is recommended for normalizing the gene expression data from OS tumors and cell lines, with a preference for *RPS5* as a highly stable reference gene in canine OS.

Abbreviations

B2M: β-2-Microglobulin; bp: base pair; CB: chondroblastic; cDNA: complementary DNA; FB: fibroblastic; GAPDH: Glyceraldehyde-3-phosphate dehydrogenase; GUSB: β-glucuronidase; HNRNPH: Heterogeneous nuclear ribonucleoprotein H; HPRT: Hypoxanthine guanine phosphoribosyl transferase; MIQE: Minimum Information for Publication of Quantitative Real-Time PCR Experiments; mRNA: messenger RNA; OB: osteoblastic; OS: osteosarcoma; PSMB6: Proteosome subunit beta type 6; qPCR: quantitative real-time PCR; RIN: RNA Integrity Number; RPL8: Ribosomal protein L8; RPS19: Ribosomal protein S19; RPS5: Ribosomal protein S5; SRPR: Signal recognition particle receptor; T_a: annealing temperature; TL: telangiectic

Acknowledgements

The authors would like to thank Adri Slob, Frank Riemers and Monique van E. Wolferen from the University of Utrecht for their laboratory and analytical assistance with this research.

Funding

The research was funded by the Malaysia Ministry of Higher Education (MOHE) and the University Putra Malaysia and the Department of Clinical Sciences of Companion Animals (DCSCA), Faculty of Veterinary Medicine of Utrecht University, The Netherlands.

Authors' contributions

GTS and FASB reviewed the clinical data from the archived tumors and performed RNA isolation, qPCR assays, analyzed data, and contributed in writing the manuscript. EPMTS was involved in quality control assessment of the data, validation, and interpretation of GeNorm data. JK and JAM were major contributors to the design of the experiment, interpretation, and reviewed the manuscript critically. All authors read and approved the final manuscript.

Consent for publication

Not applicable.

Competing interests

The authors declare that they have no competing interests.

References

1. Loukopoulos P, Robinson WF. Clinicopathological relevance of tumour grading in canine osteosarcoma. J Comp Pathol. 2007;136:65–73.
2. Kirpensteijn J, Kik M, Rutteman GR, Teske E. Prognostic significance of a new histologic grading system for canine osteosarcoma. Vet Pathol. 2002;39:240–6.
3. Selvarajah GT, Kirpensteijn J, van Wolferen ME, Rao NA, Fieten H, Mol JA. Gene expression profiling of canine osteosarcoma reveals genes associated with short and long survival times. Mol Cancer. 2009;8:72.
4. Paoloni M, Davis S, Lana S, Withrow S, Sangiorgi L, Picci P, et al. Canine tumor cross-species genomics uncovers targets linked to osteosarcoma progression. BMC Genomics. 2009;10:625.
5. Drury S, Anderson H, Dowsett M. Selection of REFERENCE genes for normalization of qRT-PCR data derived from FFPE breast tumors. Diagn Mol Pathol. 2009;18:103–7.
6. Bustin SA, Benes V, Garson JA, Hellemans J, Huggett J, Kubiasta M, et al. The MIQE guidelines: minimum information for publication of quantitative real-time PCR experiments. Clin Chem. 2009;55:611–22.
7. Derveaux S, Vandesompele J, Hellemans J. How to do successful gene expression analysis using real-time PCR. Methods. 2010;50:227–30.
8. Wood SH, Clements DN, McEwan NA, Nuttall T, Carter SD. Reference genes for canine skin when using quantitative real-time PCR. Vet Immunol Immunopathol. 2008;126:392–5.
9. Etschmann B, Wilcken B, Stoevesand K, von der Schulenburg A, Sterner-Kock A. Selection of reference genes for quantitative real-time PCR analysis in canine mammary tumors using the GeNorm algorithm. Vet Pathol. 2006;43:934–42.
10. Flint AF, U'Ren L, Legare ME, Withrow SJ, Dernell W, Hanneman WH. Overexpression of the erbB-2 proto-oncogene in canine osteosarcoma cell lines and tumors. Vet Pathol. 2004;41:291–6.
11. Fossey SL, Liao AT, McCleese JK, Bear MD, Lin J, Li PK, et al. Characterization of STAT3 activation and expression in canine and human osteosarcoma. BMC Cancer. 2009;9:81.
12. De Maria R, Miretti S, Iussich S, Olivero M, Morello E, Bertotti A, et al. Met oncogene activation qualifies spontaneous canine osteosarcoma as a suitable pre-clinical model of human osteosarcoma. J Pathol. 2009;218:399–408.
13. Takagi S, Kato Y, Asano K, Ohsaki T, Bosnakovski D, Hoshino Y, et al. Matrix metalloproteinase inhibitor RECK expression in canine tumors. J Vet Med Sci. 2005;67:761–7.
14. Takagi S, Kitamura T, Hosaka Y, Ohsaki T, Bosnakovski D, Kadosawa T, et al. Molecular cloning of canine membrane-anchored inhibitor of matrix metalloproteinase, RECK. J Vet Med Sci. 2005;67:385–91.
15. Shoieb AM, Hahn KA, Barnhill MA. An in vivo/in vitro experimental model system for the study of human osteosarcoma: canine osteosarcoma cells (COS31) which retain osteoblastic and metastatic properties in nude mice. In Vivo. 1998;12:463–72.
16. Barroga EF, Kadosawa T, Okumura M, Fujinaga T. Establishment and characterization of the growth and pulmonary metastasis of a highly lung metastasizing cell line from canine osteosarcoma in nude mice. J Vet Med Sci. 1999;61:361–7.
17. Kadosawa T, Nozaki K, Sasaki N, Takeuchi A. Establishment and characterization of a new cell line from a canine osteosarcoma. J Vet Med Sci. 1994;56:1167–9.
18. Fieten H, Spee B, Ijzer J, Kik MJ, Penning LC, Kirpensteijn J. Expression of hepatocyte growth factor and the proto-oncogenic receptor c-met in canine osteosarcoma. Vet Pathol. 2009;46:869–77.
19. Brinkhof B, Spee B, Rothuizen J, Penning LC. Development and evaluation of canine reference genes for accurate quantification of gene expression. Anal Biochem. 2006;356:36–43.
20. Schlotter YM, Veenhof EZ, Brinkhof B, Rutten VP, Spee B, Willemse T, et al. A GeNorm algorithm-based selection of reference genes for quantitative real-time PCR in skin biopsies of healthy dogs and dogs with atopic dermatitis. Vet Immunol Immunopathol. 2009;129:115–8.
21. Vandesompele J, De Preter K, Pattyn F, Poppe B, Van Roy N, De Paepa A, et al. Accurate Normalization of Real-Time Quantitative RT-PCR Data by Geometric Averaging of Multiple Internal Control Genes. Genome Biol. 2002;3:RESEARCH0034.
22. Rubie C, Kempf K, Hans J, Su T, Tilton B, Georg T, et al. Housekeeping gene variability in normal and cancerous colorectal, pancreatic, esophageal, gastric and hepatic tissues. Mol Cell Probes. 2005;19:101–9.
23. Botling J, Edlund K, Segersten U, Tahmasebpoor S, Engstrom M, Sundstrom M, et al. Impact of thawing on RNA integrity and gene expression analysis in fresh frozen tissue. Diagn Mol Pathol. 2009;18:44–52.
24. Becker C, Hammerle-Fickinger A, Riedmaier I, Pfaffl MW. MRNA and microRNA quality control for RT-qPCR analysis. Methods. 2010;50:237–43.
25. Peters IR, Peeters D. Helps CR, day MJ. Development and application of multiple internal reference (housekeeper) gene assays for accurate normalisation of canine gene expression studies. Vet Immunol Immunopathol. 2007;117:55–66.
26. Figueiredo MD, Salter CE, Andrietti AL, Vandenplas ML, Hurley DJ, Moore JN. Validation of a reliable set of primer pairs for measuring gene expression by real-time quantitative RT-PCR in equine leukocytes. Vet Immunol Immunopathol. 2009;131:65–72.
27. Nygard AB, Jorgensen CB, Cirera S, Fredholm M. Selection of reference genes for gene expression studies in pig tissues using SYBR green qPCR. BMC Mol Biol. 2007;8:67.
28. Olsvik PA, Softeland L, Lie KK. Selection of reference genes for qRT-PCR examination of wild populations of Atlantic cod Gadus Morhua. BMC Res Notes. 2008;1:47.
29. Penning LC, Vrieling HE, Brinkhof B, Riemers FM, Rothuizen J, Rutteman GR, et al. A validation of 10 feline reference genes for gene expression measurements in snap-frozen tissues. Vet Immunol Immunopathol. 2007; 120:212–22.
30. Zornhagen KW, Kristensen AT, Hansen AE, Oxboel J, Kjaer A. Selection of suitable reference genes for normalization of genes of interest in canine soft tissue sarcomas using quantitative real-time polymerase chain reaction. Vet Comp Oncol. 2015 Dec;13(4):485–93.
31. Miyajima N, Watanabe M, Ohashi E, Mochizuki M, Nishimura R, Ogawa H, et al. Relationship between retinoic acid receptor alpha gene expression and growth-inhibitory effect of all-trans retinoic acid on canine tumor cells. J Vet Intern Med. 2006;20:348–54.
32. Lallemant B, Evrard A, Combescure C, Chapuis H, Chambon G, Raynal C, et al. Reference gene selection for head and neck squamous cell carcinoma gene expression studies. BMC Mol Biol. 2009;10:78.
33. Nguewa PA, Agorreta J, Blanco D, Lozano MD, Gomez-Roman J, Sanchez BA, et al. Identification of importin 8 (IPO8) as the most accurate reference gene for the Clinicopathological analysis of lung specimens. BMC Mol Biol. 2008;9:103.
34. Greer S, Honeywell R, Geletu M, Arulanandam R, Raptis L. Housekeeping genes; expression levels may change with density of cultured cells. J Immunol Methods. 2010;355:76–9.
35. Ayers D, Clements DN, Salway F, Day PJ. Expression stability of commonly used reference genes in canine articular connective tissues. BMC Vet Res. 2007;3:7.
36. Khanna C, Lindblad-Toh K, Vail D, London C, Bergman P, Barber L, et al. The Dog as a Cancer Model. Nat Biotechnol 2006;24:1065–6.

8

Coincidence of Persistent Müllerian duct syndrome and testicular tumors in dogs

Eun Jung Park[1,2], Seok-Hee Lee[1,2], Young-Kwang Jo[1,2], Sang-Eun Hahn[1,2], Do-Min Go[3], Su-Hyung Lee[3], Byeong-Chun Lee[1,2] and Goo Jang[1,2,4*] (ID)

Abstract

Background: Persistent Müllerian duct syndrome (PMDS), a rare form of male pseudohermaphroditism in dogs, is an abnormal sexual phenotype in males that is characterized by the existence of a hypoplastic oviduct, uterus, and cranial part of the vagina. Dogs suffering from PMDS are often accompanied by cryptorchidism. To date, it has been mainly found in the Miniature Schnauzer breed.

Case presentation: In this report, two cases of PMDS with a malignant testicular tumor originating from cryptorchidism in breeds other than the Miniature Schnauzer breed are described. The patients were a seven-year-old male Maltese dog and a 17-year-old male mixed-breed dog weighing 3.8 kg. They also exhibited an enlarged prostate with or without abscess and an elevated serum estradiol level and were surgically treated to remove the testicular tumor and Müllerian duct derivatives.

Conclusions: It is recommended that PMDS should be differentially diagnosed by ultrasonography and that orchiectomy be performed at an early age in patients suspected to have cryptorchidism to prevent the ectopic testes from becoming tumorous.

Keywords: Cryptorchidism, Hyperestrogenemia, PMDS, Prostatomegaly, Testicular tumor

Background

Persistent Müllerian duct syndrome (PMDS), a type of male pseudohermaphroditism, is a known autosomal recessive inherited abnormality in the Miniature Schnauzer. This syndrome refers to male dogs presenting normal karyotypes (78, XY) that have bilateral testes with vestigial organs of the oviduct, uterus, and cranial vagina, as the Müllerian duct has failed to regress [1, 2]. The regression of the Müllerian duct is controlled by Müllerian-inhibiting factor (MIF). Sertoli cells in the testes secrete MIF in normal and PMDS-affected fetuses and neonatal dogs [3], and a single base-pair mutation in the gene coding the canine MIF receptor impairs the regression of the Müllerian duct [4]. These observations indicate that PMDS results from the refractory targeting of cells by MIF rather than from a lack of MIF secretion.

Cryptorchidism often occurs simultaneously with PMDS, and the incidence rate of cryptorchidism is approximately 50% in PMDS dogs [2, 5]. Testicular tumors occur in both scrotal and ectopic testes, but ectopic testes tend to develop tumors more frequently than scrotal testes. PMDS with simultaneously existing testicular tumor in a Miniature Schnauzer dog has been reported [6], but there have been no reports for other breeds to our knowledge. Here, we report two cases of PMDS accompanied by testicular tumor from abdominal cryptorchidism in non-Miniature Schnauzer breeds. Informed consent was obtained from the owners.

Case presentation

Case 1

A seven-year-old male Maltese dog that had been diagnosed with an abdominal mass was referred to the Veterinary Medical Teaching Hospital, Seoul National University, for medical treatment and surgical removal of the mass. An edematous, pendulous prepuce and

* Correspondence: snujang@snu.ac.kr
[1]Laboratory of Theriogenology & Biotechnology, College of Veterinary Medicine and the Research Institute of Veterinary Science, Seoul National University, Kwanak-ro 1, Daehak-Dong, Kwanak-Gu, Seoul 08826, Republic of Korea
[2]Veterinary Teaching Hospital, College of Veterinary Medicine and the Research Institute of Veterinary Science, Seoul National University, Seoul 08826, Republic of Korea
Full list of author information is available at the end of the article

enlarged nipples were observed during a physical examination. The owner reported that the dog had been castrated at 10 months old, and the veterinarian and owner agreed that both testes had been removed. In radiography and ultrasonography, prostatomegaly (1.50 × 0.94 cm) (Fig. 1a) and a round-shaped mass (2.14 × 1.36 cm) at the right cranial to the urinary bladder apex region were detected (Fig. 1b), respectively. A hypoechoic tubular structure with a diameter of 0.38 cm was found incidentally, extending from the mass to the right inguinal region (Fig. 1c and d). All the blood analysis panel values were within the normal reference intervals. Table 1 shows that the serum estradiol concentration was 19.6 pg/mL, which is slightly higher than the upper margin of the reference intervals in male dogs (<15 pg/mL [6, 7]), and the testosterone level was 0.025 ng/mL, which is much lower than in intact males (1–5 ng/mL) and similar to that of castrated dogs (<0.02 ng/mL [7]). Thus, we concluded that the mass in the abdomen secreted estradiol, not testosterone. For removing the mass, a laparotomy was performed. As the mass was exposed, it was found that a pampiniform plexus-like vascular structure and a ductus deferens-suspected tubular structure were connected to the mass (Fig. 1e). On the opposite site of the adnexa in the mass, a uterus-like smooth muscle structure with a Y shape linked to the mass was also found (Fig. 1e and f). The Y-shaped structure had vascular distribution and a rugged broad ligament, while the end of the left horn of the Y shape was suspended from the abdominal wall by fibrous tissue, and an incompletely fused body terminated at the prostate. The mass with adnexa was isolated from the abdomen and examined by a histologist. The sections confirmed the presence of malignant seminoma with tumor emboli in the testis (Fig. 1g) and thick muscle and lumen lining with epithelium, which were diagnosed as Müllerian duct derivatives (Fig. 1h). Four days after the surgery, the estradiol level decreased to less than 5 pg/mL.

Case 2

A 17-year-old male mixed-breed dog weighing 3.8 kg was transferred for diagnosis and medical treatment related to a very large abdominal mass. Hyperkeratosis, alopecia in the trunk and ear margin, a pendulous prepuce, enlarged nipples, unilateral scrotal testis, thoracolumbar kyphosis (Fig. 2a and b), and frequent urination were observed during a physical examination. A preputial swab showed an exfoliative cytology (Fig. 2d) similar to the vaginal cytology of female dogs in estrus, which is different from that of normal males (Fig. 2c). An ill-defined margin and marked homogenous soft-tissue opacity of a mass (11 × 6 cm) in the right-middle abdomen resulted in left cranial displacement of a descending, transverse colon and stomach and left caudal displacement of the intestinal loops (Fig. 3b and c). The additional relatively well-defined homogenous soft-tissue opacity of a mass (6.4 × 4.3 cm) in the caudal abdomen

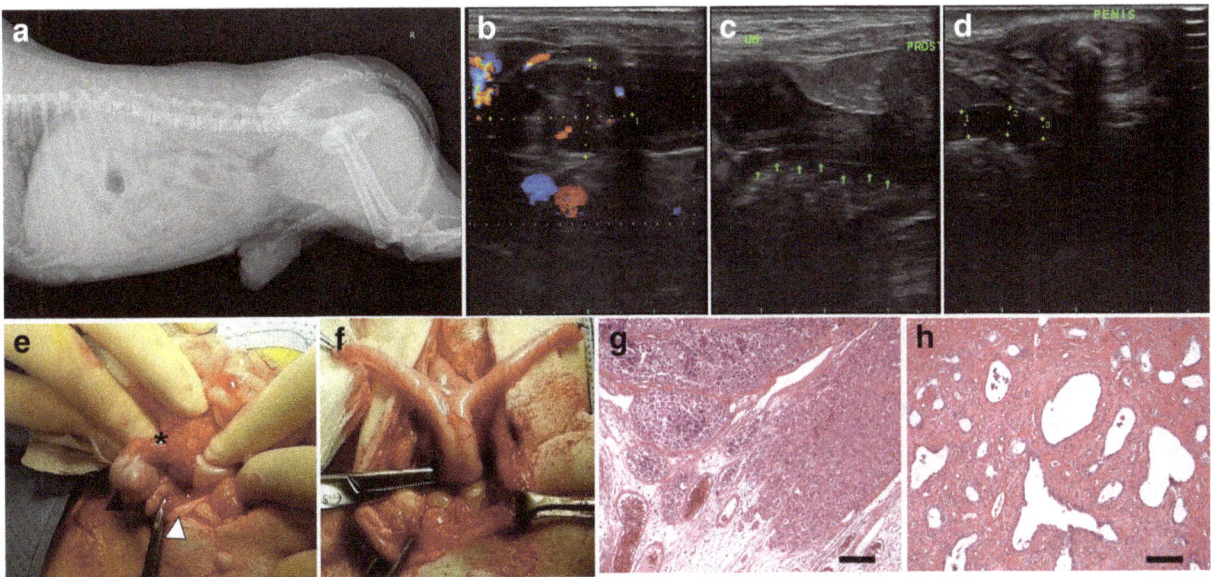

Fig. 1 Radiography and ultrasonography findings in surgery and histological examination of the testicular tumor and Müllerian duct derivatives of Case 1. **a** prostatomegaly shown in radiography; **b** abdominal mass showing mild blood signal; **c** and **d** tubular structure with hypoechoic lumen (*arrows*) extending from the mass to adjacent inguinal region; **e** the abdominal mass (*filled arrowhead*), spermatic cord-like structure (pampiniform plexus and ductus deference, *asterisk*), and tubular structure (*blank arrowhead*); **f** smooth muscle structure with Y shape linked to the mass; **g** malignant seminoma with tumor emboli (× 100); **h** Müllerian duct derivatives involving thick muscle and lumen lining with epithelium (× 100). Scale bar = 200 um

Table 1 Blood analysis and serum sex hormone levels of both cases

		Case 1	Case 2	Reference range
CBC	WBC (/μL)	9490	5840	6000–17000
	Hct (%)	41.9	24.1	37.0–55.0
	Thrombocyte (/μL)	337,000	39,000	200,000–500,000
Na+/K+/Cl- (mEq/L)		149/4.5/116	155/3.9/118	145–155/2.7–5.0/96–122
PT/APTT (s)		-	12/ 89	11–17/ 72–102
Estrogen (pg/mL)		19.6	267.8	<15 [6, 7]
Testosterone (ng/mL)		0.025	0.602	1–5 [7]

at the L5 pelvic inlet level causing cranial displacement of the intestinal loops was detected via radiography (Fig. 3b and c). Ultrasonography showed two severely enlarged, heterogenous masses in the abdomen. The larger abdominal mass included multiple cystic lesions in the parenchyma with echogenic and anechoic fluid and moderate blood signals (Fig. 3a). Information about the other abdominal organs taken from the ultrasonography was limited due to the volume of the masses. The blood analysis results presented pancytopenia (Table 1). The serum estradiol concentration was 267.8 pg/mL, which is approximately 18 times higher than the upper margin of the reference interval. The testosterone level was 0.602 ng/mL, which is lower than the normal reference interval in intact males (Table 1) and within the reference range of a dog with a Sertoli cell tumor (SCT) (0.1–2 ng/mL [7]). Therefore, the mass in the abdomen was suspected to be an SCT secreting estradiol strongly. Despite the risk of complications during and after surgery due to pancytopenia and the old age of the patient,

the owner wanted the mass to be removed to relieve the discomfort and complications caused by the mass. Thus, the coagulation time, such as PT/APTT, was analyzed for a laparotomy, and these values were in the normal range (Table 1). The mass was too large to be extracted via a routine laparotomy; accordingly, the incision line was extended to the xiphoid process cranially. The diaphragm was abnormally pushed forward by the mass which occupied almost the entire abdominal cavity. Stay sutures were applied to the mass to remove it from the abdominal cavity carefully (Fig. 3d). The mass was removed successfully, and then dissected (Fig. 3e and f). A pampiniform plexus-like vascular structure and a smooth muscle structure with a Y shape linked to the mass were found (Fig. 3g), and one of its horns was isolated from the mass. While the other horn remained intact, we moved to the caudal abdomen and found the urinary bladder was collapsed and unable to distend as well as bilateral prostatic enlargement with abscess (Fig. 3h). The dog became hypotensive during the removal of the

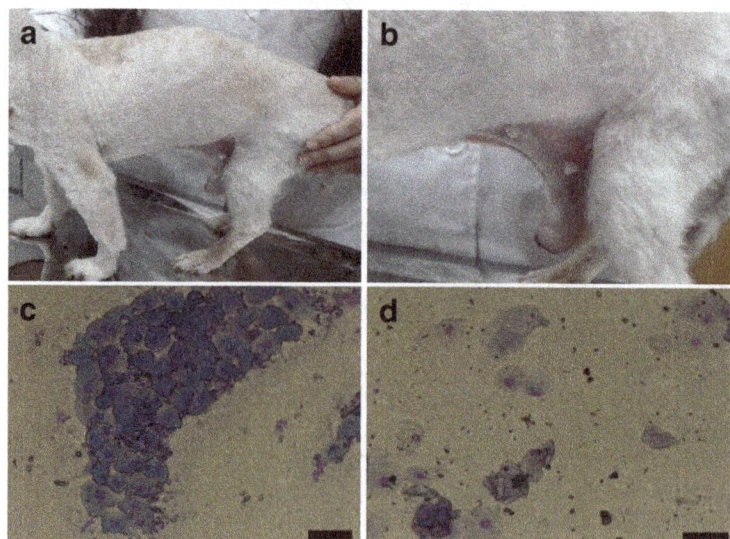

Fig. 2 Photographs from physical examination and preputial cytology of Case 2. **a** hyperkeratosis and alopecia in trunk and thoracolumbar kyphosis; **b** pendulous prepuce and enlarged nipples; **c** nucleated round epithelial cells and neutrophils in preputial cytology of normal male dog (× 200); **d** superficial epithelial cells in preputial cytology of Case 2 (× 200). Diff-quik stain was used for the cytology. Scale bar= 50 um

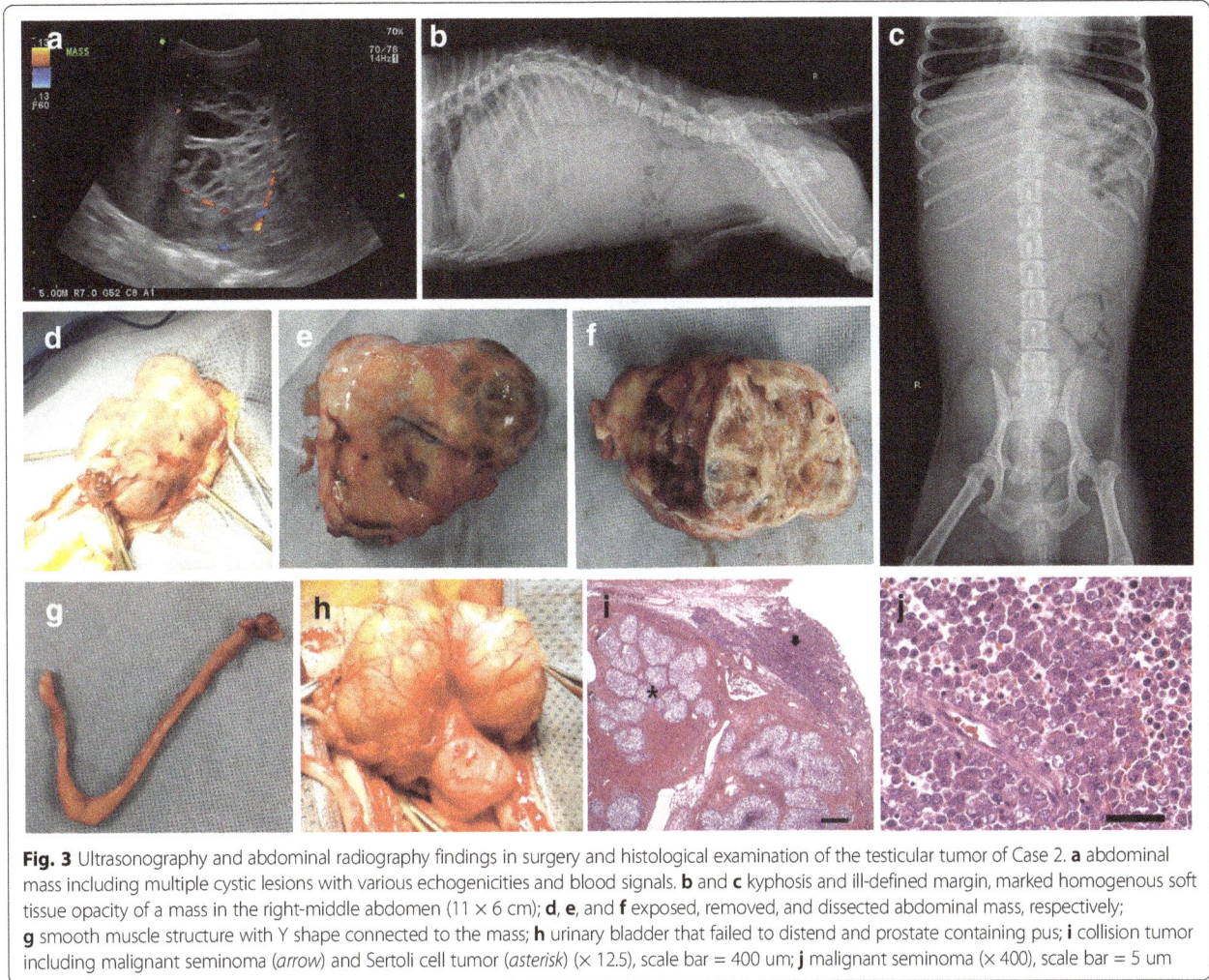

Fig. 3 Ultrasonography and abdominal radiography findings in surgery and histological examination of the testicular tumor of Case 2. **a** abdominal mass including multiple cystic lesions with various echogenicities and blood signals. **b** and **c** kyphosis and ill-defined margin, marked homogenous soft tissue opacity of a mass in the right-middle abdomen (11 × 6 cm); **d**, **e**, and **f** exposed, removed, and dissected abdominal mass, respectively; **g** smooth muscle structure with Y shape connected to the mass; **h** urinary bladder that failed to distend and prostate containing pus; **i** collision tumor including malignant seminoma (*arrow*) and Sertoli cell tumor (*asterisk*) (× 12.5), scale bar = 400 um; **j** malignant seminoma (× 400), scale bar = 5 um

prostatic abscess, so the surgical procedure, including removal of the entire uterus-suspected structure and draining of pus in the prostate, was stopped and transfusion, dopamine, dobutamine, and vasopressin were administered to overcome the hypotension. The patient recovered from hypotension, but cardiopulmonary arrest suddenly occurred 36 h after surgery. Although the cardiac and pulmonary function was recovered by cardiopulmonary cerebral resuscitation, the patient failed to recover his brain function and died within 12 h. Histologic examination of the suspected testicular tumor mass allowed diagnosis of the mass as a collision tumor of malignant seminoma with SCT (Fig. 3i and j).

Discussion

In this case report, two dogs presenting with PMDS and testicular tumor from cryptorchidism have been described. Both cases in this report exhibited elevated serum estradiol levels, testicular tumors, and feminization characteristics, including gynecomastia and a pendulous penile sheath. PMDS-affected dogs exhibit cryptorchidism frequently and may present with a fluid-filled uterus, urinary tract infection, or prostatic infection [8]. Less than 10% of seminomas produce estrogen (communicated with reviewer's comment), so it is interesting that the malignant seminoma in Case 1 produced slightly more estradiol than in normal males. However, we had the limitation of having no standard because the GnRH stimulation test and multiple-sample assays of estradiol and testosterone were not conducted in this study.

The intra-abdominal testes have a significantly higher risk of being tumorous, especially seminoma and SCT, which have an approximately nine-fold incidence rate compared with scrotal testes [9]. Among the testicular tumor types, SCT specifically secretes excess estrogen, resulting in the feminization of male dogs and bone-marrow suppression, which leads to pancytopenia. Both patients presented elevated serum estradiol levels, but the patient in Case 2 only exhibited pancytopenia following severe hyperestrogenemia. Although the complications of pancytopenia include infection, anemia, and spontaneous bleeding, there was no spontaneous bleeding or delayed coagulation in this case, which enabled us to decide to remove the mass to relieve the patient from distress. As we confirmed, however, a severe prostatic abscess existed. It is assumed that prolonged pancytopenia resulting from hyperestrogenemia caused prostatic infection, which subsequently developed into an abscess. Regarding another effect of hyperestrogenemia, the preputial cytology of Case 2 exhibited exfoliative, superficial epithelial cells similar to the vaginal cytology of female dogs in estrus, which corresponds with a report that the preputial cytology of male dogs that have hyperestrogenemia (>40 pmol/L) exhibited superficial epithelial cells [10]. Recently, it has been reported that neoplastic Sertoli cells in dogs produce a significantly high MIF level compared with healthy Sertoli cells [11, 12]. If we had detected the level of AMH in both cases, the patient in Case 2, which had SCT, might have exhibited a higher level of AMH compared with the patient in Case 1 with no SCT. MIF secretion in canine immature Sertoli cells starts from embryonic day 34, when testicular differentiation initiates, and continues until day 143 after birth. Müllerian duct regression begins shortly after testicular development at day 36–46 of gestation through MIF in canines [13]. The PMDS in both cases of this report might have arisen from the abnormal action of MIF during the embryonic Müllerian duct regression period. Meyers-Wallen et al. report that oviduct regression depends on MIF activity, but uterus regression is independent of the MIF level [13]. That is, uterine and oviductal sensitivities to MIF differ, which explains why we observed a uterus, but not an oviduct. These observations might correspond with the report of a study that described a dog with an obviously present uterine structure, despite no oviduct being observed [6].

The two dogs in this report exhibited a testicular tumor in the right abdomen and prostatomegaly. Unilateral cryptorchidism tends to occur on the right side [14] because the right testis, formed more cranially, needs to move a longer distance until it reaches the scrotum than the left one [15], and prostatomegaly is commonly present in PMDS patients [16]. PMDS is known as an inherited condition in the Miniature Schnauzer and Basset Hound breeds and has also been reported in other canine breeds [16, 17]. The coincidence of SCT that has developed from cryptorchidism with PMDS occurs almost solely in the Miniature Schnauzer breed [6, 18]. To the best of our knowledge, this is the first report to describe PMDS with coexisting malignant seminoma or collision tumor in the testes in breeds other than the Miniature Schnauzer.

Conclusions

It is recommended that Müllerian duct derivatives should be examined in cryptorchidism through ultrasonography and that orchiectomy be performed at an early age for patients that have cryptorchidism to prevent the intra-abdominal testes from becoming tumorous.

Abbreviations
APTT: Activated Partial Thromboplastin Time; MIF: Müllerian-inhibiting factor; PMDS: Persistent Müllerian duct syndrome; PT: Prothrombin Time; SCT: Sertoli cell tumor

Acknowledgements
Not applicable.

Funding
This study was financially supported by the Research Institute of Veterinary Science, Biogreen (PJ0090962014) and the BK21 PLUS Program for Creative Veterinary Science Research.

Authors' contributions
EJ attended the surgery and carried out the conception, design, acquisition, and analysis of data and drafted the manuscript. SH contributed to the design and acquisition of data. YK and SE assisted the surgery and assisted in data mining. DM and SH carried out the acquisition and analysis of data. BC has been involved in drafting the manuscript or revising it critically for important intellectual content. G attended the surgery as the main surgeon and participated in the design of the study, drafted the manuscript, and gave final approval of the version to be published. All authors read and approved the final manuscript.

Competing interests
The authors declare that they have no competing interests.

Consent for publication
Not applicable.

Author details
[1]Laboratory of Theriogenology & Biotechnology, College of Veterinary Medicine and the Research Institute of Veterinary Science, Seoul National University, Kwanak-ro 1, Daehak-Dong, Kwanak-Gu, Seoul 08826, Republic of Korea. [2]Veterinary Teaching Hospital, College of Veterinary Medicine and the Research Institute of Veterinary Science, Seoul National University, Seoul 08826, Republic of Korea. [3]Veterinary Pathology, College of Veterinary Medicine and the Research Institute of Veterinary Science, Seoul National University, Seoul 08826, Republic of Korea. [4]Emergence Center for Food-Medicine Personalized Therapy System, Advanced Institutes of Convergence Technology, Seoul National University, Gyeonggi-do 443-270, Republic of Korea.

References
1. Lyle SK. Disorders of sexual development in the dog and cat. Theriogenology. 2007;68(3):338–43. doi:10.1016/j.theriogenology.2007.04.015.
2. Romagnoli S, Schlafer DH. Disorders of sexual differentiation in puppies and kittens: a diagnostic and clinical approach. Vet Clin North Am Small Anim Pract. 2006;36(3):573–606, vii. doi:10.1016/j.cvsm.2005.12.007.
3. Meyers-Wallen VN, Donahoe PK, Ueno S, Manganaro TF, Patterson DF. Mullerian inhibiting substance is present in testes of dogs with persistent mullerian duct syndrome. Biol Reprod. 1989;41(5):881–8.
4. Wu X, Wan S, Pujar S, Haskins ME, Schlafer DH, Lee MM, et al. A single base pair mutation encoding a premature stop codon in the MIS type II receptor is responsible for canine persistent Mullerian duct syndrome. J Androl. 2009; 30(1):46–56. doi:10.2164/jandrol.108.005736.

5. Poth T, Breuer W, Walter B, Hecht W, Hermanns W. Disorders of sex development in the dog-Adoption of a new nomenclature and reclassification of reported cases. Anim Reprod Sci. 2010;121(3–4):197–207. doi:10.1016/j.anireprosci.2010.04.011.

6. Matsuu A, Hashizume T, Kanda T, Nagano M, Sugiyama A, Okamoto Y, et al. A case of persistent Mullerian duct syndrome with sertoli cell tumor and hydrometra in a dog. J Vet Med Sci. 2009;71(3):379–81.

7. Feldman and Nelson. Canine and feline endocrinology and reproduction, 3rd ed. St. Louis: Saunders; 2004.

8. Meyers-Wallen V. Inherited abnormalities of sexual development in dogs and cats. Recent advances in small animal reproduction Ithaca, International Veterinary Service (www.ivis.org). 2001.

9. Hayes HM Jr, Wilson GP, Pendergrass TW, Cox VS. Canine cryptorchism and subsequent testicular neoplasia: case-control study with epidemiologic update. Teratology. 1985;32(1):51–6. doi:10.1002/tera.1420320108.

10. Dreimanis U, Vargmar K, Falk T, Cigut M, Toresson L. Evaluation of preputial cytology in diagnosing oestrogen producing testicular tumours in dogs. J Small Anim Pract. 2012;53(9):536–41. doi:10.1111/j.1748-5827.2012.01261.x.

11. Holst BS, Dreimanis U. Anti-Müllerian hormone: a potentially useful biomarker for the diagnosis of canine Sertoli cell tumours. BMC Vet Res. 2015;11:166. doi:10.1186/s12917-015-0487-5.

12. Ano H, Hidaka Y, Katamoto H. Evaluation of anti-Müllerian hormone in a dog with a Sertoli cell tumour. Vet Dermatol. 2014;25(2):142–5. e41

13. Meyers-Wallen VN, Donahoe PK, Manganaro T, Patterson DF. Mullerian inhibiting substance in sex-reversed dogs. Biol Reprod. 1987;37(4):1015–22.

14. Post K, Kilborn SH. Canine sertoli cell tumor: a medical records search and literature review. Can Vet J. 1987;28(7):427–31.

15. Moulton JE. Tumors in domestic animals. California: University of California Press; 1978.

16. Lim CK, Heng HG, Hui TY, Thompson CA, Childress MO, Adams LG. Ultrasonographic features of uterus masculinus in six dogs. Vet Radiol Ultrasound. 2015;56(1):77–83. doi:10.1111/vru.12189.

17. Kuiper H, Wagner F, Drogemuller C, Distl O. Persistent Mullerian duct syndrome causing male pseudohermaphroditism in a mixed-breed dog. Vet Rec. 2004;155(13):400–1.

18. Vegter AR, Kooistra HS, van Sluijs FJ, van Bruggen LW, Ijzer J, Zijlstra C, et al. Persistent Mullerian duct syndrome in a Miniature Schnauzer dog with signs of feminization and a Sertoli cell tumour. Reprod Domest Anim. 2010;45(3):447–52. doi:10.1111/j.1439-0531.2008.01223.x.

9

Solid type primary intraosseous squamous cell carcinoma in a cat

Darja Pavlin[1]* (iD), Tamara Dolenšek[2], Tanja Švara[2] and Ana Nemec[1]

Abstract

Background: Squamous cell carcinoma (SCC) is the most common nonodontogenic oral tumor in cats. In the jaw, it usually presents as an ulceroproliferative lesion associated with enlargement of the affected bone.

Case presentation: This report describes the case of a cat in which clinical and radiographic findings of a mandibular swelling were suggestive of an aggressive process, but the oral mucosa was unaffected. The results of histopathological and immunohistochemical examination of the samples obtained from the intraosseous lesion were consistent with SCC. The animal was euthanized 5 months after initial presentation as a result of the severe progression of the disease, and no other primary tumors were identified at necropsy.

Conclusions: Based on the clinicopathological, microscopic, and immunohistochemical staining features, as well as the absence of a primary tumor at a distant site, we propose that the term, solid type primary intraosseous SCC (PIOSCC), be used to describe this neoplasia, as it shares similar features with human PIOSCC.

Keywords: Primary intraosseous squamous cell carcinoma, Squamous cell carcinoma, Cat, Odontogenic oral tumors

Background

Mandibular swelling can occur in cats as a result of tumors, osteomyelitis or cysts [1, 2]. Of the oral tumors, squamous cell carcinoma (SCC) is the most common tumor, representing approximately 60–70% of all feline oral malignancies [3]. SCC is a tumor of older cats with a mean age at presentation of 12.5 years [4]. There is no known breed or sex predisposition in cats.

SCC is a nonodontogenic oral tumor of epithelial origin, typically presenting as an ulceroproliferative lesion in the sublingual area or on the mandibular or maxillary gingiva, which is associated with enlargement of the affected bone. Other less common sites include the buccal mucosa, lips and pharynx. Characteristic clinical signs include excessive salivation, hemorrhagic or purulent oral discharge, pain, difficulty eating and tooth loss. Radiographs frequently reveal significant bone lysis, although new bone formation can also be observed. Due to the rapid and invasive growth of these tumors, SCC in cats is often very advanced at the time of initial presentation [4]. The previously presumed low metastatic rate of these

tumors appears to be an underestimate, since up to 37.5% of these tumors metastasized to regional lymph nodes in a study by Gendler et al. [5]. However, the majority of cats die due to the primary disease prior to development of clinically evident metastatic disease [3]. Despite considerable efforts to develop effective treatments, prognosis for feline patients with oral SCC is poor, since none of the therapeutic options currently available are curative or result in long-term control of the disease [4]. The median survival time (MST) with palliative treatment (nonsteroidal anti-inflammatory drugs, antibiotics, and corticosteroids) is approximately 1.5 months [3, 4]. Surgery, when feasible, increases the MST to 6 months, which can be extended to up to approximately one year with multimodal therapy (different combinations of surgery, radiotherapy and chemotherapy) [4].

In humans with swelling of the jaw, primary intraosseous squamous cell carcinoma (PIOSCC) is considered as a possible differential diagnosis. PIOSCC is a very rare invasive tumor, and in contrast to the more common "classical" oral SCC, it is an odontogenic tumor. It develops within the mandible or maxilla without any initial connection to the oral mucosa. The diagnostic criteria, differentiating PIOSCC from other similar tumors (e.g., oral SCC, alveolar carcinoma, or metastatic bone lesions), include

* Correspondence: darja.pavlin@vf.uni-lj.si
[1]University of Ljubljana, Veterinary faculty, Small Animal Clinic, Gerbičeva, 60 Ljubljana, Slovenia

undamaged oral mucosa and the absence of a primary tumor at a distant site. The WHO classification categorizes PIOSCC into three subtypes: solid de novo tumors that originate from remnants of odontogenic epithelium or, rarely, dedifferentiation from a benign ameloblastoma, tumors originating from odontogenic cysts and those originating from keratocystic odontogenic tumors [6].

Case presentation

A 14-year-old 3.5 kg female spayed strictly indoor domestic shorthair cat was admitted to the Small animal clinic, Veterinary faculty Ljubljana, Slovenia, for evaluation of a facial skin lesion of approximately two weeks duration. The history and general physical examination were unremarkable, except for a small superficial autotraumatic skin lesion in the right mandibular region (ventrally at the level of the right mandibular canine tooth). A brief dermatologic examination of the cat revealed no other abnormalities of the skin or coat and no evidence of ectoparasites. The right rostral mandible appeared swollen. On a brief oral examination, several missing teeth, a severely mobile right mandibular canine tooth and moderate generalized plaque, calculus and gingivitis affecting the remaining of the teeth were noted.

Informed consent was obtained from the client to perform a detailed oral and dental examination under general anesthesia with dental radiographs and biopsy, as indicated. A basic preanesthetic bloodwork panel was within normal limits (Table 1). The three-view thoracic radiographs were unremarkable and other diagnostic imaging procedures (e.g., CT scan) were declined by the owner. The detailed oral and dental examination revealed swelling and palpable instability of the rostral mandibles

with severe mobility of all of the mandibular incisor teeth and the right mandibular canine tooth. No excessive probing depth, gingival recession or any other soft tissue lesions were diagnosed for any of the teeth (Fig. 1). Several teeth were missing, gingivitis was present on all of the remaining teeth and tooth resorption of various stages was diagnosed at several of the remaining teeth. The dental radiographs of the rostral mandibles are presented in Fig. 2. The mandibular lymph nodes were palpably within normal limits.

Based on the clinical and radiographic features, an aggressive process, such as osteomyelitis or cancer, was suspected, and a biopsy was recommended. The oral cavity was rinsed with a 0.12% chlorhexidine solution, and left and right inferior alveolar nerve blocks were performed with 0.2 ml of 2.5 mg/ml levobupivacaine prior to performing a professional dental cleaning. A full-thickness triangular flap was created to remove the remnants of the right mandibular canine tooth and to obtain soft tissue and bony samples for histopathology (Fig. 3). The flap was sutured back in place with 5–0 resorbable monofilament suture material, and other dental treatments were postponed pending the biopsy results. The cat was discharged from the hospital with oral meloxicam (0.1 mg/kg/day), which was to be administered once daily until the re-check examination.

The incisional biopsies that were collected for histopathology were fixed in 10% buffered formalin, embedded in paraffin, sliced into 4 μm sections and stained with hematoxylin and eosin stain. Samples containing a large

Table 1 Preanesthetic bloodwork results

Parameter	Result	Reference value
Complete blood count		
WBC	5.02×10^9/L	6.3–19.6
% Neutrophils	66.2	29.5–74.5
% Lymphocytes	27.7	20.0–61.2
% Eosinophils	2.3	3.4–11.4
% Monocytes	3.8	0.2–5
% Basophils	0	0–1.0
RBC	8.95×10^{12}/L	6.0–10.1
Ht	0.45	0.28–0.47
PLT	219×10^9/L	156.4–626.4
Pct	0.31	0.3–0.8
Biochemistry		
Urea	8.9 mmol/L	5.3–12.1
Creatinine	126 μmol/L	70.7–140

WBC white blood cells, *RBC* red blood cells, *Ht* hematocrit, *PLT* platelets, *Pct* plateletcrit

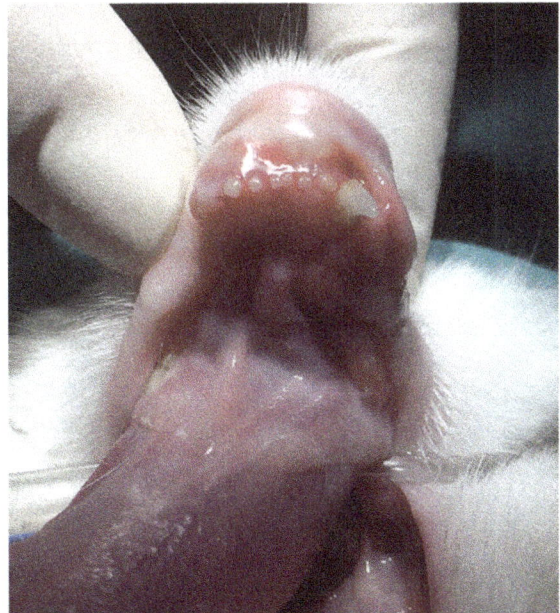

Fig. 1 The rostral mandibles of the cat in dorsal recumbency under general anesthesia. Swelling of the rostral mandibles is notable, but there is no oral soft tissue lesion

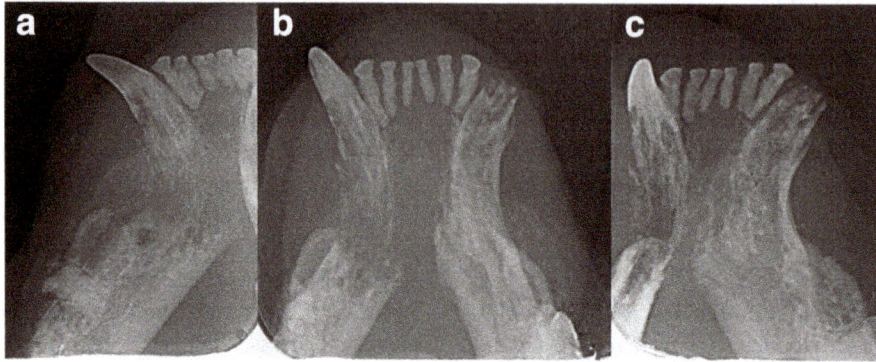

Fig. 2 Right lateral (**a**), occlusal (**b**) and left lateral (**c**) dental radiographs of the rostral mandibles of the cat. Geographic bone loss is evident at the right rostral mandible and symphyseal area, combined with permeative bone loss in the apical region of the right mandibular canine tooth. Mild inflammatory root resorption is present in all of the incisor teeth. The left mandibular canine and third premolar tooth are affected by stage 5 tooth resorption. The right mandibular canine tooth is affected by stage 4c tooth resorption and there is a complete loss of hard tissues in the apical area. The right mandibular third premolar tooth is affected by stage 5 tooth resorption and there is a retained mesial root of the right mandibular fourth premolar tooth

amount of bony tissue were decalcified with OSTEO-MOLL® (Merck Millipore) before further processing.

The histopathological examination of the biopsies revealed an infiltrative lesion, composed of islands and cords of oval to polyhedral cells, which exhibited marked anisocytosis and had lightly eosinophilic, nongranulated cytoplasm and round to oval nuclei with moderate anisokaryosis and one to two prominent nucleoli. The mitotic index was 20 mitotic figures per 10 high power fields. Some of the neoplastic cells were binucleated or trinucleated. Foci of dyskeratotic neoplastic cells were evident, but true keratinization was not present. There was a moderate amount of fibrous stroma, which was

multifocally infiltrated with lymphocytes. The neoplastic cells infiltratively grew into the surrounding bony tissue, but no blood or lymph vessel invasion was noted (Fig. 4a).

Additionally, immunohistochemistry was conducted on formalin-fixed, paraffin-embedded tissue sections to confirm the epithelial origin of the neoplastic cells. Mouse monoclonal antibody raised against human cytokeratin (clone MNF116; Dako, Glostrup, Denmark), which was diluted 1:100, was used for the immunolabelling. The antigen retrieval was performed by microwave treatment at medium power (550 W) for 20 min in a 0.1 M citrate buffer (pH 6.0). The remaining immunohistochemical procedure was performed using a previously described protocol [7]. Sections of normal feline skin were used as a positive control, and sections not treated with primary antibodies served as a negative control. Immunohistochemically, a moderate to marked positive cytoplasmic reaction for cytokeratin was observed in almost all of the neoplastic cells (Fig. 4b).

A two-week re-check examination revealed progression of clinical signs with a more pronounced mandibular swelling. Soft tissue proliferation at the biopsy site and hemorrhagic oral discharge were present at this time. The client declined further procedures and elected palliative pain medications. Five months after the initial presentation, the client elected humane euthanasia of the animal due to the rapid deterioration of its health. An extensive oral lesion was found on necropsy (Fig. 5) and the mandibular lymph nodes were mildly to moderately enlarged. No other tumors were detected elsewhere in the body. Histopathology revealed multiple islands of carcinomatous cells bilaterally in the mandibular lymph nodes, but no other primary tumor or metastases were discovered.

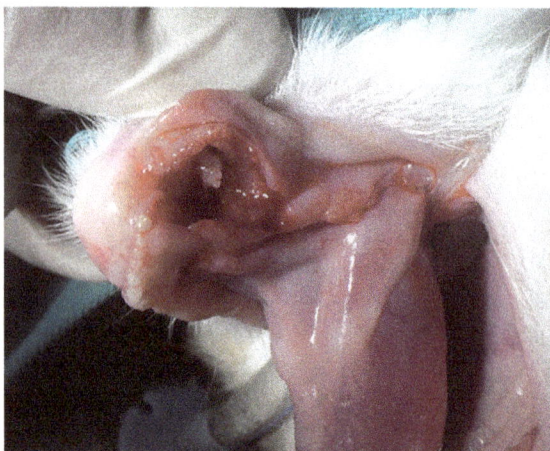

Fig. 3 An intraoperative photograph of the right rostral mandible after a full-thickness triangular flap was created and the crown of the right mandibular canine tooth was removed. Proliferative soft tissue is visible filling the alveolus of the right mandibular canine tooth

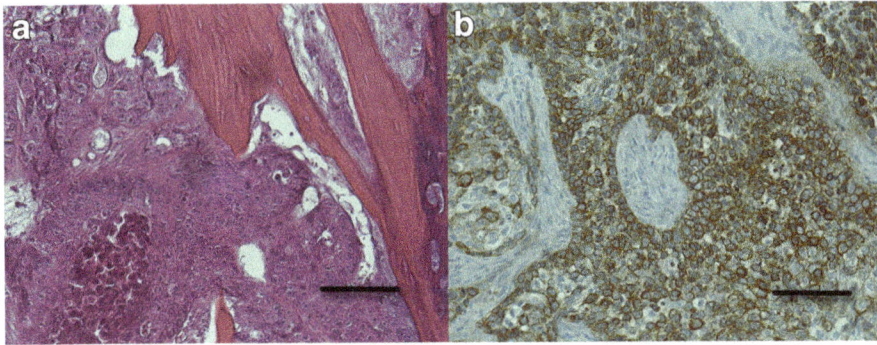

Fig. 4 Primary intraosseous squamous cell carcinoma (PIOSCC) of the mandible in the cat. **a** Sheets of polygonal neoplastic cells with eosinophilic, nongranulated cytoplasm and round to oval nuclei with prominent nucleoli are evident infiltrating the bony tissue. A focus of dyskeratotic neoplastic cells is present in the left bottom corner. HE. Bar = 100 μm **b** The neoplastic cells exhibit a moderate to marked positive cytoplasmic reaction for cytokeratin. Immunohistochemistry for cytokeratin. Bar = 100 μm

Discussion and conclusions

Based on the clinicopathological, microscopic, and immunohistochemical staining features and the absence of a primary tumor at a distant site, we propose that the lesion in this cat be diagnosed as a solid type PIOSCC. In

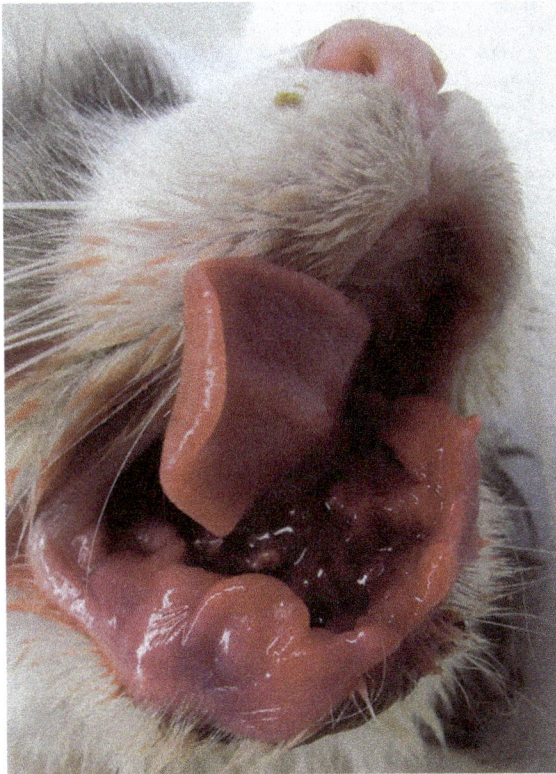

Fig. 5 The rostral mandibles of the cat at necropsy. The majority of the right rostral mandible, symphysis and a 1.5 cm long segment of the left rostral mandible are severely thickened with the right rostral mandible demonstrating segmental osteolysis. The lower lip is severely swollen and deformed. There is extensive and deep mucosal ulceration extending into the sublingual mucosa

human medicine, PIOSCC is a rare oral tumor, representing less than 2% of all oral SCCs in people [8–10]. The majority of PIOSCCs arise from other benign odontogenic tumors or cysts, while solid de novo type PIOSCC is extremely rare [11, 12]. Although PIOSCC has not yet been described in cats, in the clinical case presented here, the radiographic and microscopic features were very similar to those described for human solid type PIOSCC. Namely, the cat presented with very non-specific clinical signs in which the major complaint was an autotraumatic superficial skin lesion on the chin. Given the findings of the extensive oral examination, it was considered likely that the lesion was a result of pain or discomfort arising from the oral cavity. Although solid type PIOSCCs in humans are frequently asymptomatic, pain and jaw swelling without oral soft tissue involvement, as observed in this cat, is considered to be the main clinical features of solid type PIOSCC in humans [6, 13, 14].

The proposed diagnosis of solid type PIOSCC in this cat was further supported by the radiographic findings, which revealed an osteolytic lesion associated with tooth resorption; this outcome was similar to the typical radiographic appearance of human solid type PIOSCC [6, 15, 16].

The histopathological findings were consistent with oral SCC in cats [17] and SCC [18] and solid type PIOSCC in humans [6]. Given the clinicopathological features in this cat, and since prominent features including cellular atypia, moderate mitotic activity and no true keratinization were observed in the sections examined; this tumor was further classified as a poorly differentiated nonkeratinizing solid type PIOSCC [13, 19, 20].

Immunohistochemically, a moderate to marked positive cytoplasmic reaction for pancytokeratin was observed in almost all of the neoplastic cells. Cytokeratins are intermediate filaments found in epithelial cells of all types and are therefore specific markers for an epithelial cell lineage

[21]. This immunohistochemical finding confirmed an epithelial origin of the tumor in our case.

Although there have already been five cases reported in the literature describing SCC in cats that presented with mandibular swelling without oral soft tissue lesions [22, 23], there is an important difference in the radiographic appearance of our case and the previously described cases. The skull radiographs performed in three of the previously described five cases exhibited a predominant mixed pattern of osteoproduction and osteolysis mimicking osteosarcoma. Quigley et al. even described a "sunburst appearance" of the affected mandible, while our case demonstrated only an osteolytic lesion radiographically [22]. Additionally, the microscopic appearance of our case differs from those previously described cases. Both of the previous reports emphasized osteoblastic and fibrous proliferation, whereas in our case, these features were absent. This leads us to believe that our case differs from the previously reported cases in cats in some important respects and may therefore represent a different pathological entity. Since the pathological entity described in our case resembles the features of human solid type PIOSCC, we propose that the term solid type PIOSCC be used to describe this condition in cats.

Abbreviations
MST: median survival time; PIOSCC: Primary intraosseous squamous cell carcinoma; SCC: Squamous cell carcinoma

Acknowledgments
Not applicable

Funding
Part of the funding (cost of immunohistochemical staining) was provided by Slovenian Research Agency through grants P4-0053 and P4-0092; other costs were covered by the patient's owner during the clinical workup of the case.

Authors' contributions
DP and AN were the attending clinicians of the presented patient responsible for the diagnosis, therapy and monitoring of the patient. TD and TŠ performed histopathological and immunohistological examinations of the tumor samples, as well as the necropsy. All authors contributed to the preparation of the manuscript and read and approved the final version.

Consent for publication
The owners of the cat gave oral consent for publication of the presented case.

Competing interests
The authors declare that they have no competing interests.

Author details
[1]University of Ljubljana, Veterinary faculty, Small Animal Clinic, Gerbičeva, 60 Ljubljana, Slovenia. [2]University of Ljubljana, Veterinary faculty, Institute of Pathology, Wild Animals, Fish and Bees, Gerbičeva, 60 Ljubljana, Slovenia.

References
1. Kapatkin AS, Manfra Maretta S, Patnaik AK, Burk RL, Matus RE. Mandibular swellings in cats: prospective study of 24 cats. J Am Anim Hosp Assoc. 1991;27:575–80.
2. LaDouceur EE, Walker KS, Mohr FC, Murphy B. Odontogenic keratocyst in a cat. J Comp Pathol. 2014;151:212–6.
3. Bilgic O, Duda L, Sánchez MD, Lewis JR. Feline oral squamous cell carcinoma: Clinical manifestations and literature review. J Vet Dent. 2015;32:30–40.
4. Mc E. Clinical behavior of nonodontogenic tumors. In: FJM V, Lommer MJ, editors. Oral and maxillofacial surgery in dogs and cats. Edinburgh: Saunders Elsevier; 2012. p. 387–402.
5. Gendler A, Lewis JR, Reetz JA, Schwartz T. Computed tomographic features of oral squamous cell carcinoma in cats: 18 cases (2002 – 2008). J Am Vet Med Assoc. 2010;235:319–25.
6. Eversole LR, Siar CH, van der Waal I. Primary intraosseous squamous cell carcinomas. In: Barnes L, Evson JW, Reichart P, Sidransky D, editors. World Health Organization Classification of Tumors. Pathology and Genetics Head and Neck Tumors. Lyon: IARC Press; 2005. p. 290–1.
7. Cociancich V, Gombač M, Švara T, Pogačnik M. Malignant Mesenchymoma of the aortic valve in a dog. Slov Vet Res. 2013;50:83–8.
8. Jing W, Xuan M, Lin Y, Wu L, Liu L, Zheng X, et al. Odontogenic tumours: a retrospective study of 1642 cases in a Chinese population. Int J Oral Maxillofac Surg. 2007;36:20–5.
9. Adebayo ET, Ajike SO, Adekeye EO. A review of 318 odontogenic tumors in. Kaduna, Nigeria. J Oral Maxillofac Surg. 2005;63:811–9.
10. Naruse T, Yanamoto S, Sakamoto Y, Ikeda T, Yamada SI, Umeda M. Clinicopathological study of primary intraosseous squamous cell carcinoma of the jaw and a review of the literature. J Oral Maxillofac Surg. 2016;74:2420–7.
11. Bodner L, Manor E, Shear M, van der Waal I. Primary intraosseous squamous cell carcinoma arising in an odontogenic cyst: a clinicopathologic analysis of 116 reported cases. J Oral Pathol Med. 2011;40:733–8.
12. Saxena C, Aggarwal P, Wadhwan V, Bansal V. Primary intraosseous squamous cell carcinoma in odontogenic keratocyst: a rare entity. J Oral Maxillofac Pathol. 2015;19:406.
13. Chaisuparat R, Coletti D, Kolokythas A, Ord RA, Nikitakis NG. Primary intraosseous odontogenic carcinoma arising in an odontogenic cyst or de novo: a clinicopathologic study of six new cases. Oral Surg Oral Med Oral Pathol Oral Radiol Endod. 2006;101:194–200.
14. Choi YJ, Oh SH, Kang JH, Choi HY, Kim GT, Yu JJ, et al. Primary intraosseous squamous cell carcinoma mimicking periapical disease: a case report. Imaging Sci Dent. 2012;42:265–70.
15. Alotaibi O, Al-Zaher N, Alotaibi F, Khoja H, Qannam A. Solid-type primary intraosseous squamous-cell carcinoma in the mandible: report of a rare case. Hematol Oncol Stem Cell Ther. 2016;9:118–22.
16. Matsuzaki H, Katase N, Matsumura T, Hara M, Yanagi Y, Nagatsuka H, et al. Solid-type primary intraosseous squamous cell carcinoma of the mandible: a case report with histopathological and imaging features. Oral Surg Oral Med Oral Pathol Oral Radiol. 2012;114:e71–7.
17. Head KW, Cullen JM, Dubielzig RR, et al. Histological classification of tumors of the alimentary system of domestic animals. Washington: AFIP and CL Davis DVM foundation and WHO collaborating Center for Worldwide Reference on comparative Oncology; 2003.
18. Johnson N, Franceschi S, Ferlay J, Ramadas K, Schmid S, MacDonald DG, et al. Squamous cell carcinoma. In: Barnes L, Evson JW, Reichart P, Sidransky D, editors. World Health Organization classification of tumors. Pathology and genetics of head and neck tumors. Lyon: IARC Press; 2005. p. 168–75.
19. Huang JW, Luo HY, Li Q, Li TJ. Primary intraosseous squamous cell carcinoma of the jaws. Clinicopathologic presentation and prognostic factors. Arch Pathol Lab Med. 2009;133:1834–40.
20. Wenguang X, Hao S, Xiaofeng Q, Zhiyong W, Yufeng W, Qingang H, et al. Prognostic factors of primary intraosseous squamous cell carcinoma (PIOSCC): a retrospective review. PLoS One. 2016;11:e0153646.

21. Painter JT, Clayton NP, Herbert RA. Useful immunohistochemical markers of tumor differentiation. Toxicol Pathol. 2010;38:131–41.
22. Quigley PJ, Leedale A, Dawson IM. Carcinoma of mandible of cat and dog simulating osteosarcoma. J Comp Pathol. 1972;82:15–8.
23. Takagi S, Mori T, Watanabe K, Kadosawa Tm Ochiai K, Trigoe S, et al. Mandibular squamous cell carcinoma with reactive bone proliferation in two cats. Jpn J Vet Anesth & Surg. 2004;35:89–94.

10

Pulmonary carcinoma with metastasis in a long-finned pilot whale (*Globicephala melas*)

Cristian M. Suárez-Santana*, Carolina Fernández-Maldonado, Josué Díaz-Delgado, Manuel Arbelo, Alejandro Suárez-Bonnet, Antonio Espinosa de los Monteros, Nakita Câmara, Eva Sierra and Antonio Fernández

Abstract

Background: Lung cancer is the most commonly diagnosed neoplasm in humans, however this does not apply to other animal species. Living in an aquatic environment the respiratory system of cetaceans had to undergo unique adaptations in order to them to survive and cope with totally different respiratory pathogens and potentially carcinogens from those affecting humans.

Case presentation: This article discusses not only macroscopical, histopathological and immunohistochemical features of a pulmonary carcinoma with disseminated metastases in a long-finned pilot whale (*Globicephala melas*), as well as the immunohistochemical analysis performed on various tissues of cetaceans belonging to the genus *Globicephala*. On the necropsy examination of the carcass, multiple pulmonary nodules and generalised thoracic lymphadenomegaly were noted. Histologically, a malignant epithelial neoplasia was identified in the lung, thoracic lymph nodes, and adrenal gland. Immunohistochemical analysis revealed a pulmonary carcinoma. Vasculogenic mimicry and epithelial-to-mesenchymal transition phenotype, as suggested by cytomorphological and immunohistochemical characteristics, were observed.

Conclusions: A diagnosis of metastatic pulmonary carcinoma was determined, which to the author's knowledge, appears to be not previously recorded in long-finned pilot whale species. This is also the first report of vasculogenic mimicry and epithelial-to-mesenchymal transition event in a spontaneous cancer from a cetacean species.

Keywords: Pulmonary carcinoma, Pilot whale, Cetacean, Neoplasia, Tumour, Vasculogenic mimicry, Epithelial-to-mesenchymal transition

Background

In order to survive in an aquatic environment, the respiratory system of cetaceans has undergone a complex series of morphologic adaptive changes. Some of those include pulmonary resilience and collapse during diving, presence of myoelastic sphincters, cartilaginous reinforcement of the terminal bronchi and lacking of type III brush cells, among others [1]. These adaptive capabilities may be disrupted by different pulmonary disease processes. Inflammatory conditions are one of the most prevalent disturbances affecting the lungs of free-ranging and captive cetaceans [2–4]. Other conditions, such as neoplasia, are rarely documented in this species. The only two reported cases of primary pulmonary carcinomas are one in an Amazon River dolphin (*Inia geoffrensis*)

[5] and another one on a bottlenose dolphin (*Tursiops truncatus*) [6]. In humans, lung cancer is the most frequently diagnosed malignancy worldwide, encompassing mainly carcinomas (90–95 % of cases) [7]. Whilst in domestic animals, carcinoma is the most commonly reported primary pulmonary neoplasm, with two major groups: adenocarcinomas (ACA) and bronchioloalveolar carcinomas [8].

Case presentation

This report describes gross, histopathological and immunohistochemical features of a pulmonary carcinoma with disseminated metastases in a long-finned pilot whale (LFPW) (*Globicephala melas*).

A 404 cm-long, adult, female LFPW stranded in Algeciras (36°05′49.5″N-5°26′33.0″W; Spain). The Stranding Network of Andalucía (Junta de Andalucía) assisted the animal but it died shortly after. A complete necropsy was performed supported by the public regional organism (Junta de

* Correspondence: cristian.ss104@gmail.com
Division of Histology and Animal Pathology, Institute for Animal Health and Food Security, Veterinary School, University of Las Palmas de Gran Canaria, C/ Transmontana, 35413 Canary Islands, Spain

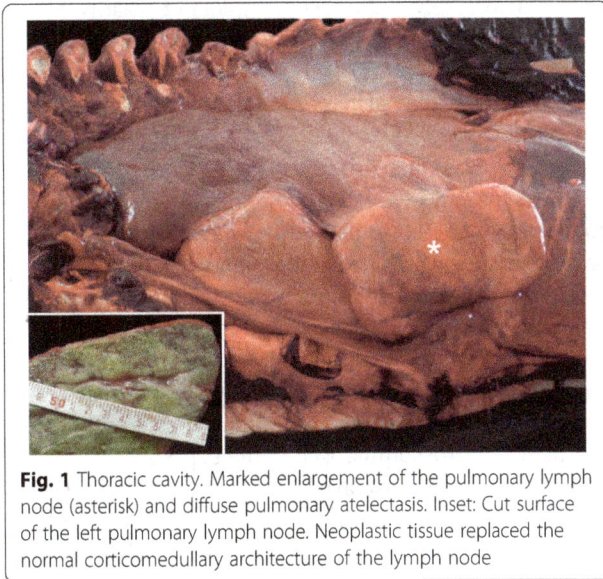

Fig. 1 Thoracic cavity. Marked enlargement of the pulmonary lymph node (asterisk) and diffuse pulmonary atelectasis. Inset: Cut surface of the left pulmonary lymph node. Neoplastic tissue replaced the normal corticomedullary architecture of the lymph node

For histopathological analysis, samples from skin, skeletal muscle, brain, hypophysis, thyroid gland, lungs, trachea, heart, prescapular, mediastinal and lung-associated lymph nodes, spleen, tongue, esophagus, liver, stomach, small and large intestine, pancreas, adrenal gland, uterus, ovary and mammary gland were collected and fixed in 10 % neutral buffered formalin. These samples where submitted to the Division of Histology and Animal Pathology of the Institute for Animal Health and Food Security (IUSA) in the Canary Island for processing and histopathological diagnosis. They were embedded in paraffin wax, sectioned at 5 μm and stained with haematoxylin and eosin. For immunohistochemistry, 4 μm sections of lung and LALN were obtained and immunolabeled with pancytokeratin, cytokeratins 5,7,8,18 and 20 and vimentin primary antibodies and visualized using the Dako EnVision™ system (Dako, Denmark). The immunohistochemical methodology is summarised in Table 1. Canine skin and mammary tissue were used as positive control for cytokeratin panel, whereas *Globicephala* sp. arteriolar smooth muscle was used as positive control for vimentin. Additionally, different *Globicephala* sp. tissues (*Globicephala melas* and *Globicephala macrorhynchus*) were tested for these antibodies (Table 2).

Histologically, the pulmonary parenchyma, mediastinal and LALN, and most of the right adrenal cortex were infiltrated and replaced by a multifocally coalescing, poorly demarcated, non-encapsulated, and highly infiltrative epithelial neoplasm. This displayed a complex structure with several histologic patterns encompassing adenocarcinomatous, bronchioloalveolar and adenosquamous differentiation, with areas of solid growth (Fig. 2). The tumour was characterized by epithelial cells arranged in disorganized acini, tubules and variably dilated, intercommunicating glands, resting on a thin collagenous basement membrane, and supported by thick bundles of desmoplastic (schirrous) stroma (Fig. 2). Neoplastic epithelium was monolayered ranging from flattened, cuboidal, columnar to pseudostratified (resembling bronchial epithelium) and occasionally

Andalucía). The animal was in poor body condition. Externally, multiple, parallel cutaneous lacerations (intra/interspecific interactions) and moderate infestation by *Syncyamus* sp. were noticed. Upon dissection of the thoracic cavity, multifocal 1.6 to 4.2 cm, moderately well-defined, pale to white, firm nodules were noted throughout the lung parenchyma, while adjacent alveolar spaces were atelectatic. The mediastinal and lung-associated lymph nodes (LALN) were markedly enlarged, up to 16 × 22.5 × 12 cm (3 kg) (Fig. 1). On section, the cortex and medulla were severely replaced by a multilobulated mass of identical features to the ones found in the lung nodules. Additionally, a focal, locally extensive, lesion of 5.2 × 4.1 cm, with similar characteristic to those described in the lungs was found in the right adrenal gland, expanding the remaining non-affected glandular parenchyma. Additional gross findings included: hydropericardium, right ventricle dilatation, and severe intestinal parasitization by *Bolbosoma* sp.

Table 1 Summary of immunohistochemical methodology

Antibody	Source	Host	Type	Clone	Antigen retrieval	Dilution
Pancytokeratins	Dako[a]	Mouse	Monoclonal	AE1/AE3	10 % pronase[b]	1 in 100
CK 5 + 8	Euro-Diagnostica[c]	Mouse	Monoclonal	RCK-102	10 % pronase	1 in 20
CK 8 + 18	Euro-Diagnostica	Mouse	Monoclonal	NCL-5D3	Citrate buffer[d]	1 in 20
CK7	Dako	Mouse	Monoclonal	OV-TL 12/30	Citrate buffer	1 in 50
CK 20	Dako	Mouse	Monoclonal	Ks 20.8	Citrate buffer	1 in 25
Vimentin	Dako	Mouse	Monoclonal	Vim 3B4	Citrate buffer	1 in 100

CK cytokeratin
[a]Dako, Glostrup, Denmark
[b]10 % pronase, 10 min at room temperature
[c]Euro-Diagnostica, Arnhem, The Netherlands
[d]Citrate buffer, pH 6.0, 20 min at 95

Table 2 Summary of immunohistochemical analysis of various tissues from genus Globicephala

Tissue	Specie	Cytokeratin profile
Epidermis	*G.macr*	CK5+, CK7-, CK8-, CK18-, CK20-
Bronchial/bronchiolar epithelium	*G.m and G.macr*	CK 7-, CK8-, CK18-, CK20+
Gastric epithelium	*G.macr*	CK20-
Duodenal epithelium	*G.macr*	CK20+
Arterioles (smooth muscle)	*G.macr*	Vimentin+
Pulmonary neoplasia	*G.m*	CK5+, CK7-, CK8-, CK18-, CK20+, Vimentin+

CK cytokeratin, G.m Globicephala melas, G.macr Globicephala macrorhynchus

multi-layered, with frequent papillary projections. Tumour cells had small to moderate amounts of eosinophilic, finely vacuolated cytoplasm with variably distinct borders, apical brush borders with cilia and cytoplasmic blebbing. Nuclei were irregularly round, basal to parabasal, with vesicular euchromatin and typically one prominent nucleolus. Aniso-cytosis and anisokaryosis were marked, and mitotic count was seven per ten 400x fields in more mitotically active areas. Karyomegaly, multinucleation, loss of polarity, vascu-logenic mimicry (VM) and single cell necrosis were fre-quent features among tumour cells, while bizarre mitoses were scarce. Tubuloacinar and glandular lumena were filled with sloughed, degenerating and necrotic tumour cells, neutrophils, karyorhectic cellular debris, erythrocytes and proteinaceous fluid. The desmoplastic tumour stroma contained moderate numbers of lymphocytes, macro-phages and few neutrophils, intermingled with areas of ne-crosis and haemorrhage. Vascular invasion was frequent. VM was more frequently observed in the LALN, medias-tinal lymph nodes and adrenal gland metastasis, with approximately 6–10 VM-like figures per 10 high power field (40x). Histological and immunohistochemical charac-teristic of VM are summarized in the Fig. 3a-d.

Neoplastic cells displayed moderate intracytoplasmic and membranous immunolabeling for AE1/AE3 and CK 5 in approximately 90 % of neoplastic cells, whereas CK20 displayed weaker immunopositivity in about 60 % of the tumour cells. Vimentin immunolabeling was variable, showing intracytoplasmic, frequently yuxtanuc-lear, mild-to-moderate positivity in about 15 to 30 % of cancerous cells in the more labelled areas. Results of the

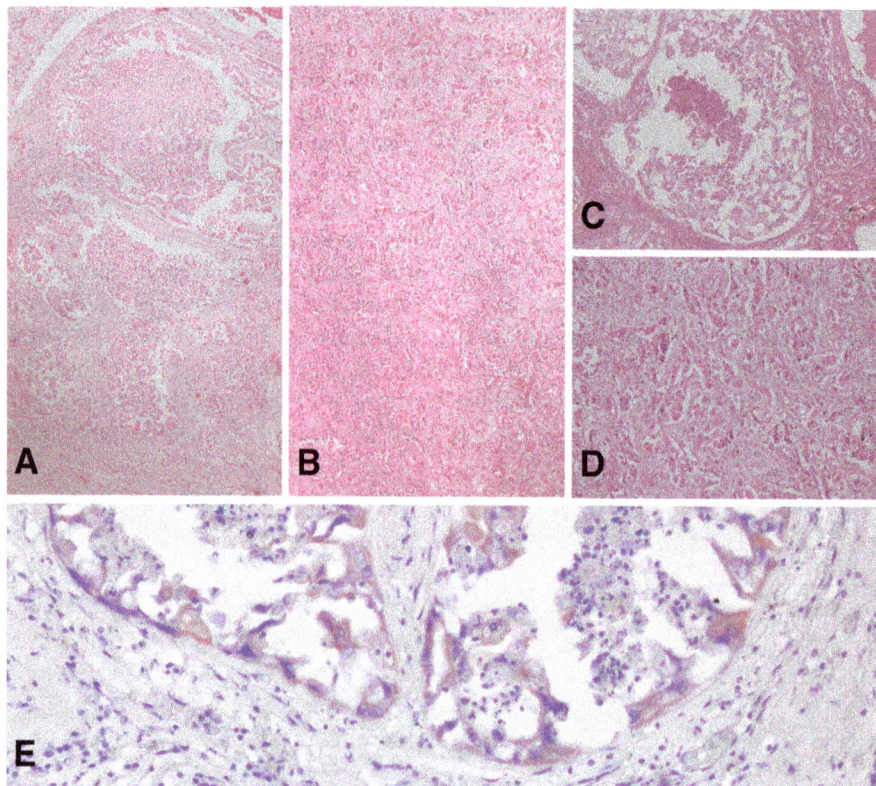

Fig. 2 Histological and immunohistochemical characteristics of the neoplasia. Images A to D represent examples of the complex structure of the tumour: **a** bronchioloalveolar pattern (H&E, 4x); **b** adenocarcinomatous pattern (H&E, 4x). **c** Higher magnification of image A (H&E, 20x). **d** Higher magnification of image B (H&E, 20x). **e** About 90 % of neoplastic epithelial cells displayed mild, cytoplasmic and membranous labelling for cytokeratin 5 (CK 5 + 8 IHC, 40x)

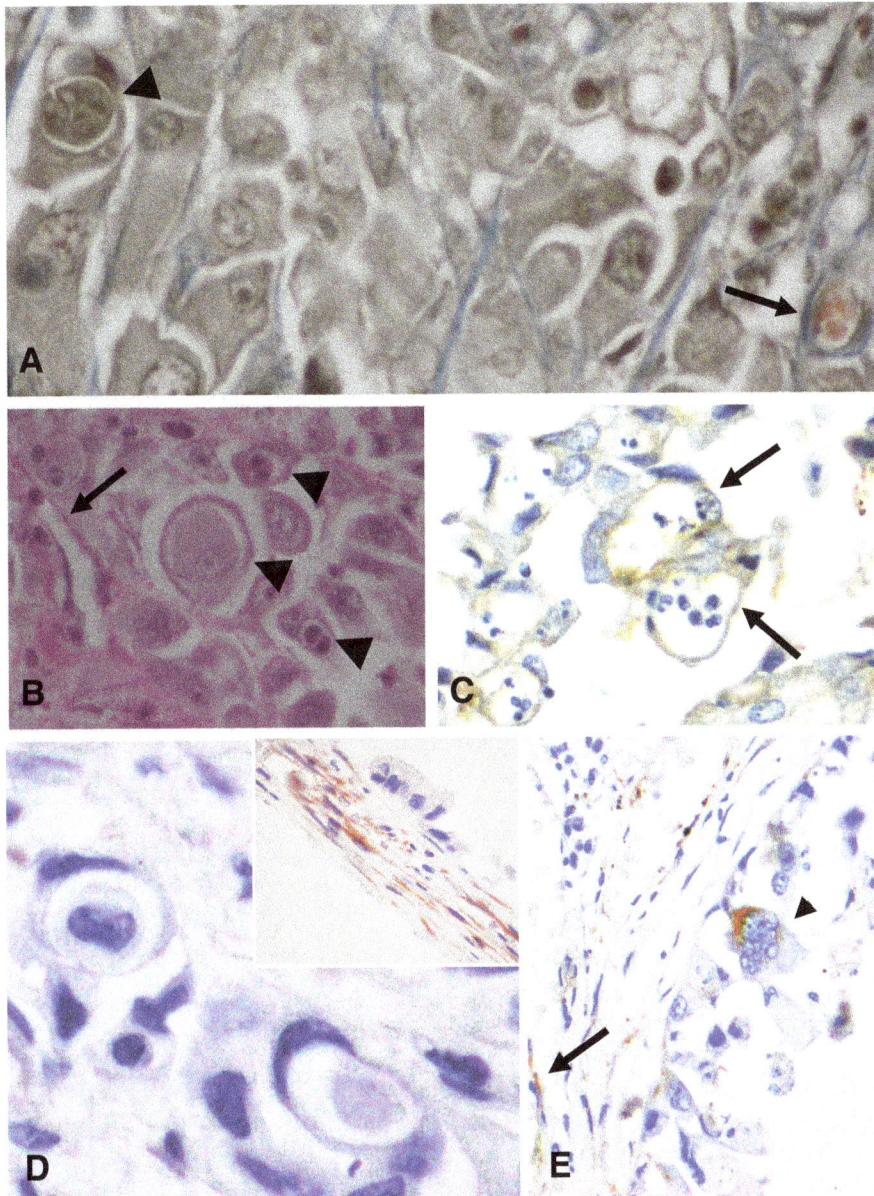

Fig. 3 Histochemical and immunohistochemical (IHC) characteristics of vasculogenic mimicry (VM) and Epithelial-to-mesenchymal transition (EMT). **a** Masson's Trichrome stain reveals a thin layer of stroma sustaining intratumoral capillaries (arrow), whereas VM-figures lack this support (Masson's Trichrome, 60x). **b** The same can be visualized with the Periodic Acid-Schiff (PAS) stain, in which the basal membrane of the vessels stains PAS positive (arrow), but do not in VM-figures (PAS staining, 60x). **c** Intracytoplasmic labelling for pancytokeratin in cells forming VM, confirming their epithelial origin (AE1/AE3 IHC, 40x). **d** Intratumoral vascular endothelium consistently express vimentin (inset), whereas VM-figures do not (Vimentin IHC, 60x). **e** A multinucleated neoplastic epithelial cell displayed intracytoplasmic immunolabelling for vimentin (arrow head), feature typical of EMT. Note the staining of the vascular endothelium (arrow) functioning as internal positive control. (Vimentin IHC, 40x)

immunohistochemical study of non-neoplastic tissues from genus *Globicephala* are depicted in Table 2. Both neoplastic cells and normal bronchial and bronchiolar epithelial cells expressed CK20, while appearing negative for CK7, CK8 and CK18 (Table 2).

Attending to gross, histological and immunohistochemical findings a primary pulmonary neoplasia with widespread metastasis was determined. Primary pulmonary

epithelial neoplasia has been rarely identified in cetaceans with only two descriptions of squamous cell carcinoma (SCC) in an Amazon River dolphin (*Inia geoffrensis*) [5] and in a bottlenose dolphin (*Tursiops truncatus*) [6]. Other primary pulmonary neoplasms reported in those species include: haemangioma in bottlenose dolphin [9], common dolphin (*Delphinus delphis*) [10] and beluga whales (*Delphinapterus leucas*) [11]; fibroma in a blue whale (*Balaenoptera musculus*) and in a fin whale (*Balaenoptera physalus*) [12]; and a chondroma and lipoma in a beluga whale [13].

In veterinary medicine, adenocarcinoma is the most prevalent malignant lung tumour in dogs, cats and cattle [8]. Bronchioloalveolar carcinoma is the most prominent pattern found in sheep induced by Jaagsiekte sheep retrovirus. Whereas granular cell tumour is the most common primary lung neoplasm in horses. In humans, ACA and SCC, especially in smokers, are the most frequent lung cancers, with relatively frequent metastasis to the adrenal gland [7]. Up to 10 % of human pulmonary carcinomas display mixtures of histologic patterns (adenocarcinomatous, bronchioloalveolar and/or adenosquamous) [7], as in our case. Associated premalignant changes in humans include epithelial hyperplasia, squamous metaplasia and dysplasia which may lead to carcinoma in situ and invasive carcinoma [7]. Squamous metaplasia of the bronchial and bronchiolar epithelium has been observed in lungworm infestation in bottlenose dolphins [14] and has been speculated to be involved in neoplastic transformation in cetaceans [6]. In the present case, lungworm infestation was not grossly nor histologically apparent; however, cannot entirely be ruled out, as they may not be identifiable with chronicity or resolution [14].

Epithelial tumour cells occasionally switch from an epithelial phenotype to a mesenchymal phenotype, a phenomenon defined as epithelial-to-mesenchymal transition (EMT). In EMT, dedifferentiation with loss of epithelial characteristics and polarity occurs, frequently accompanied by vimentin expression, and acquisition of a motile mesenchymal phenotype with increased migratory behaviour and metastatic capability [15]. This phenomenon has been more widely investigated in humans than in veterinary species, and is generally associated with a poor prognosis and chemoresistence [16, 17]. Furthermore, it has not been previously reported in marine mammal neoplasia. VM is a relatively new discovered mechanism in cancer biology that consists in the formation of channels lined by neoplastic cells, adopting a pseudo-vascular disposition in order to canalize nutrients and oxygen. This contribute for tumour growth and metastasis, as cells can use these channels to colonize new locations [18]. VM can imitate blood vessels (with erythrocytes within) or more frequently lymphatic vessels (transporting white blood cells, plasma and other neoplastic cells) [18]. This feature has been noted in highly aggressive human tumours such as melanoma, inflammatory breast cancer and large cell pulmonary carcinoma [18, 19], but in animals it has only been reported in spontaneous canine mammary carcinomas [20]. In the present case, the histological and immunohistochemical characteristics of the tumour cells support VM and EMT events [15, 18], and represent the first description of these features in marine mammals' neoplastic diseases.

Conclusions

In conclusion, we describe a naturally occurring, highly aggressive, primary pulmonary carcinoma with adenocarcinomatous, bronchioloalveolar and adenosquamous differentiation, EMT and VM phenomena, and multiple metastases. It also represents the first primary pulmonary carcinoma described in LFPW, and contributes to expand the body of knowledge on pulmonary carcinomas biology in non-human species.

Abbreviations

ACA: Adenocarcinoma; CK: Cytokeratin; EMT: Epithelial-to-mesenchymal transition; LALN: Lung-associated lymph node; LFPW: Long-finned pilot whale; SCC: Squamous cell carcinoma; VM: Vasculogenic mimicry

Acknowledgements

We want to thank all the people who indirectly participated in the elaboration of this work, therefore a very special thanks particularly to La Junta de Andalucía, our laboratory staff, and to all volunteers who collaborated in the necropsy.

Funding

This study is part of a PhD program supported by the Universidad de Las Palmas de Gran Canaria (ULPGC) through a student formation predoctoral grant (Contrato Predoctoral Convocatoria del 2012 programa propio de la ULPG, BOULPGC Año VI num. 6).

Author' contributions

CMS-S: This author wrote the article, and contributed to the gross, histological, and immunohistological diagnosis of the case. CF-M: This author performed the necropsy of the animal. JD-D: This author contributed towards the histological descriptions and diagnosis and helped writing the article. MA: This author contributed to the gross and histological diagnosis of the case. AS-B: This author contributed towards the histological diagnosis and immunohistochemical analysis of the case and helped writing the article. AEM: This author contributed towards the histological diagnosis of the case. NC: This author contributed towards the immunohistochemical analysis of the case and helped writing the article. ES: This author contributed towards the histological diagnosis of the case and performed supplementary diagnostic tests (data not shown). AF: This author contributed towards the gross and histological diagnosis of the case guided the first author during the drafting and publication process. All authors read and approved the final manuscript.

Competing interests

The authors declare that they have no competing interests.

Consent for publications

Not applicable.

References

1. Piscitelli MA, Raverty SA, Lillie MA, Shadwick RE. A review of cetacean lung morphology and mechanics. J Morphol. 2013;274:1425–40.
2. Arbelo M, De Los Monteros AE, Herraez P, Andrada M, Sierra E, Rodriguez F, Jepson P, Fernandez A. Pathology and causes of death of stranded cetaceans in the Canary Islands (1999–2005). Dis Aquat Organ. 2013;103:87–99.
3. Venn-Watson S, Daniels R, Smith C. Thirty year retrospective evaluation of pneumonia in a bottlenose dolphin Tursiops truncatus population. Dis Aquat Organ. 2012;99:237–42.

4. Jepson PD, Baker JR, Kuiken T, Simpson VR, Kennedy S, Bennett PM. Pulmonary pathology of harbour porpoises (Phocoena phocoena) stranded in England and Wales between 1990 and 1996. Vet Rec. 2000;146:721–8.

5. Geraci JR, Palmer JP, Aubin DJ. Tumors in cetaceans: analysis and new findings. Can J Fish Aquat Sci. 1897;44:1289–300.

6. Ewing RY, Mignucci-Giannoni AA. A poorly differentiated pulmonary squamous cell carcinoma in a free-ranging Atlantic bottlenose dolphin (Tursiops truncatus). J Vet Diagn Invest. 2003;15:162–5.

7. Husain AN. The lung. In: Kumar V, Abbas AK, Aster JC, editors. Robbins and cotran pathologic basis of disease. Philadelphia: Elsevier Saunders; 2015. p. 669–726.

8. Caswell LJ, Williams KJ. Respiratory system. In: Grant MM, editor. Jubb, kennedy & palmer's pathology of domestic animals. 5th ed. Edinburgh: Elsevier; 2007. p. 523–74.

9. Turnbull BS, Cowan DF. Angiomatosis, a newly recognized disease in Atlantic bottlenose dolphins (Tursiops truncatus) from the Gulf of Mexico. Vet Pathol. 1999;36:28–34.

10. Diaz-Delgado J, Arbelo M, Sacchini S, Quesada-Canales O, Andrada M, Rivero M, Fernandez A. Pulmonary angiomatosis and hemangioma in common dolphins (Delphinus delphis) stranded in Canary Islands. J Vet Med Sci. 2007;74:1063–6.

11. Lair S, Martineau D, Measures LN. Causes of mortality in St. Lawrence Estuary beluga (Delphinapterus leuca) from 1983 to 2012. DFO Can Sci Advis Sec Res Doc. 2014. http://www.dfo-mpo.gc.ca/csas-sccs/publications/resdocs-docrech/2013/2013_119-eng.pdf.

12. Mawdesley-Thomas LE. Some aspects of neoplasia in marine mammals. In: Russel FS, Yonge B, editors. Advances in marine biology. New York: Academic; 1971. p. 151–231.

13. De Guise S, Lagacé A, Béland P. Tumors in St. Lawrence beluga whales (Delphinapterus leucas). Vet Pathol. 1994;31(4):444–9.

14. Fauquier DA, Kinsel MJ, Dailey MD, Sutton GE, Stolen MK, Wells RS, Gulland FM. Prevalence and pathology of lungworm infection in bottlenose dolphins Tursiops truncatus from southwest Florida. Dis Aquat Organ. 2009;88:85–90.

15. Sureban SM, May R, Lightfoot SA S, Hoskins AB, Lerner M, Brackett DJ, Postier RG, Ramanujam R, Mohammed A, Rao CV, Wyche JH, Anant S, Houchen CW. DCAMKL-1 regulates epithelial-mesenchymal transition in human pancreatic cells through a miR-200a-dependent mechanism. Cancer Res. 2011;71:2328–38.

16. Li M, Luan F, Zhao Y, Hao H, Yu Z, Han W, Fu X. Epithelial-mesenchymal transition: an emerging target in tissue fibrosis. Exp Biol Med. 2015;241(1):1–13.

17. Fonseca-Alves CE, Kobayashi PE, Rivera-Calderon LG, Laufer-Amorim R. Evidence of epithelial-mesenchymal transition in canine prostate cancer metastasis. Res Vet Sci. 2015;100:176–81.

18. Folberg R, Maniotis AJ. Vasculogenic mimicry. APMIS. 2004;112:508–25.

19. Li Y, Sun B, Zhao X, Zhang D, Wang X, Zhu D, Yang Z, Qiu Z, Ban X. Subpopulations of uPAR+ contribute to vasculogenic mimicry and metastasis in large cell lung cancer. Exp Mol Pathol. 2015;98:136–44.

20. Clemente M, Perez-Alenza MD, Illera JC, Pena L. Histological, immunohistological, and ultrastructural description of vasculogenic mimicry in canine mammary cancer. Vet Pathol. 2010;47:265–74.

11

Extracellular matrix remodeling in equine sarcoid: an immunohistochemical and molecular study

Manuela Martano[1*], Annunziata Corteggio[2], Brunella Restucci[1], Maria Ester De Biase[1], Giuseppe Borzacchiello[1] and Paola Maiolino[1]

Abstract

Background: Equine sarcoids are locally invasive, fibroblastic benign skin tumors. Bovine papillomavirus type-1 (BPV-1) and/or Bovine papillomavirus type-2 (BPV-2) are believed to be the causative agent of sarcoids, although the mechanisms by which the virus induce the tumor are still poorly understood. We hypothesized that in genetically predisposed equines latent BPV infection may be reactivated by immunosoppression and/or mechanical injury leading to a form of pathologic wound which may transform into a sarcoid. In this study, we investigated in 25 equine sarcoids and in five normal skin samples the histological features and evaluated the immunohistochemical and molecular expression of type I and type III Collagen, vimentin (VIM), alfa Smooth Muscle Actin (α-SMA), Matrix Metalloproteinase (MMPs) -2, 9, 14 and tissue inhibitor of metalloproteinase 2 (TIMP-2).

Results: In 64 % of investigated sarcoids, type I collagen staining was stronger than that of type III collagen. In 80 % of sarcoids, SFs were strongly positive for vimentin and negative for α-SMA; the remaining sarcoid samples (20 %) showed 70–80 % of SFs labeled for vim and approximately 20–30 % labeled for α-SMA. Moreover, all sarcoid specimen showed a variable staining pattern (weak to moderate) for MMP-9 and MMP-14, and a moderate to strong staining for MMP-2 and TIMP-2. Biochemical analysis confirmed immunohistochemical results and showed in sarcoids, for the first time, the cleaved form of MMP9, the 35 KDa active species for MMP-9.

Conclusions: This study revealed that in equine sarcoids exhibit an altered turnover of the Extracellular Matrix (ECM) deposition and degradation, as result of an altered expression of MMPs and TIMPs. Therefore, these observations seem to confirm that the basic mechanism for growth of equine sarcoids could be a neoplastic transformation during wound healing.

Keywords: BPV, ECM, Equine sarcoid, MMPs

Background

Equine sarcoids are locally invasive, fibroblastic benign skin tumors and represent the most common skin tumor in equidae worldwide [1, 2]. They can occur as single lesion, or, more commonly, as multiple lesions, frequently at sites of previous injury and scarring; although they can develop anywhere on the integument sites of predilection are in particular the paragenital region, the thorax–abdomen and the head [3, 4]. Equine sarcoids

rarely regress, are notoriously difficult to treat and are associated with a high recurrence rate following surgical intervention [5–7]; these features are likely due to the invasiveness of sarcoid fibroblasts (SFs) [8, 9]. BPV-1 and less commonly BPV-2 are widely recognized as the causative agents of the disease. Although the viral etiology, the biology, the morphology and the epidemiology of equine sarcoids are known [4, 10, 11], the pathogenic events leading to the development of tumour and the mechanisms used by BPV to induce the tumour are less understood. Sarcoid formation is known as one of the main long-term complications in the wound healing of horses [12, 13]. We hypothesized that in healthy

* Correspondence: manuela.martano@unina.it
[1]Department of Veterinary Medicine and Animal Productions, Naples University "Federico II", Via F. Delpino 1, 80137 Naples, Italy

genetically predisposed horses, BPV-1/BPV2 may be responsible for abnormal fibroblast proliferation on one hand, and on the other for alterations in dynamics of the extracellular matrix (ECM) and its main components (e.g. collagen). These changes could induce an alteration of the wound healing process and may therefore be an important factor in the pathogenesis of equine sarcoids. The hypothesis that cancer may be "a wound that won't heal" has been supported by numerous studies [14–16] suggesting that wound healing and tumorigenesis share consistently similarities in terms of histological features and signaling molecules; those are among others Matrix Metalloproteinases (MMPs), a family of at least 25 zinc-dependent endopeptidases, and their inhibitors (TIMPs) all essentially capable of degrading Extracellular Matrix (ECM), including collagen. Besides participating in normal connective tissue homeostasis and remodeling, MMPs activity is involved in remodeling of ECM and the migration of numerous cell types during various pathological conditions, such as wound healing, keloid formation, chronic inflammatory diseases, and as well as in tumour invasion [17–19]. In this study, we speculate that changes of the expression levels and of the enzymatic activity of MMP-2, MMP-9, MMP-14 (MMP1-MMT) and TIMP-2 may play an important role in the pathogenesis of sarcoids, being responsible for ECM turnover. Of the growing family of MMPs, MMP-2 (gelatinase A, 72-kDa type IV collagenase,) and MMP-9 (gelatinase B, 92-kDa type IV collagenase) are unique for their fibronectin-like collagen binding domains and are responsible of degradation of type IV collagen in the basement membranes and in fibrillar collagens, which are essential features of tissue repair and remodeling processes. Their activity is controlled by a group of protein inhibitors, the TIMPs. MMP-14 is a trans-membrane protease, capable of degrading different ECM components such as collagen types I, II, and III, as well as fibronectin and laminin [20]. The main interest in this enzyme is due to its ability to activate different proteases, particularly MMP-2 and MMP-9 [21]. Recently, Yuan et al. (2010) [8] have shown that BPV-1 induce overexpression of MMPs contributing to invasiveness of SFs in vitro. Our in vivo study aimed at gaining new insights into the pathogenetic mechanisms of equine sarcoids, by employing immunohistochemistry and western blot analysis to investigate their histological features, as well as the expression of type I and type III collagen, MMP-2, MMMP-9, MMP-14 and their inhibitors, such as TIMP-2. Moreover, the enzymatic activities of MMP-2 and MMP-9 were quantified by gelatin-zymography of the same homogenized tumour tissues.

Results

Histological features

Examined sarcoids showed the typical histological changes in their epidermal (when present) and dermal component such as hyperkeratosis and epidermal hyperplasia often accompanied by rete pegs extending deep into the proliferating dermal connective tissue. Dermal proliferation consisted of tightly whirling plump spindle cells, proliferating in an ECM which appeared more developed than normal. The superficial dermal fibroblasts were usually oriented perpendicular to the basilar epidermal layer in a 'picket fence' pattern (Fig.1a). Ulceration as well as inflammation (infiltration of polymorphonuclear cells) were commonly seen. Van Gieson's stain of sarcoids confirmed an increase in the amount of deep red color collagen fibers in the dermis, identified as mature collagen (Type I), compared with pink color collagen fibers, identified as immature collagen (Type III) (Fig.1b), as compared to normal skin.

Immunohistochemistry

The expression patterns of Vimentin (VIM), alpha-Smooth Muscle Actin (α-SMA), type I Collagen, type III Collagen, MMP-2, MMP-9, MMP-14, and TIMP-2 in 25 equine sarcoids and five normal skin samples are summarized in Table 1.

Normal skin

All normal skin samples showed positive immunostaing for type I and III Collagen, which was light brown stained with a widely distributed staining pattern within the dermal layer. Moreover, a weak and finely granular cytoplasmic MMP-2 and MMP-9 reactivity was observed in the epidermis. TIMP-2 and MMP-14 immunoexpression was present in the epidermis but also in vascular endothelial cells, inflammatory cells and fibroblastic cells.

Sarcoid samples

Type I and Type III collagen appeared as fine discontinuous individual fibers in a loose network, and showed a moderate immunosignal in 36 % of sarcoid samples (Fig. 2: a-b). Type I Collagen staining was stronger than type III collagen in the remaining samples (64 %). In 80 % of sarcoids, SFs were strongly positive for vimentin and negative for α-SMA; in the remaining samples (20 %), 70–80 % of SFs were labeled for vimentin (Fig. 3a) and approximately 20–30 % were strongly labeled for α-SMA (Fig. 3b). Furthermore, sarcoid specimens showed a variable (64 % moderate; 36 % strong) and finely granular staining pattern for MMP-2 in 30–50 % of SFs, as well as in the cytoplasm of epidermal cells (Fig. 4a). Sarcoids featured a weak (52 %) to moderate (48 %) staining for MMP-9, which appeared highly and finely granular in the cytoplasm of epidermal cells and rarely (often lacking) in the rete peg epithelium. A moderate to strong cytoplasmic staining for MMP-9 was observed in 30–70 % of SFs, inflammatory cells and vascular endothelial cells (Fig. 5a). TIMP-2 showed

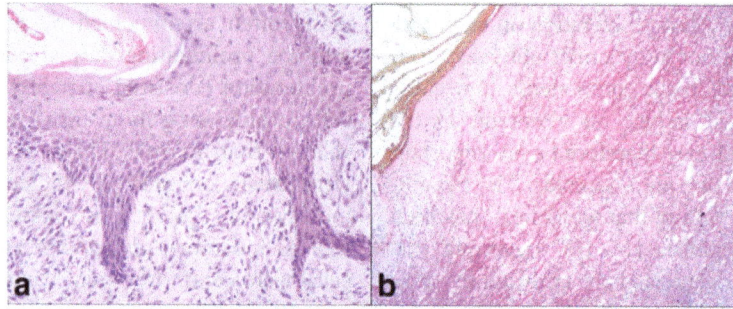

Fig. 1 a Equine sarcoid. Epidermal hyperplasia, rete peg and picket fence formation. Hematoxylin-eosin. 20X. **b** Equine sarcoid. Red color collagen fibers (collagen I) in equine sarcoid. Van Gieson Stain. 10X

Table 1 Immunoreactivity scoring of VIM, α-sma, Type I collagen, Type III collagen, MMP-2, MMP-9, MMP14, TIMP-2 in 25 equine sarcoids and 5 normal skin

Samples[a]	Location	VIM[b]	A-SMA[b]	Type I collagen[b]	Type III collagen[b]	MMP-2[b]	MMP-9[b]	MMP14[b]	TIMP-2[b]
T1	Abdomen	++	-	+	+	+	+	+/−	++
T2	Limbs	++	-	+	+	++	+	+/−	++
T3	Neck	++	-	+	+	+	+	+/−	++
T4	Abdomen	++	-	+	+	+	+/−	+/−	++
T5	Paragenit region	++	-	+	+	++	+	+	++
T6	Pectoral region	++	-	+	+	+	+/−	+	++
T7	Paragenit region	++	-	+	+	+	+/−	+	++
T8	Neck	++	-	+	+	++	+	+	++
T9	Neck	++	-	+	+	+	+/−	+/−	++
T10	Pectoral region	++	-	++	+	+	+	+/−	++
T11	Paragenit region	++	-	++	+	++	+	+/−	++
T12	Limbs	++	-	++	+	++	+	+/−	++
T13	Neck	++	-	++	+	+	+/−	+	++
T14	Abdomen	++	-	++	+	+	+/−	+	++
T15	Limbs	++	-	++	+	++	+	+/−	++
T16	Pectoral region	++	-	++	+	+	+/−	+/−	++
T17	Pectoral region	++	-	++	+	+	+/−	+/−	++
T18	Limbs	++	-	++	+	++	+	+	++
T19	Abdomen	++	-	++	+	+	+/−	+	+
T20	Pectoral region	++	-	++	+	+	+/−	+/−	+
T21	Limbs	++	++	++	+	++	+	+/−	+
T22	Neck	++	++	++	+	++	+	+/−	+
T23	Abdomen	++	++	++	+	+	+/−	+	+
T24	Paragenit region	++	++	++	+	+	+/−	+	+
T25	Pectoral region	++	++	++	+	+	+/−	+	+
N1	Limbs	n.a.	n.a.	+/−	+/−	+	+/−	-	-
N2	Abdomen	n.a.	n.a.	+/−	+/−	+	+/−	+/−	+/−
N3	Pectoral region	n.a.	n.a.	+/−	+/−	+	+/−	-	+/−
N4	Neck	n.a.	n.a.	+/−	+/−	+	+/−	+/−	-
N5	Limbs	n.a.	n.a.	+/−	+/−	+	+/−	+/−	+/−

[a]*T* tumour sample, *N* normal skin sample, [b]- negative staining; +/− weak immunolabelling; + moderate immunolabelling; ++ extensive and strong immunolabelling; *n.a.* not assessed

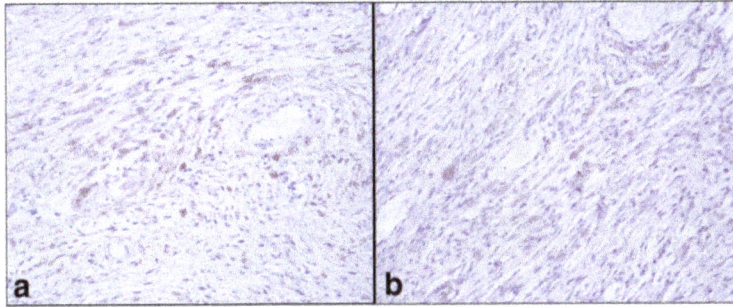

Fig. 2 a Type I Collagen and **b** Type III collagen immunostaining in equine sarcoids. Streptavidin-biotin-peroxidase stain 20X

extensive and strong cytoplasmic positivity in epidermal cells and in 50–70 % of SFs in almost every sample (72 %) (Fig. 6a). In all tumors, MMP-14 expression was observed in epidermis and in 50–70 % of SFs, with variable (56 % weak; 44 % moderate) cytoplasmic immunolabelling (Fig. 7a).

Biochemical analysis

To further confirm our findings, six sarcoid samples, which were available for biochemical analysis and two skin samples from healthy horses were subjected to western blot analysis. Hela cell line was also analyzed as positive control for the antibodies used (data not shown). The anti-Collagen I and anti-Collagen III antibodies yielded a band of the expected molecular weight in the neoplastic tissues and normal skin. An increase in the amount of both collagen type protein levels in all tumour samples compared with normal skin was observed, albeit in different amounts among the samples (Fig. 8). The analysis of MMP-2 showed that 50 % of sarcoid samples (T3, T4 and T5) had a high level of protein, above all in its active (cleaved) form (62 kDa). In addition, an increase in the expression level of MMP9 in all tumour samples versus healthy skin samples was observed. The sarcoids showed the overexpression of the cleaved form of MMP9, the 35 KDa active species which was an autocatalytic product of the 82KDa pre-form.

We analyzed the expression of MMP-14 and TIMP-2, in order to evaluate their involvement in MMP2 activity. There was no significant up-regulation of MMP14 protein in the sarcoids compared to normal skin samples, even if in one sarcoid sample (T1) it was present at a very high level. TIMP2 was overexpressed in sarcoids when compared to normal skin. Actin was shown as control for ensuring the equal loading of protein extracts (Fig. 9). Finally, we examined gelatinase MMP's activity in sarcoid tumors using zymography, which has been extensively used to detect both latent and active form of MMPs. Gelatine zymography was employed to specifically detect MMP-2 and MMP-9 protease activity. As shown in Fig. 10, all the examined sarcoids expressed the pro- and active form of MMP2. However, sarcoids showed higher expression levels than normal skin samples. In addition, the MMP9 was present in the activated form in all the analyzed sarcoids. Interestingly, four out of six the sarcoid samples (80 %) overexpressed a cleaved form of 35 kDa MMP9, thus demonstrating the strong activity of MMP9 during sarcoids tumorigenesis.

Discussion

Sarcoids are the most common equine skin tumours, characterized by neoplastic fibroblasts intermingled in a collagenous stroma, frequently associated to epidermal hyperplasia [2, 22]. BPV-1/BPV-2 are believed to be the

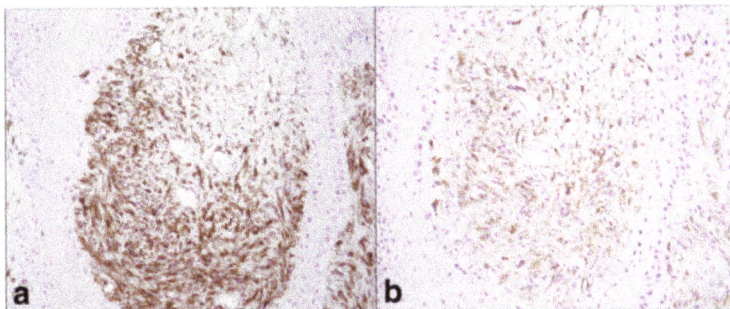

Fig. 3 VIM and Alfa-sma immunostaining in equine sarcoid. **a** 70–80 % of SFs show strong vimentin immunostaining; **b** 20–30 % of SFs show strong Alfa-sma immunostaining. Streptavidin-biotin-peroxidase stain 20X

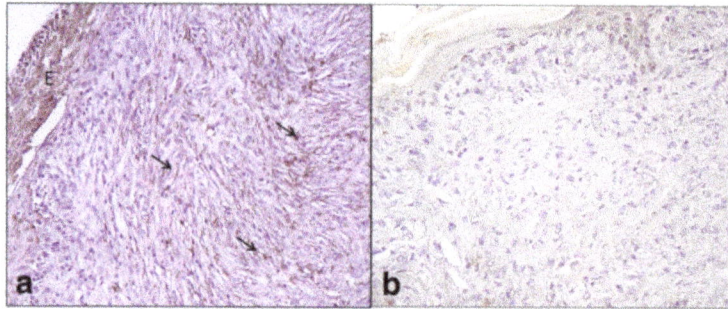

Fig. 4 a MMP-2 immunostaining in equine sarcoid. SFs (*arrows*) show a strong immunostaining, the epidermis (E) is also strongly MMP-2 positive. **b** Secondary-only negative control. Streptavidin-biotin-peroxidase stain. 20X

causative agent of equine sarcoid. This is based on the fact that: 1) BPV-1/-2 DNA is detected in the majority of sarcoid tumors [7, 23–27]; 2) BPV genes are expressed in sarcoids [10, 28–30]; 3) experimental inoculation of equine skin with BPV induces sarcoid-like lesions in horses [31]; 4) BPV- 1 DNA can transform primary equine fibroblasts in vitro [8, 32]. Interestingly, BPV DNA presence has also been reported in normal skin and the virus has been found to be transcriptionally active in some cases of equine inflammatory skin lesions [33, 34]. It is noteworthy that very recently BPV has been found also in exuberant granulation tissue [35]. It is widely accepted that equine sarcoids may develop subsequently to injury and scarring in genetically predisposed equines [24]. For this reason we hypotized that latent BPV infection may be reactivated by chronic physical trauma, leading to development of a form of pathologic wound healing (e.g. keloid); thus, the scar producing process may be altered during the maturation phase of wound healing allowing transformation of scar tissue (keloids) into sarcoids.

In fact, our immunohistochemical results showed that, in most sarcoids (20/25), fibroblasts represented the principal cellular population, the remainder was composed of fibroblasts and myofibroblasts.

Furthermore, in our sample tissues collagen content was elevated and disorganized when compared to normal skin and, in contrast to what Williams et al. reported [36], the ratio of type I (mature collagen) to type III collagen (immature collagen) seemed to be slightly higher, which was as also demonstrated by Van Gieson stain. Also, and in line with the immunohistochemical results, western blotting analysis confirmed that collagen I and III were present in higher amounts in tumour samples when compared to normal skin samples. It is known tissue of normal wound repair contains primarily type III collagen with abundant myofibroblasts. In contrast, abnormal wound repair tissue, (for instance keloid), consists of type I and III bundles with few myofibroblasts [37]. Combining these data strongly suggests that these sarcoid tumours actually originate in abnormal wound repair tissue [38].

We hypothesized that the basic mechanism for the development of equine sarcoids could be an imbalance of ECM deposition and degradation as seen also during pathologic wound healing.

This process is mediated by ECM degrading enzymes, such as MMPs, and we believe that these changes are likely the result of altered expression levels between these enzymes and their inhibitors (TIMPs). The MMPs

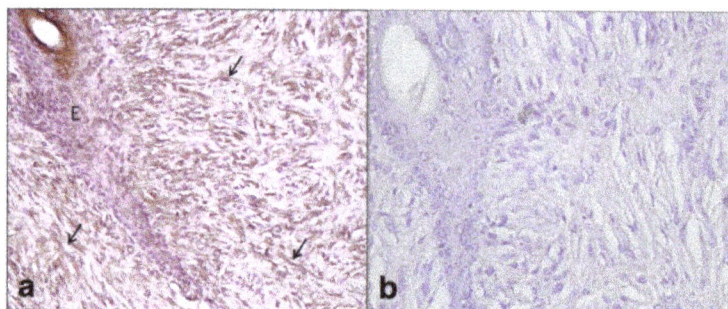

Fig. 5 a MMP-9 immunostaining in equine sarcoid. The epidermis (E) shows strong positivity except for rete peg epithelium, SFs are strongly MMP-9 positive (*arrows*). **b** Secondary-only negative control. Streptavidin-biotin-peroxidase stain. 20X

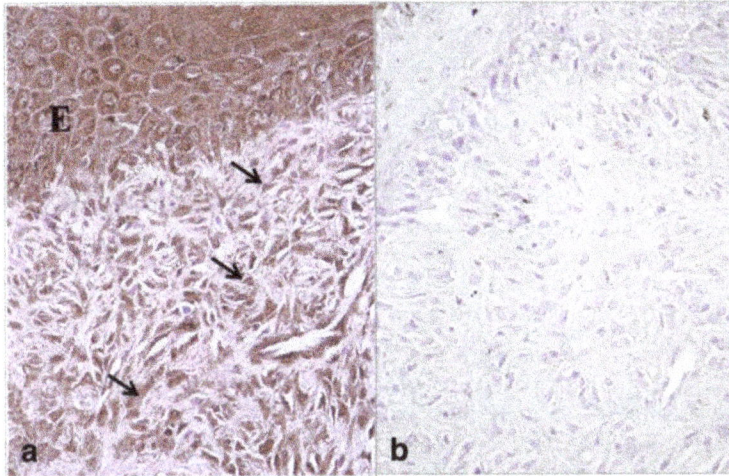

Fig. 6 a TIMP-2 immunostaining in equine sarcoid. TIMP-2 is strongly expressed by epidermis (E) and by 50–70 % of SFs (*arrows*). **b** Secondary-only negative control. Streptavidin-biotin-peroxidase stain. 40X

are usually not detectable or at very low levels in healthy resting tissue and are instead induced in wound repair and in keloid formation in response to cytokines, growth factors and/or cell contact with ECM [17–19]. It has been shown that the over-expression and activation of MMPs is induced by BPV oncoproteins in equine sarcoid fibroblasts and, recently, MMPs expression has been confirmed also in vivo [8, 9, 32]. These previous observations are in line with the results of our study in which we also found that both MMP-9 and MMP-2 were consistently expressed by epidermal and dermal cells and with different intensity.

MMP-9 is secreted as pro-MMP-9 (92 kDa) and is activated into the functional form (82 kDa).

In equine sarcoids our data show for the first time, the overexpression of a 35 KDa super-active form of MMP-9, an auto-catalytic product of the 82KDa proform, which possesses highly efficient proteolytic activity for different ECM proteins (gelatins, fibronectin and collagen type IV) [39]. In our sarcoid samples, MMP-9 was expressed by

SFs and keratinocytes, strongly suggesting its role in the formation of long rete pegs [40, 41]; this in turn promotes keratinocyte detachment from the basement zone through controlled digestion of type IV collagen.

Thus, sarcoid development could be the result of fibroblast stimulated proliferation of overlying epithelial cells (with rete peg formation), which in turn stimulate the fibroblasts in the underlying dermis to proliferate and to produce more collagen.

In our study, MMP-2 showed a variable and finely granular staining pattern in 30–50 % of SFs, confirming that fibrillar collagens, rather that collagen IV, are its specific substrate.

Normally, MMP-2 is secreted as pro-MMP-2 (72 kDa) and is activated into the functional form (66 kDa). Biochemical analysis showed that MMP-2 was overexpressed and hyper-activated in 50 % of sarcoid samples, when compared to normal skin. Moreover, in sarcoids MMP-2 expression was associated with a weak to moderate expression of MMP-14, which is considered its

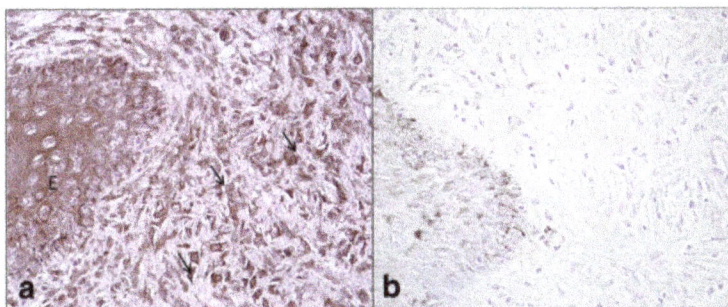

Fig. 7 a MMP-14 immunostaining in equine sarcoid. MMP-14 is strongly stained by epidermis (E) and by 50–70 % of SFs (*arrows*). **b** Secondary-only negative control. Streptavidin-biotin-peroxidase stain. 40X

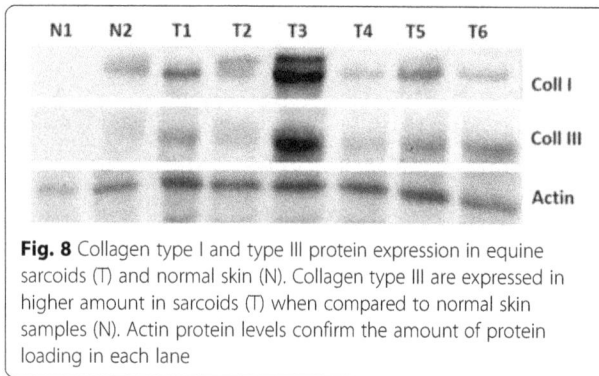

Fig. 8 Collagen type I and type III protein expression in equine sarcoids (T) and normal skin (N). Collagen type III are expressed in higher amount in sarcoids (T) when compared to normal skin samples (N). Actin protein levels confirm the amount of protein loading in each lane

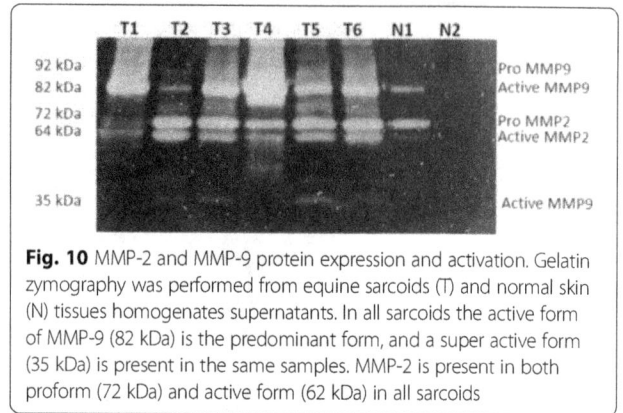

Fig. 10 MMP-2 and MMP-9 protein expression and activation. Gelatin zymography was performed from equine sarcoids (T) and normal skin (N) tissues homogenates supernatants. In all sarcoids the active form of MMP-9 (82 kDa) is the predominant form, and a super active form (35 kDa) is present in the same samples. MMP-2 is present in both proform (72 kDa) and active form (62 kDa) in all sarcoids

main activator; this, with a strong expression of TIMP-2, which is considered its main inhibitor [42]. Although MMP-14 expression seems increased, the higher level of TIMP-2, could lead to a decrease in MMP2 collagenolytic activity, which in turn causes insufficient degradation of collagen produced in excess by SFs. In fact, in our sarcoid samples a high content of collagen(s) was observed, suggesting that ECM deposition continues with insufficient degradation.

Therefore, we postulate that excessive and progressive deposition of connective tissue (collagen) in sarcoids, as well as in keloids [43], might not only be the result of elevated synthesis by SFs, but also caused by a deficiency in matrix degradation due to an altered expression of MMPs and TIMPs. This imbalance between production and degradation of collagen could play an important role in the pathogenesis of the equine sarcoid. Therefore, it may be suggested that, in genetically predisposed equines with latent BVP infection, an altered wound healing process creates a microenvironment that activates the latent infection, leading to neoplastic transformation and sarcoid formation.

Conclusions

Currently, there is no efficient curative therapy for equine sarcoids. The commonly employed treatments include cryotherapy, surgical excision and local immune modulation [44]. The present findings include the identification of the main cellular effectors of sarcoid growth, that is, the key cytokines regulating the scar formation process, and the regulators of ECM turnover; these findings therefore open the avenue for a number of potential therapeutic approaches that are likely to be developed in the near future.

Methods

Tumour samples

Ethics approval was obtained from the Ethical Animal Care and Use Committee of the University of Naples Federico II (Prot. N° 125861; 23/12/2015).

Twenty-five samples of equine sarcoid (each from a different horse), were clinically identified based on their gross morphology according to Pascoe and Knottenbelt (1999) [45]. Tumors were localized on the abdomen (5), neck (5), (para)-genital (4), pectoral region (6), and limbs (5) (Table 1). The length of time the sarcoids were present was variable (from 1 month to over 6 years), and often not precisely known.

No history of previous skin lacerations (wounds) could be determined due to lack of informations from both owners and practioneers. Sarcoid tissues used in this study were known to be positive for BPV 1- BPV 2 DNA ([28]; personal observations). Tumors, together with five normal skin samples from healthy horses, were either surgically excised or a representative biopsy was taken under local anesthesia. In all cases, owners signed a written consent form following a detailed verbal explanation of the study protocol. Samples were 10 % formalin fixed,

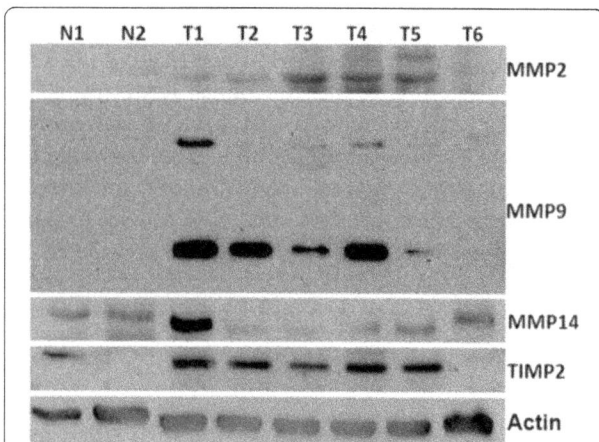

Fig. 9 MMP-2, MMP-9, MMP-14 and TIMP-2 protein expression in equine sarcoids (T) and normal skin (N). MMP-2 and MMP-9 are expressed in higher amount in sarcoids. MMP9 is present in two different forms, a 82 kDa band and 35 kDa band (super active form). MMP-9 is expressed at similar levels in all the analyzed samples, albeit in T1 samples is present at very higher level. TIMP-2 is expressed in higher amount in sarcoids (T) when compared to normal skin samples (N). Actin protein levels confirm the equal amount of protein loading in each lane

paraffin-embedded for routine histological processing and stained with haematoxylin and eosin for light microscopy study and Verhoeff-Van Gieson (VVG) method to asses collagen content.; six out of 25 sarcoid samples were perfused thoroughly with cold 0.9 % NaCl and frozen at −80 °C for western blotting analysis.

Immunohistochemistry

Paraffin sections of 25 sarcoids and five normal skin from healthy horses were dewaxed in xylene, dehydrated in graded alcohols and washed in 0.01 M phosphate-buffered saline (PBS), pH 7.2–7.4. Endogenous peroxidase was blocked with hydrogen peroxide 0.3 % in absolute methanol for 30 min. The immunohistochemical procedure (streptavidin biotin- peroxidase method, (LSAB Kit; Dako, Glostrup, Denmark) was the same as that used by the authors in a previous study [46]. Primary antibodies, used in this study are listed in Table 2. Antibodies were diluted in an antibody diluent (Dako, Glostrup, Denmark) and applied overnight at 4 °C. The immunolabelling procedure included negative control sections incubated with PBS instead of the primary antibody. A mixture of biotinylated anti-mouse and anti-rabbit immunoglobulins (LSAB Kit; Dako), diluted in PBS, was used as secondary antibody, and applied for 30 min. After washing in PBS, the sections were incubated in streptavidin conjugated to horseradish peroxidase in Tris–HCl buffer containing sodium azide (LSAB Kit; Dako) 0.015 %, for 30 min. To reveal immunolabelling, diaminobenzidine tetrahydrochloride was used as a chromogen, and haematoxylin was used as counterstain.

Scoring of immunoreactivity

The intensity of immunolabelling in each specimen, for each antibody, was scored by two independent observers (PM, MM) under blinded conditions, as performed in a previous study [47]. For each tumor 20 fields were examined at 200X magnification (20X objective 10X ocular), and immunosignal was scored from absent to strong, as follows: n.a., not assessed; − negative staining; +/− weak immunolabelling; + moderate immunolabelling; ++ extensive and strong immunolabelling.

Protein extraction and SDS PAGE/Western blotting

Six sarcoids (T1, T2, T3, T4, T5, T6), two samples of normal skin (N1, N2) and Hela cells line (positive control) were available for molecular analysis. Tissues were snap frozen in liquid nitrogen and homogenized in ice-cold lysis buffer (50 mM tris PH 7.5, 150 mM NaCl, 1 % Triton, 0.25 % Deoxicolic acid, 1 mM EDTA) added with protease inhibitor cocktail (Sigma, Milan, Italy). HeLa cell lines were grown for 2 days in 60-mm dishes, washed with ice-cold phosphate saline buffer two times and lysed for 20 min in ice-cold lysis buffer. Tissue homogenates and cell lysates were clarified by centrifugation and protein concentration was determined by Bradford protein assay performed according to manufacturer protocol (Bio-Rad Laboratories, Milan, Italy). 50 µg of total protein were boiled at 100° for 5′ in Laemmli sample buffer (Bio-Rad Laboratories, Hercules, CA) and analyzed by SDS polyacrylamide gel electrophoresis (PAGE). The proteins were blotted from the gel onto nitrocellulose membranes. The membranes were blocked for 1 h with 5 % bovine serum albumin (BSA) at room temperature and incubated with anti-MMP2 (1:500), anti-MMP9 (1:1000), anti-MMP14 (1:500), anti-TIMP-2 (1.200), anti-collagen I (1:5000), and anti-collagen III (1:5000) antibodies (Table 2). After appropriate washing steps, peroxidase-conjugated anti-rabbit or anti-mouse IgG (1:2000, Santa Cruz Biotechnology), were applied for 1 h at room temperature. After washing, bound

Table 2 List of primary antibodies used for immunohistochemistry and western blotting analysis

Antibody	Manufacturer	Clone	Specificity	Host species	Antigen retrieval	IHC Dilution	WB Dilution
VIMENTIN	Dako cytomation	V-9	man, cow, dog, hamster, horse, rabbit, rat	mouse	No antigen retrieval	1:50	-
SMOOTH MUSCLE ACTIN	Dako cytomation	1-a-4	chicken, cow, rat	mouse	Citrate, ph 6.0, 30 min, steamer	1:50	1:5000
TYPE I COLLAGEN	Ab-cam	Col-1	rat, rabbit, cow, human, pig, deer	mouse	Citrate, ph 6.0, 30 min, steamer	1:100	1:5000
TYPE III COLLAGEN	Millipore	le7-d7	rabbit, human	mouse	Citrate, ph 6.0, 30 min, steamer	1:100	1:5000
MMP-2	Thermo-scientific	Ab-7	human, mouse, rat, cow	rabbit	Citrate, ph 6.0, 30 min, steamer	1:200	1:500
MMP-9	Millipore	56-2a4	human, rat, rabbit, guinea pig	mouse	Citrate, ph 6.0, 30 min, steamer	1:200	1:1000
MT1-MMP (MMP-14)	Millipore	113-5b7	human	mouse	Citrate, ph 6.0, 30 min, steamer	1:200	1:500
TIMP-2	Millipore	2TMP05	bovine, guinea pig, human, mouse, rat, rabbit	mouse	Citrate, ph 6.0, 30 min, steamer	1:200	1:200

antibody was visualized on enhanced chemiluminescence (ECL) film (Amersham Pharmacia Biotech). The blots were stripped and reprobed against mouse anti-actin antibody (Santa Cruz Biotechnology) at 1:5000 to confirm equal loading of proteins in each lane. For collagen I and III protein detection the SDS-PAGE procedure was performed in non-denaturing conditions.

Gelatinase zymography

Substrate-specific zymography for determination of gelatinolytic activity of MMP-2 and MMP-9 was performed as previously described [48]. Briefly, 20 µg of each protein extract were subjected to gel electrophoresis using 10 % Zymogram (Gelatin) pre cast Gel and zymogram gel was developed according to manufacturer protocol (Bio-Rad Laboratories, Milan, Italy). After electrophoresis, the gel was washed twice 2.3 % triton X-100 for 30 min and incubated in development buffer (50 mM tris, 200 mM NaCl, 5 mM $CaCl_2$, 0.02 % Brij-35 at 37 °C for 20 h. Gel was then stained with 0.5 % coomassie blue R-250 in staining solution (40 % methanol, 10 % acetic acid, 0.5 % coomassie blue, 100 ml deionized water) at room temperature (RT) for 1 h and was de-stained in destaining solution (40 % methanol, 10 % acetic acid, 250 ml deionized water), until clear lysis bands appeared. To quantify the intensities of the degradated bands, zymogram gel was scanned using ChemiDoc gel scanner (Bio-Rad Laboratories).

Abbreviations

ECM: extracellular matrix; MMP: matrix metalloproteinase; TIMP: tissue inhibitor of metalloproteinase; SFs: sarcoid fibroblasts; BPV-1: bovine papillomavirus type-1; BPV-2: bovine papillomavirus type2; VIM: vimentin; α-SMA: alpha-smooth muscle actin; T: sarcoid samples; N: normal skin.

Competing interests

The authors declare that they have no competing interests.

Authors' contributions

PM has conceived the study, coordinated the group and drafted the manuscript; MM together with PM, has participated in the conception and design of the study, in analysis and interpretation of histological and immunohistochemical data and drafted the manuscript; GB and BR have been involved in revising the manuscript for important intellectual content; AC and MEDB carried out the molecular genetic studies, taking part in western blotting analysis, and zymography; AC helped with interpretation of molecular data and drafted the manuscript. All authors read and approved the final manuscript.

Authors' information

MM is employed as a researcher at the Department of Veterinary Medicine and Animal Production; BR and GB are employed as associate professors at the Department of Veterinary medicine and animal production; PM is employed as a full professor at the Department of Veterinary medicine and animal production; MEDB is a student trainee for the degree thesis; AC is a post-doc research fellowship at Institute of Protein Biochemistry (IBP)National Research Council (CNR), Via Pietro Castellino 111, 80131 Naples, Italy.

Acknowledgment

The authors acknowledge Mr. Raffaele Ilsami for its technical support during microscopy analysis. This research was financially supported by Department of Veterinary Medicine and Animal Production, University of Naples, Italy.

Author details

[1]Department of Veterinary Medicine and Animal Productions, Naples University "Federico II", Via F. Delpino 1, 80137 Naples, Italy. [2]Present Address: Institute of Protein Biochemistry (IBP) National Research Council (CNR), Via Pietro Castellino 111, 80131 Naples, Italy.

References

1. Borzacchiello G, Corteggio A. Equine sarcoid: state of the art. Ippologia. 2009;20:7–14.
2. Nasir L, Brandt S. Papillomavirus associated diseases of the horse. Vet Microbiol. 2013;167(Suppl 1–2):159–67.
3. Torrontegui BO, Reid SJ. Clinical and pathological epidemiology of the equine sarcoid in a referral population. Eq Vet Educ. 1994;6:85–8.
4. Nasir L, Campo MS. Bovine papillomaviruses: their role in the aetiology of cutaneous tumours of bovids and equids. Vet Dermatol. 2008;19:243–54.
5. Knottenbelt DC. A suggested clinical classification of the equine sarcoid. Clin Tech in Eq Pract. 2005;4:278–95.
6. Tarwid JN, Fretz PB, Clark EG. Equine sarcoids: A study with emphasis on pathological diagnosis. Compend Contin Educ. 1985;7:293–300.
7. Martens A, De Moor A, Demeulemeester J, Peelman L. Polymerase chain reaction analysis of the surgical margins of equine sarcoids for bovine papilloma virus DNA. Vet Surg. 2001;30:460–7.
8. Yuan Z, Gobeil PA, Campo MS, Nasir L. Equine sarcoid fibroblasts over-express matrix metalloproteinases and are invasive. Virol. 2010;396:143–51.
9. Mosseri S, Hetzel U, Hahn S, Michaloupoulou E, Sallabank HC, Knottenbelt DC, et al. Equine sarcoid: In situ demonstration of matrix metalloproteinase expression. Vet J. 2014;202(Suppl2):279–85.
10. Chambers G, Ellsmore VA, O'Brien PM, Reid SWJ, Love S, Campo MS, et al. Sequence variants of bovine papillomavirus E5 detected in equine sarcoids. Virus Res. 2003;96(Suppl 1–2):141–5.
11. Martens A, Moor ADE, Demeulemeester J, Ducatelle R. Histopathological characteristics of five clinical types of equine sarcoid. Res Vet Sci. 2000;69(Suppl3):295–300.
12. Cochrane AC. Models in vivo of wound healing in the horse and the role of growth factors. Vet Dermatol. 1997;8:259–72.
13. Hansen RR. Complications of EquineWound Management and Dermatologic Surgery. Vet Clin Eq. 2009;24:663–96.
14. Haddow A. Molecular repair, wound healing, and carcinogenesis: tumor production a possible overhealing? Adv Cancer Res. 1972;16:181–234.
15. Dvorak HF. Tumors: wounds that do not heal. Similarities between tumor stroma generation and wound healing. N Engl J Med. 1986;315:1650–9.
16. Schäfer M, Werner S. Cancer as an overhealing wound: an old hypothesis revisited. Nat Rev Mol Cell Biol. 2008;9 Suppl 8:628–38.
17. Imaizumi R, Akasaka Y, Inomata N, Okada E, Ito K, Ishikawa Y, et al. Promoted activation of matrix metalloproteinase (MMP)-2 in keloid fibroblasts and increased expression of MMP-2 in collagen bundle regions: implications for mechanisms of keloid progression. Histopathol. 2009;54(Suppl6):722–30.
18. Pilcher BK, Dumin JA, Sudbeck BD, Krane SM, Welgus HG, Parks WC. The activity of collagenase-1 is required for keratinocyte migration on a type I collagen matrix. J Cell Biol. 1997;137:1445–57.
19. Allen DL, Teitelbaum DH, Kurachi K. Growth factor stimulation of matrix metalloproteinase expression and myoblast migration and invasion in vitro. Am J Physiol Cell Physiol. 2003;284 Suppl 4:C805–15.
20. Giantin M, Aresu L, Benali S, Aricò A, Morello EM, Martano M, et al. Expression of matrix metalloproteinases, tissue inhibitors of metalloproteinases and vascular endothelial growth factor in canine mast cell tumours. J Comp Pathol. 2012;147 Suppl 4:419–29.
21. Osenkowski P, Toth M, Fridman R. Processing, shedding, and endocytosis of membrane type 1-matrix metalloproteinase (MT1-MMP). J Cell Physiol. 2004;200 Suppl 1:2–10.
22. Borzacchiello G, Mogavero S, De Vita G, Roperto S, Della Salda L, Roperto F. Activated platelet-derived growth factor beta receptor expression, PI3K-AKT

pathway molecular analysis, and transforming signals in equine sarcoids. Vet Pathol. 2009;46 Suppl 4:589–97.

23. Brandt S, Tober R, Corteggio A, Burger S, Sabitzer S, Walter I, et al. BPV-1 infection is not confined to the dermis but also involves the epidermis of equine sarcoids. Vet Microbiol. 2011;150(Suppl 1–2):35–40.

24. Chambers G, Ellsmore VA, O'Brien PM, Reid SW, Love S, Campo MS, et al. Association of bovine papillomavirus with the equine sarcoid. J Gen Virol. 2003;84:1055–62.

25. Martens A, De Moor A, Ducatelle R. PCR detection of bovine papilloma virus DNA in superficial swabs and scrapings from equine sarcoids. Vet J. 2001;161:280–6.

26. Otten N, von Tscharner C, Lazary S, Antczak DF, Gerber H. DNA of bovine papillomavirus type 1 and 2 in equine sarcoids: PCR detection and direct sequencing. Arch Virol. 1993;132:121–31.

27. Reid SW, Smith KT, Jarrett WF. Detection, cloning and characterisation of papillomaviral DNA present in sarcoid tumours of Equus asinus. Vet Rec. 1994;135:430–2.

28. Borzacchiello G, Russo V, Della Salda L, Roperto S, Roperto F. Expression of platelet-derived growth factor-b receptor and bovine papillomavirus E5 and E7 oncoproteins in equine sarcoid. J Comp Pathol. 2008;139:231–7.

29. Carr EA, Théon AP, Madewell BR, Griffey SM, Hitchcock ME. Bovine papillomavirus DNA in neoplastic and non-neoplastic tissues obtained from horses with and without sarcoids in the western United States. Am J Vet Res. 2001;62:741–4.

30. Nasir L, Reid SW. Bovine papillomaviral gene expression in equine sarcoid tumours. Virus Res. 1999;61:171–5.

31. Ragland WL, Spencer GR. Attempts to relate bovine papillomavirus to the cause of equine sarcoid: Equidae inoculated intradermally with bovine papillomavirus. Am J Vet Res. 1969;30:743–52.

32. Yuan ZQ, Gault EA, Gobeil P, Nixon C, Campo MS, Nasir L. Establishment and characterization of equine fibroblast cell lines transformed in vivo and in vitro by BPV-1: model systems for equine sarcoids. Virol. 2008;373:352–61.

33. Bogaert L, Martens A, De Baere C, Gasthuys F. Detection of bovine papillomavirus DNA on the normal skin and in the habitual surroundings of horses with and without equine sarcoids. Res Vet Sci. 2005;79 Suppl 3:253–8.

34. Yuan ZQ, Philbey AW, Gault EA, Campo MS, Nasir L. Detection of bovine papillomavirus type 1 genomes and viral gene expression in equine inflammatory skin conditions. Virus Res. 2007;124(Suppl1-2):245–9.

35. Wobeser BK, Hill JE, Jackson ML, Kidney BA, Mayer MN, Townsend HG, et al. Localization of Bovine papillomavirus in equine sarcoids and inflammatory skin conditions of horses using laser microdissection and two forms of DNA amplification. J Vet Diagn Invest. 2012;24 Suppl 1:32–41.

36. Williams IF, Heaton A, McCullagh KG. Connective tissue composition of the equine sarcoid. Eq Vet J. 1982;14 Suppl 4:305–10.

37. Bran GM, Goessler UR, Hormann K, Riedel F, Sadick H. Keloids: Current concepts of pathogenesis (Review). Int J Mol Med. 2009;24:283–93.

38. Theoret CL, Olutoye OO, Parnell LK, Hicks J. Equine exuberant granulation tissue and human keloids: a comparative histopathologic study. Vet Surg. 2013;42 Suppl 7:783–9.

39. Ries C, Pitsch T, Mentele R, Zahler S, Egea V, Nagase H, et al. Identification of a novel 82 kDa proMMP-9 species associated with the surface of leukemic cells: (auto-) catalytic activation and resistance to inhibition by TIMP-1. Biochem J. 2007;405(Suppl3):547–58.

40. Mohan R, Chintala SK, Jung JC, Villar W, McCabe F, Russo L, et al. Matrix metalloproteinase gelatinase B (MMP-9) regulates and effects epithelial regeneration. J Biol Chem. 2002;277:2065–72.

41. O'Toole EA, van Koningsveld R, Chen M, Woodley DT. Hypoxia induces epidermal keratinocyte matrix metalloproteinase-9 secretion via the protein kinase C pathway. J Cell Physiol. 2008;214 Suppl 1:47–55.

42. Klein T, Bischoff R. Physiology and pathophysiology of matrix metalloproteases. Amino Acids. 2011;41(Suppl2):271–90.

43. Butler PD, Longaker MT, Yang GP. Current progress in keloid research and treatment. J Am Coll Surg. 2008;206 Suppl 4:731–41.

44. Bergvall KE. Sarcoids. Vet Clin North Am Eq Pract. 2013;29(Suppl3):657–71.

45. Pascoe RR, Knottenbelt DC. Manual of Eq Dermatol pub. London: WB Saunders; 1999. p. 244–50.

46. Restucci B, Martano M, Maiolino P. Expression of endothelin-1 and endothelin-1 receptor A in canine mammary tumours. Res Vet Sci. 2015;100:182–8.

47. Martano M, Carella F, Squillacioti C, Restucci B, Mazzotta M, Lo Muzio L, et al. Metallothionein expression in canine cutaneous apocrine gland tumors. Anticancer Res. 2012;32 Suppl 3:747–52.

48. Kleiner DE, Stetler-Stevenson WG. Quantitative zymography: detection of picogram quantities of gelatinases. Anal Biochem. 1994;218(2):325–9.

12

Identification of immunologic and clinical characteristics that predict inflammatory response to C. Novyi-NT bacteriolytic immunotherapy

Amy E. DeClue[1]* (iD), Sandra M. Axiak-Bechtel[2], Yan Zhang[1], Saurabh Saha[3], Linping Zhang[3], David D. Tung[3] and Jeffrey N. Bryan[2]

Abstract

Background: Clostridium novyi-NT (CNV-NT), has shown promise as a bacterolytic therapy for solid tumors in mouse models and in dogs with naturally developing neoplasia. Factors that impact the immunologic response to therapy are largely unknown. The goal of this pilot study was to determine if plasma immune biomarkers, immune cell function, peripheral blood cytological composition and tumor characteristics including evaluation of a PET imaging surrogate of tumor tissue hypoxia could predict which dogs with naturally developing naïve neoplasia would develop an inflammatory response to CNV-NT.

Results: Dogs that developed an inflammatory response to CNV-NT had a higher heart rate, larger gross tumor volume, greater tumor [^{64}Cu]ATSM SUV$_{Max}$, increased constitutive leukocyte IL-10 production, more robust NK cell-like function and greater peripheral blood lymphocyte counts compared to dogs that did not develop an inflammatory response to CNV-NT. Of these, unstimulated leukocyte IL-10 production, heart rate, and gross tumor volume appeared to be the best predictors of which dogs will develop an inflammatory response to CNV-NT.

Conclusions: Development of inflammation in response to CNV-NT is best predicted by pretreatment unstimulated leukocyte IL-10 production, heart rate, and gross tumor volume.

Keywords: Immunology, Cancer, Canine, Immunotherapy

Background

For centuries it has been recognized that certain bacterial infections could induce tumor regression. In more modern times, the controlled use of bacteriolytic immunotherapy has been evaluated in both induced and spontaneous tumor models [1]. One such proposed bacterolytic immunotherapy, Clostridium novyi-NT (CNV-NT), has shown promise as a therapy for solid tumors [2, 3]. The advantage of CNV-NT over other types of bacterolytic immunotherapy is that CNV-NT is a strict anaerobe and thus is restricted to growing in the relatively hypoxic regions of tumor tissue and not

in healthy tissues. This should, theoretically, maximize local immune stimulation and inflammation in the tumor microenvironment while minimizing systemic effects [4].

C. novyi-NT bacteriolytic immunotherapy has successfully cured induced neoplasia in mouse models and resulted in objective tumor responses in naturally developing neoplasia in the dog [1–3]. However, the response rate in dogs with naturally developing neoplasia has been less than 40%, thus strategies to optimize response rates are needed [2]. Proposed explanations for the limited response rate include a lack of appropriate immune response to infection or variability in the degree of hypoxic tissue in the tumor leading to reduced CNV-NT germination. Dogs with various forms of neoplasia have altered immune function which could impact the efficacy

* Correspondence: decluea@misssouri.edu
[1]Department of Veterinary Medicine and Surgery, Comparative Internal Medicine Laboratory, University of Missouri, College of Veterinary Medicine, 900 E. Campus Dr, Columbia, MO 65203, USA
Full list of author information is available at the end of the article

of immunotherapies like induced infection and little is known about the regional blood flow distribution in solid tumors in this species [5–8].

The purpose of this pilot investigation is to identify possible immunologic, tumor or clinical characteristics pre-treatment that would predict which dogs are more likely to successfully develop immunologically pertinent inflammation after administration of CNV-NT. To evaluate this, plasma immune biomarkers, immune cell function, peripheral blood cytological composition and tumor characteristics including evaluation of a PET imaging surrogate of tumor tissue hypoxia were measured in dogs with naturally developing naïve neoplasia prior to administration of CNV-NT; following CNV-NT treatment the development of inflammation was recorded. Baseline parameters were compared between dogs that developed inflammation and those that did not. Parameters that were significantly different between groups were then used to develop a predictive model.

Methods

Population

Client owned dogs presented to the University of Missouri Veterinary Health Center with histologically or cytologically confirmed soft-tissue sarcoma, oral or cutaneous malignant melanoma, oral squamous cell carcinoma, or other cutaneous carcinomas were eligible for enrollment with written informed client consent (IACUC protocol #7386). Eligibility criteria included tumors greater than 2 cm in diameter, tumor size and location where surgical excision with at least marginal resection was a viable option, and body weight of > 10 kg. Dogs were excluded if comorbidities were present that suggested survival expectation of less than 6 weeks, evidence of metastasis outside of the local draining lymph node, tumor location where abscess development would be catastrophic (e.g., CNS), persistent neutropenia or thrombocytopenia, grade 2 increases in plasma ALT, BUN or creatinine, administration of antimicrobial therapy within the 7 days preceding enrollment, concurrent infection requiring systemic antimicrobial therapy, chemotherapy, radiation therapy, or other immunotherapy within the 3 weeks preceding enrollment, pregnancy or potential pregnancy, enrollment in another clinical trial, cardiac disease severe enough that a balanced crystalloid solution administered at 4 mL/kg/h would likely induce congestive heart failure, and unavailability during the full study duration.

Baseline evaluations included medical history, physical examination, complete blood count, plasma biochemical profile, complete urinalysis, thoracic radiographs, and cytologic evaluation of the draining lymph bed if accessible. Prior to therapy, tumors were evaluated using PET/CT to evaluate tumor size, estimate glucose metabolism with [18F]FDG, and estimate relative tumor hypoxia using [64Cu]ATSM (some data not presented in this manuscript).

Treatments

Dogs received CNV-NT (BioMed Valley Discoveries Inc., Kansas City, MO) either intravenous (IV) or intratumoral (IT) on day 0. The change from IV to IT was based on a programmatic decision by the sponsor.

Intravenous administration CNV-NT (1×10^9) spores were administered in 50 mls of physiologic saline through an intravenous catheter. Initially, 5 mL was administered over 2 min; dogs' vital parameters were monitored for 30 min. If the dog's vital parameters were within 10% of baseline after 30 min, the remaining 45 mL was administered over a 5 min time period. Following completion of CNV-NT infusion, intravenous fluids were administered for 2 h and dogs were discharged to their owners if no signs of a reaction was noted.

Intratumoral administration CNV-NT was provided in 3 mL of saline at a dose of 1×10^8 spores. Following sedation, the tumor was clipped and aseptically prepped, and CNV-NT was administered directly into the tumor with 0.75 mL injected into 4 total sites evenly distributed within the tumor. Vital parameters were monitored for 3 h following injection.

Groups

The primary outcome measure used to group the dogs was the development of clinically identifiable inflammation within 28 days of treatment for the IV group and within 56 days of treatment for the IT group. In the IV CNV-NT group, dogs that developed fever (rectal temperature > 39.2 °C (102.5 °F)) and lethargy were placed in the inflammation group while dogs that developed no clinical signs following infusion were classified as having not developed inflammation. In the IT group, dogs that developed clinical evidence of abscess formation including edema, erythema, and/ or mucopurulent discharge were placed in the inflammation group. Dogs that had no evidence of abscess formation were placed in the no evidence of inflammation group.

Sample collection and processing

At baseline (pre-treatment), blood was collected from the jugular vein and placed in either EDTA, sodium heparin, lithium heparin or evacuated tubes for immunologic evaluation. Lithium heparinized blood was immediately cooled and centrifuged within 1 hour of collection. Plasma or serum was collected and stored at − 80 °C for batch analyses of immune protein evaluation. The remainder of the blood was processed immediately for PBMC isolation, CBC, phagocytic function and leukocyte cytokine production assays as indicated below.

Clinical/tumor characteristics

Dogs were evaluated prior to therapy utilizing rectal temperature, heart rate, complete blood count, plasma globulin concentration (total protein- albumin = globulin), CT scan measurement of tumor volume and PET scan with [^{18}F]FDG to characterize tumor metabolism and [^{64}Cu]ATSM to characterize tumor hypoxia. [^{64}Cu]ATSM is reduced and trapped in hypoxic cells, localizing for imaging with positron emission tomography (PET). Dogs were injected with 74 MBq (2 mCi) of [^{64}Cu]ATSM 45 min prior to scanning. Dogs were anesthetized and maintained on a propofol infusion breathing room air. Scans were acquired with a Philips C-PET+ with attenuation correction. Reconstructed images were evaluated using MIMfusion software. Maximum standard uptake value (SUV_{Max}) and threshold volume with SUV > 1.0 were calculated.

Plasma immune biomarkers

Plasma was collected centrifuged at 400 g for 15 min and then stored at − 80 °C for batch analysis. Thirteen immune markers: IL-6, CXCL-8, IL-2, IL-7, TNF-α, GM-CSF, IL-18, CXCL-1, IP-10, IL-15, IL-10 and MCP-1 were evaluated in undiluted plasma as previously described using canine specific multiplex bead-based, ELISA assay (Millipore Sigma, Burlington, MA), a MAGPIX Multiplexing instrument and analyzed using MILLPLEX Analyst 5.1 software [9]. Serum HMGB-1 (IBL International, Toronto, ON) and CRP (ICL Inc., Portland OR) were measured using commercially available ELISAs according to the manufacturers' recommendations [10, 11].

Immune cell function

Immune cell function was assessed by evaluating granulocyte phagocytic and respiratory burst function, leukocyte cytokine production capacity and NK-like cell function.

Phagocytic function was determined using the Phagotest® commercial test kit (Orpegen Pharma, Heidelberg, Germany) which evaluates phagocytosis of FITC-labeled, opsonized E. coli. The assay has been previously validated in dogs and was performed as previously described [5, 7]. Samples were analyzed by flow cytometry using the CyAn ADP flow cytometer (Beckman Coulter, Brea, CA) and associated data analysis software (Summit V 5.2.0.7477, Brea, CA) within 30 min and a minimum of 15,000 events were recorded for each sample. DNA stain positive cells were gated and placed on a forward and side scat plot. Phagocytes were identified using standard forward and side scatter characteristics. Then, FITC positive phagocytes were identified on a histogram. Both the relative number of E. coli-positive cells as well as the mean fluorescence intensity (MFI) of positive cells indicating the number of bacteria per cell were recorded.

The quantification of oxidative burst of PMNs was performed using a Phagoburst® kit (ORPEGEN Pharma, Heidelberg, Germany) which evaluates E.coli and PMA–induced oxidative burst using dihydrorhodamine 123 as a fluorogenic substrate. The assay has been previously validated in dogs and was performed as previously described [5, 7]. Samples were analyzed by flow cytometry using the CyAn ADP flow cytometer and associated data analysis software within 30 min and a minimum of 15,000 events were recorded for each sample. DNA stain positive cells were gated and placed on a forward and side scatter plot. Phagocytes were identified using standard forward and side scatter characteristics. Then, a FLI histogram was used to identify positive phagocytes. The percentage of positive cells indicating recruitment and the MFI indicating the intensity of oxidative burst were recorded.

Leukocyte cytokine production capacity was determined by stimulating whole blood with lipopolysaccharide (LPS) from Escherichia coli 0127:B8 (final concentration, 100 ng mL^{-1}; Sigma-Aldrich, St. Louis, MO), lipoteichoic acid (LTA) from Streptococcus faecalis (final concentration, 1000 ng mL^{-1}; Sigma-Aldrich), or phosphate buffered saline (PBS; unstimulated control) and then measuring cytokine concentrations in the cell culture supernatant as previously described [12]. Blood was diluted 1:2 with media and samples were cultured on 12 well plates with LPS, LTA or PBS and then incubated for 24 h at 37 °C in 5% CO_2. Cell supernatant was collected at end of incubation and stored in − 80 °C for analysis. Quantification of TNF-α, IL-6 and IL-10 was accomplished using a canine specific multiplex bead-based, ELISA assay (Millipore Sigma) and a MAGPIX Multiplexing instrument as stated for the plasma immune markers.

NK-like cell function was determined using a thyroid adenocarcinoma cytotoxicity assay as previously described [8]. Canine thyroid adenocarcinoma (CTAC) cells were used as target cells. Prior to the assay, CTAC cells were labeled with 3 mM green fluorescent 3,3′-Dioctadecyloxacarbocyanine (DiO) for 20 min at 37 °C in 5% CO_2. Cytotoxicity of cancer cells was assessed by co-incubating PBMC with DiO-labeled CTAC cells for 24 h at 37 °C with 5% CO_2. Cells were comingled in different PBMC to Dio-CTAC cell ratios: 1:1, 10:1, 25:1 and 50:1. Single cell population of PBMC or Dio-CTAC were used as controls. At end of incubation, cells were incubated with propidium iodide (PI). Samples were analyzed using the CyAn ADP flow cytometer and associated data analysis software. A minimum of 10,000 events were recorded for each sample. Data were analyzed as previously described [8]. Briefly, the CTAC cells were gaited on a forward/side scatter plot and then applied to a plot comparing DiO and PI. DiO and PI positivity were determined using unstained cells as controls. Cells positive for DiO and PI were defined as dead CTAC cells. Baseline cell death was established using DiO/PI stained CTAC cells alone. The NK-like cell killing index was calculated by dividing the % death from the PBMC+CTAC cell mixture by the CTAC cells alone.

Peripheral blood immune cell composition

Peripheral blood immune cell composition was determined by performing a complete blood count to determine the number of total white blood cells, neutrophils, monocytes and lymphocytes in the peripheral blood and flow cytometry to determine lymphocyte phenotype. A complete blood count was performed by the University of Missouri Veterinary Diagnostic Laboratory. Antibodies used for PBMC phenotype assay were rat anti-mouse CD3-PE (abcam, Cambridge, UK; Clone KT3), mouse anti-dog CD21-Alexa Fluor 647 (AbD Serotec, Raleigh, NC; Clone: CA2.1D6), rat anti-mouse/rat FoxP3-APC (eBioscience, San Diego, CA; Clone: FJK-16 s), rat-anti-dog CD4-FITC (AbD Serotec; Clone: YKIX302.9), mouse anti-human CD25-PE (Dako; Clone: ACT-1), rat anti-human CD3-Alexa Fluor 647 (AbD Serotec; Clone: CD3-12), rat anti-dog CD8-APC (eBioscience; Clone: YCATE55.9), anti-human CD56-PE (Dako, Santa Clara, CA; Clone: MOC-1), Rat IgG2a APC isotype control, Mouse IgG1 PE isotype control and Rat IgG2a FITC isotype control (eBioscience). PBMCs were harvested and 200 µl of 10^6 PBMC per sample were added to a 96 well round bottom plate. Plates were centrifuged at 300 g for 6 min and supernatant removed. 50 µl of FACS buffer was added to each sample and then samples were stained for the following markers: CD4 T cell (CD3$^+$/CD4$^+$), CD8 T cell (CD3$^+$/CD8$^+$), NK-like cell (CD3$^-$/CD56$^+$) and B cell (CD21$^+$) for 30 min on ice protected from light. At end of incubation cells were washed twice with PBS and fixed with 2% paraformaldehyde. T regulatory cells (CD4$^+$/CD25$^+$/FoxP3$^+$) were detected using surface CD4 and CD25 stains and incubating for 30 min as previously described [13]. Cells were washed with PBS, then fixed and permeabilized with fix/perm FoxP3 staining buffer (eBioscience) for 30 min to detect intracellular FoxP3. At the end of incubations, cell were washed and collected into FACS tubes; all samples were then analyzed at the University of Missouri Cell and Immunology Core Facility using CyAn ADP and Summit software (Summit V 5.2.0.7477, CA, USA). A minimum of 15,000 events were recorded for each sample. Unstained cells and matched isotype controls from the same manufacturer were used for negative antibody controls for analyses. Lymphocytes were identified and gated using a forward and side scatter plot. To evaluate CD3$^+$/CD4$^+$ or CD3$^+$/CD8$^+$ T cells, the gated lymphocytes were then applied to PE (CD3) vs FITC (CD4) or PE (CD3) vs APC (CD8) plots, respectively, and double positive cells were identified (Fig. 1).

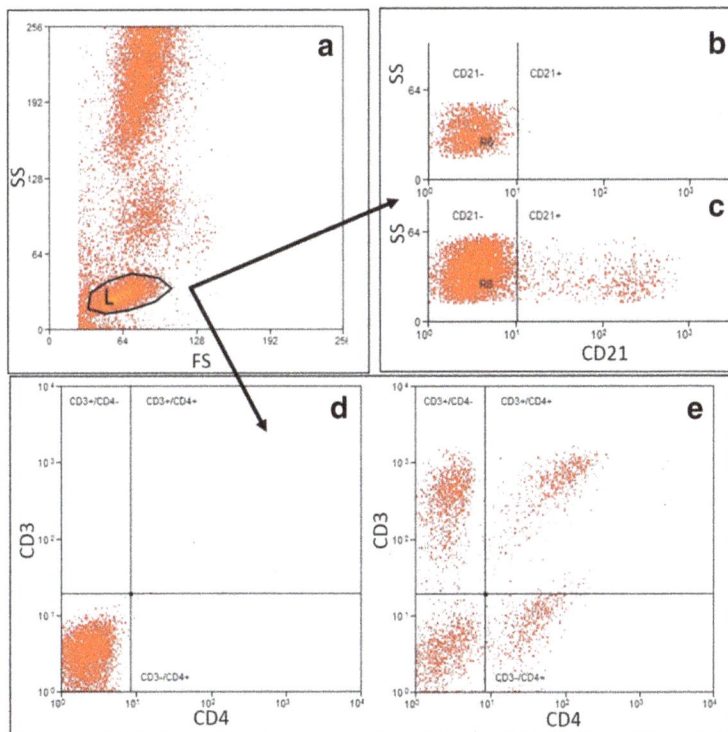

Fig. 1 Example gating scheme for identification of CD3$^+$/CD4$^+$ lymphocytes and CD21$^+$ lymphocytes. Lymphocytes were identified and gated using a forward and side scatter plot (**a**). Gated lymphocytes were applied were then applied to PE (CD3) vs FITC (CD4) plots or an Alexa Fluor 647 (CD21) histogram, respectively. Unstained cells and matched isotype controls from the same manufacturer were used to determine cut offs for negative (**b** and **d**) versus positive (**c** and **e**) cells. CD3$^+$/CD4$^+$ or CD21 positive cells were then identified. CD3$^+$/CD8$^+$ cells were selected in the same manner as the CD3$^+$/CD4$^+$ cells

To identify B cells, lymphocytes were applied to an Alexa Fluor 647 (CD21) histogram (Fig. 1). NK-like cells were identified by applying the gated lymphocytes to an Alexa Fluor 647 (CD3) vs side scatter plot and selecting for the Alexa Fluor 647 negative cells. The CD3 negative cells were then applied to a PE (CD56) vs side scat plot and the PE positive cells were selected (Fig. 2). T regulatory cells were identified by applying the gated lymphocytes to a FITC (CD4) vs PE (CD25). Then FITC and PE double positive cells were applied to an APC (Fox P3) vs side scatter plot as previously described [13].

Statistical analysis

Statistical analysis was accomplished using SigmaPlot software (SigmaStat; Systat Software Inc., San Jose, CA). To construct the initial model, variables were compared using a univariate analysis to identify parameters that differed between dogs that developed inflammation and those that did not. A Mann-Whitney Rank Sum test was used in initial comparison of variables between groups. Because the goal of this pilot investigation was to identify markers that would predict which dogs developed inflammation at the tumor site and we did not want to inappropriately exclude markers due to type II statistical error, a p-value of < 0.10 was considered statistically significant and variables with a p-value less than this cut-off were included in predictive modeling. Parameters that were significantly associated with the development of inflammation were then entered into a best subsets regression model. Best subsets were developed based on R squared as the best criterion. The final model selection

was determined by selecting the model with the greatest R squared with the smallest Mallows Cp value, significant contribution from all variables ($p < 0.05$) and minimal multicollinearity based on a variance inflation factor of < 1.50. Data are presented as median and range unless otherwise noted.

Results

Patient population

Twenty dogs were enrolled, 10 dogs received IV and 10 dogs received IT administration of CNV-NT. The median age of dogs enrolled was 9.5 years (range 5-13 years, age of one dog unknown) and the median weight was 28.2 kg (range 14.4-70 kg). The sexes included intact male ($n = 2$), neutered male ($n = 10$), and spayed female ($n = 8$). Breeds of dogs enrolled were Labrador retriever ($n = 5$), Golden retriever ($n = 3$), Husky ($n = 3$), and one each of the following breeds: Standard Poodle, American Staffordshire terrier, English setter, Pug, Beagle, Bloodhound, Border Collie, Pointer, and mixed breed. Tumor types were soft tissue sarcoma (STSA) ($n = 10$), oral sarcoma ($n = 6$), oral melanoma ($n = 3$), and carcinoma ($n = 1$). One dog in the IV group was excluded from analysis due to development of gastric dilation and volvulus 9 days post-infusion, necessitating surgery and subsequent antibiotic therapy. This dog was withdrawn from trial and 19 dogs were included in the immunologic analysis. Of the dogs with evaluable data, 14 were classified as having developed inflammation, six in the IV group and eight in the IT group; 5 did not develop

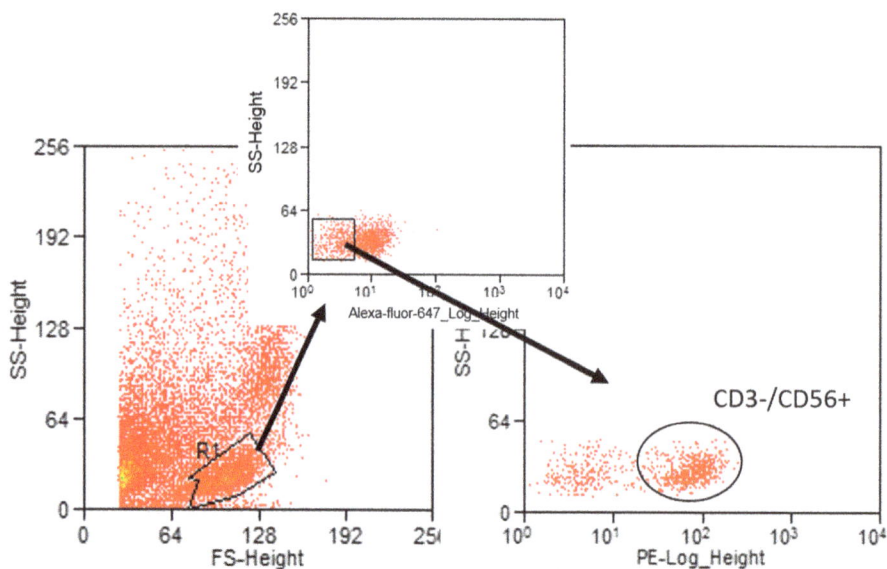

Fig. 2 Example gating scheme for identification of CD3-/CD56+ lymphocytes. Lymphocytes were identified and gated using a forward and side scatter plot. Gated lymphocytes were applied to an Alexa Fluor 647 (CD3) vs side scatter plot and selecting for the Alexa Fluor 647 negative cells. Then PE positive cells were selected on a PE (CD56) vs side scat plot

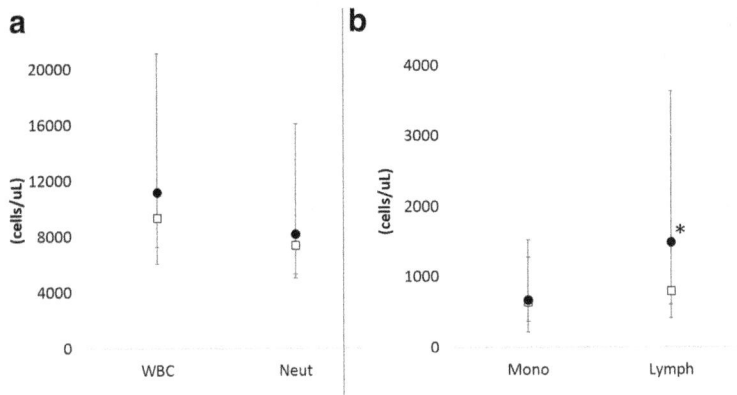

Fig. 3 Comparison of median and range of (**a**) peripheral blood white blood cell (WBC), neutrophil (Neut), (**b**) monocyte (Mono) and lymphocyte (Lymph) counts between dogs that developed inflammation (closed circles) and those that did not (open squares). *$p = 0.087$

inflammation. There was no difference in body weight between the groups.

Clinical/Tumor parameters

Peripheral blood white blood cell, neutrophil and monocyte counts did not differ between groups (Fig. 3). However, peripheral blood lymphocyte count was significantly greater in the dogs that developed inflammation compared to those that did not ($p = 0.087$). Heart rate was significantly higher in dogs that developed inflammation compared to those that did not (Fig. 4, $p = 0.055$). Gross tumor volume was significantly larger for dogs that developed inflammation compared to those that did not (Fig. 4, $p = 0.058$). [^{64}Cu]ATSM scan SUV$_{Max}$ was significantly greater for dogs that developed inflammation (Fig. 4, $p = 0.092$), but there was no difference in the threshold volume of tissue with SUV > 1.0 between groups. There was no difference in initial rectal temperature between groups (data not shown).

Serum/plasma immune biomarkers

Plasma concentrations of IL-6, IL-2, IL-7, GM-CSF, IL-18, IL-15, MCP-1, TNF-α, IL-10 and IP-10 fell below the lower limit of detection for ≥50% of the samples and thus were not statistically analyzed (data not shown). Serum HMGB-1 and CRP and plasma CXCL-8 and CXCL-1 concentrations were not significantly different between groups (Fig. 5).

Immune cell function

Unstimulated leukocyte IL-10 (Fig. 6, $p = 0.060$) production was significantly greater in the dogs that developed an inflammatory response compared to those that did not. Unstimulated leukocyte TNF-α and IL-6 production and LPS or LTA-stimulated leukocyte TNF-α, IL-6 and IL-10 production did not significantly differ between groups (Fig. 6). NK cell function was significantly greater in the dogs that developed an immune response compared to those that did not (Fig. 7, $p = 0.043$). There was no difference in the percentage of cells undergoing phagocytosis or the number of bacteria phagocytized, nor was there a

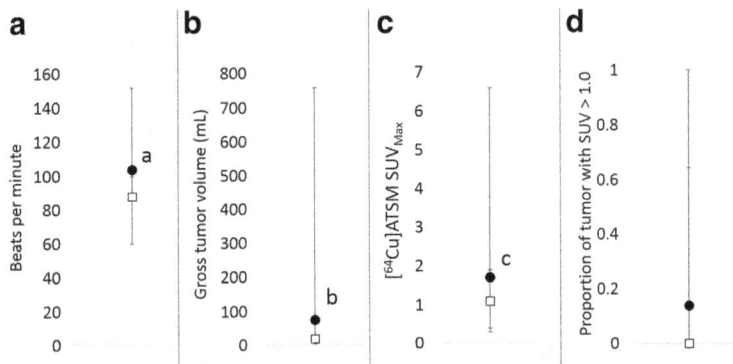

Fig. 4 Comparison of median and range of heart rate (**a**), gross tumor volume (**b**), [^{64}Cu]ATSM SUV$_{Max}$ (**c**) and threshold volume of tissue with SUV > 1.0 (**d**) between dogs that developed inflammation (closed circles) and those that did not (open squares). $^{a}p = 0.055$. $^{b}p = 0.058$, $^{c}p = 0.092$

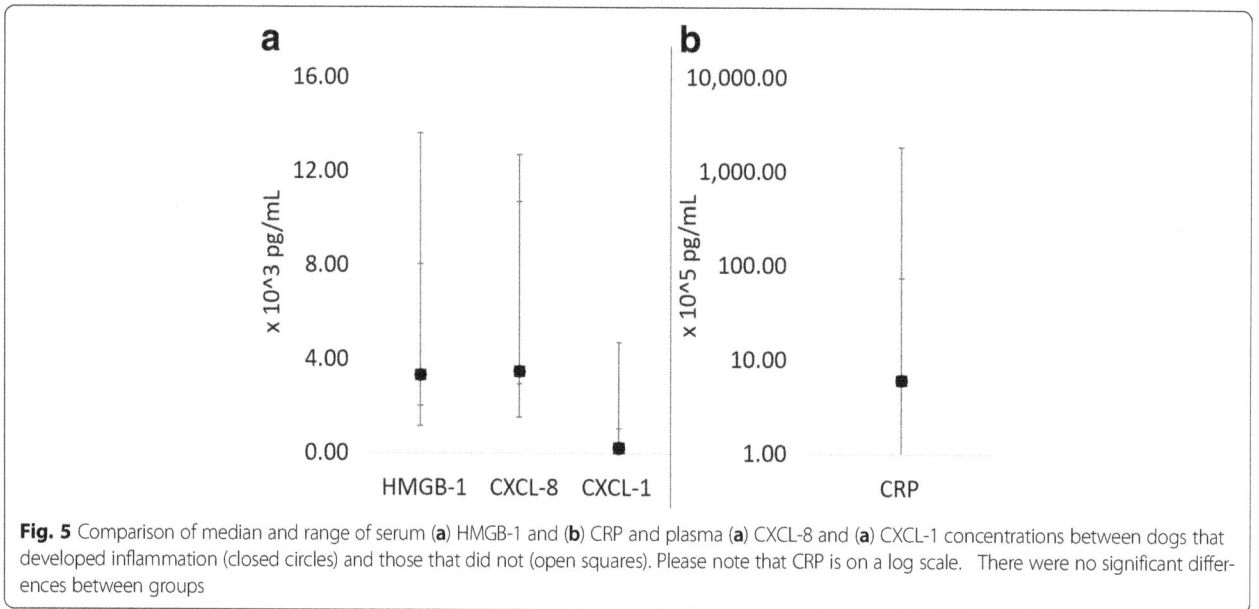

Fig. 5 Comparison of median and range of serum (**a**) HMGB-1 and (**b**) CRP and plasma (**a**) CXCL-8 and (**a**) CXCL-1 concentrations between dogs that developed inflammation (closed circles) and those that did not (open squares). Please note that CRP is on a log scale. There were no significant differences between groups

difference in the percentage of cells performing oxidative burst stimulated by *E. coli* or PMA or the intensity of the oxidative burst between groups (Fig. 8).

Peripheral lymphocyte composition

While peripheral blood lymphocyte count was significantly greater in the dogs that developed inflammation compared to those that did not, there were no differences in peripheral blood lymphocyte phenotype (CD4, CD8, CD21, Treg) between groups (Fig. 9).

Predicting inflammation

Best subsets regression was used to evaluate the variables unstimulated leukocyte IL-10 production, leukocyte NK-like activity, heart rate, lymphocyte count, gross tumor volume and [64Cu]ATSM scan SUV_{Max} max for prediction of inflammation. The model containing a combination of unstimulated leukocyte IL-10 production, heart rate, and gross tumor volume appeared to be the best predictor of inflammation (Adjusted R squared 0.553; Cp 2.405; $p <$ 0.034).

Discussion

Dogs that developed an inflammatory response to CNV-NT had a higher heart rate, larger gross tumor volume, greater tumor [64Cu]ATSM SUV_{Max}, increased constitutive leukocyte IL-10 production, more robust NK cell-like function and greater peripheral blood lymphocyte counts compared to dogs that did not develop an inflammatory response to CNV-NT. Of these, unstimulated leukocyte

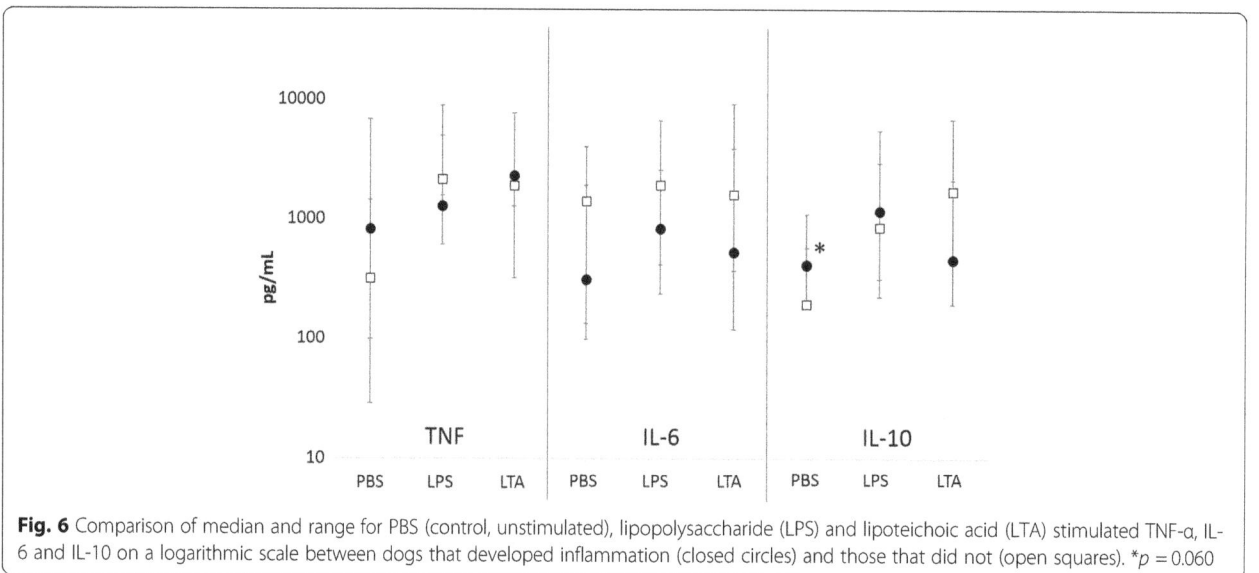

Fig. 6 Comparison of median and range for PBS (control, unstimulated), lipopolysaccharide (LPS) and lipoteichoic acid (LTA) stimulated TNF-α, IL-6 and IL-10 on a logarithmic scale between dogs that developed inflammation (closed circles) and those that did not (open squares). *$p = 0.060$

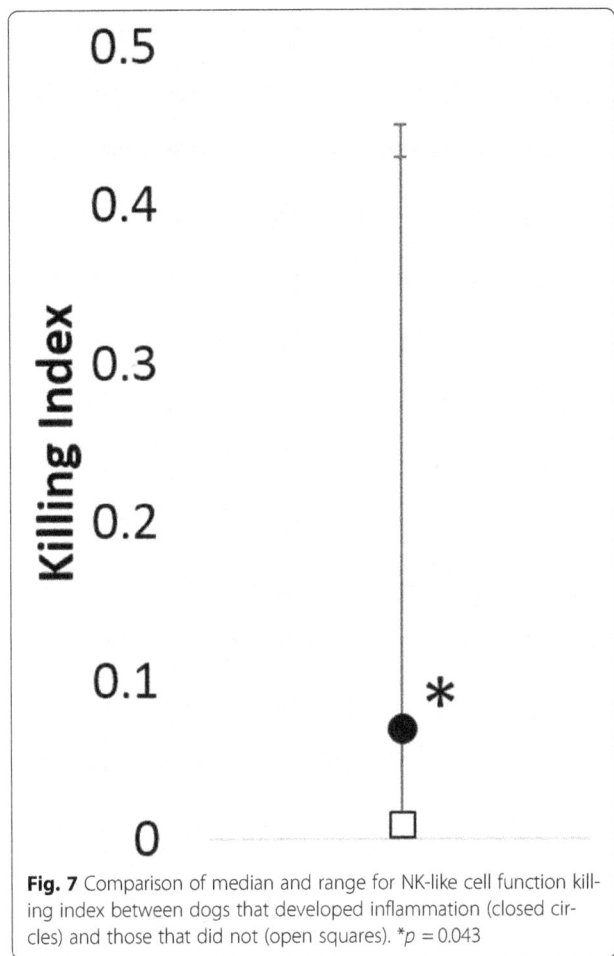

Fig. 7 Comparison of median and range for NK-like cell function killing index between dogs that developed inflammation (closed circles) and those that did not (open squares). *p = 0.043

IL-10 production, heart rate, and gross tumor volume appeared to be the best predictors of which dogs will develop an inflammatory response to CNV-NT.

Ideally, we would use routinely measured clinical parameters to identify which dogs are more likely to have an inflammatory response to CNV-NT. In this study, we evaluated clinical and tumor characteristics including gross tumor volume, [64Cu]ATSM uptake, heart rate, rectal temperature, hematocrit, peripheral white blood cell count and plasma globulin concentrations as possible clinical biomarkers. However, only heart rate, peripheral leukocyte cell count, [64Cu]ATSM uptake and gross tumor volume were significantly different between groups. Of these, heart rate and gross tumor volume were predictors of development of inflammation in response to CNV-NT administration in our best subsets model. Tachycardia could be caused by activation of the sympathetic nervous system which has been associated with more severe inflammatory responses to infection. This might explain why dogs that developed inflammation had higher heart rates. It has traditionally been expected that as tumor volume increases, the relative percentage of hypoxic tissue increases. Germination of CNV-NT appears to be more robust in tumors with larger volumes and greater hypoxic regions [14]. Therefore, it was expected that a greater [64Cu]ATSM SUV_{Max} and larger tumor volume would be associated with greater germination and a more intense inflammatory response.

Failure to generate an appropriate immune response to infection could impact the efficacy of CNV-NT bacteriolytic immunotherapy. Immunodysfunction has been identified in dogs and people with cancer. Altered neutrophil phagocytosis, respiratory burst function, cytokine production, peripheral circulating lymphocyte phenotype distribution and NK-cell like function have all been reported in dogs and people with cancer [5–8]. Whether these changes represent a paraneoplastic syndrome or primary immunodysfunction is unclear and it is likely that both mechanisms are observed in the dog and human population. In evaluating baseline immune system characteristics, we found that constitutive leukocyte IL-10 production, NK cell-like function and greater peripheral blood lymphocyte counts were significantly different

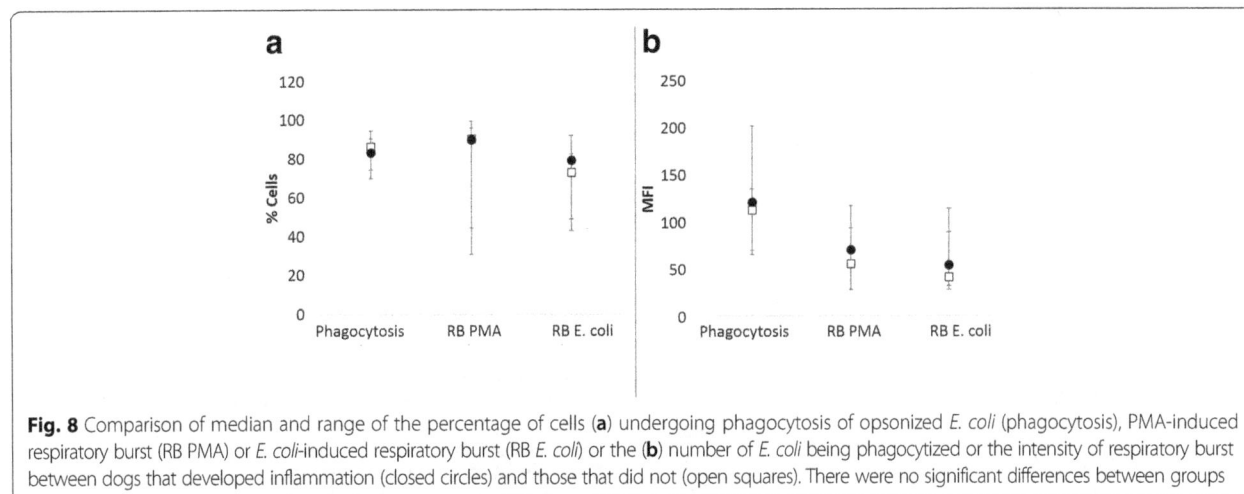

Fig. 8 Comparison of median and range of the percentage of cells (**a**) undergoing phagocytosis of opsonized *E. coli* (phagocytosis), PMA-induced respiratory burst (RB PMA) or *E. coli*-induced respiratory burst (RB *E. coli*) or the (**b**) number of *E. coli* being phagocytized or the intensity of respiratory burst between dogs that developed inflammation (closed circles) and those that did not (open squares). There were no significant differences between groups

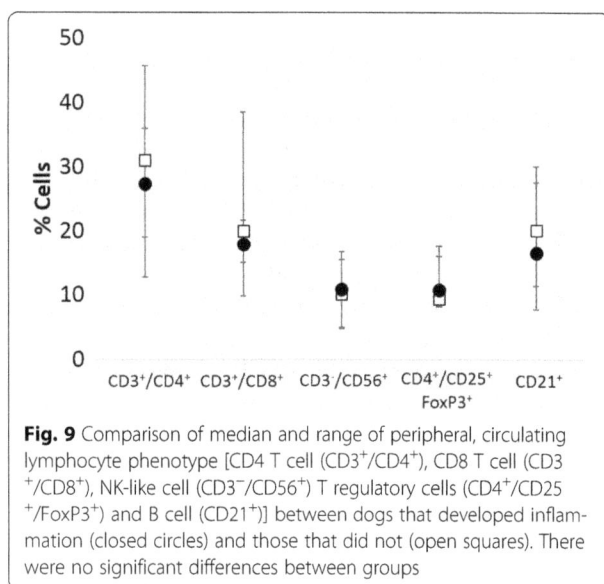

Fig. 9 Comparison of median and range of peripheral, circulating lymphocyte phenotype [CD4 T cell (CD3$^+$/CD4$^+$), CD8 T cell (CD3$^+$/CD8$^+$), NK-like cell (CD3$^-$/CD56$^+$) T regulatory cells (CD4$^+$/CD25$^+$/FoxP3$^+$) and B cell (CD21$^+$)] between dogs that developed inflammation (closed circles) and those that did not (open squares). There were no significant differences between groups

between dogs that developed inflammation in response to CNV-NT and those that did not. Of these, only constitutive leukocyte IL-10 production was selected as a predictor of development of inflammation in response to CNV-NT administration in our best subsets model. This was an unexpected finding since production of IL-10 is an immunosuppressive cytokine that has been implicated in cancer-associated immunodysfunction. It is possible that dogs with greater constitutive IL-10 production were immunosuppressed at the time of CNV-NT administration. This immunosuppression allowed CNV-NT germination to go unchecked by the immune system initially, allowing for a larger bacterial dose than dog with less IL-10 and a competent immune system. This greater bacterial dose eventually provided enough stimulus to overcome the immunosuppression and allow for the measurable inflammatory response.

We identified differences in NK cell-like function and peripheral blood lymphocyte counts between the dogs that developed inflammation and those that did not, however, these characteristics were not identified as good predictors of the development of inflammation. Stress-induced lymphopenia is a common finding in clinically ill dogs. This physiologic response is mediated by glucocorticoids, which also have direct immunosuppressive effects. It is possible that dogs with lymphopenia had greater circulating concentrations of glucocorticoids which resulted in suppression of the inflammatory response to CNV-NT. NK-like cells are important in anti-tumor and cytotoxic immune responses. NK-cells are also thought to be important effector cells during clostridium infection [15]. Greater baseline NK-like cell function might have allowed for a greater immune response to CNV-NT germination.

Larger-scale studies focused on the impact of stress hormones and baseline NK-like cell function are needed to tease out the importance of these markers.

There were several limitations to this study. First, this was a pilot study and therefore the number of dogs enrolled was limited and the cut-off point for determining significance was a $p < 0.10$. The rationale for this was to avoid type II statistical error and insure that any possible candidate biomarker would be identified to assist with development of future studies in a larger patient population. We also did not compare difference between IV and IT administration. Prior to clinical use of these biomarkers, they must be studied in a larger population and comparisons made between IV and IT administration. We did not correlate induction of inflammation with tumor response or with definitive germination of CNV-NT in this study, but this is needed to understand the full importance of these biomarkers. Further, while this study focused on solid tumors, there were three histologic tumor types in multiple anatomic locations. It is possible that this heterogeneity impacted our results. The lower limit of detection of the plasma immune markers are relatively high due to the relative analytical insensitivity of the currently available assays for dogs. In the future, more analytically sensitive assays should be developed.

Conclusion

In this pilot study, we identified several parameters that might help identify dogs with cancer that are more likely to have an inflammatory response to CNV-NT. In the future, investigators should consider evaluating if heart rate, tumor volume, surrogate markers of tumor hypoxia, IL-10 production, NK-like cell function and circulating lymphocyte count could be useful markers for patient selection or stratification of patients in clinical trials evaluating CNV-NT for the treatment of cancer.

Acknowledgements
The authors thank Juliana Amorim and Debbie Tate for their technical assistance.

Funding
Funding was provided by Biomed Valley Discoveries. Biomed Valley Discoveries provided monetary support and NT-CNV spores. Some of the authors (SS, LZ, DT) are employed by Biomed Valley Discoveries. These individuals contributed to the initial study design, interpretation of the data analysis and final manuscript review.

Authors' contributions
AD developed the study design, analyzed and interpreted the data and was a major contributor in writing the manuscript. SB developed the study design, managed the clinical trial, analyzed and interpreted the data and was a contributor in writing the manuscript. YZ performed the immunologic assays and interpreted the data. SS, LZ and DT developed the study design

Identification of immunologic and clinical characteristics that predict inflammatory response...

99

and interpreted the data. JB developed the study design, managed the clinical trial, and analyzed and interpreted the data. All authors read, edited and approved the final manuscript.

Consent for publication
NA

Competing interests
Some of the authors (SS, LZ, DT) are employed by the company which provided CNV-NT and the funding for this clinical trial.

Author details
[1]Department of Veterinary Medicine and Surgery, Comparative Internal Medicine Laboratory, University of Missouri, College of Veterinary Medicine, 900 E. Campus Dr, Columbia, MO 65203, USA. [2]Department of Veterinary Medicine and Surgery, Comparative Oncology Radiobiology and Epigenetics Laboratory, University of Missouri, College of Veterinary Medicine, 900 E. Campus Dr, Columbia, MO 65203, USA. [3]Biomed Valley Discoveries, 4435 Main Street, Suite 550, Kansas City, MO 64111, USA.

References
1. Agrawal N, Bettegowda C, Cheong I, Geschwind JF, Drake CG, Hipkiss EL, Tatsumi M, Dang LH, Diaz LA Jr, Pomper M, et al. Bacteriolytic therapy can generate a potent immune response against experimental tumors. Proc Natl Acad Sci U S A. 2004;101(42):15172–7.
2. Roberts NJ, Zhang L, Janku F, Collins A, Bai RY, Staedtke V, Rusk AW, Tung D, Miller M, Roix J, et al. Intratumoral injection of Clostridium novyi-NT spores induces antitumor responses. Sci Transl Med. 2014;6(249):249ra111.
3. Krick EL, Sorenmo KU, Rankin SC, Cheong I, Kobrin B, Thornton K, Kinzler KW, Vogelstein B, Zhou S, Diaz LA Jr. Evaluation of Clostridium novyi-NT spores in dogs with naturally occurring tumors. Am J Vet Res. 2012;73(1): 112–8.
4. Diaz LA Jr, Cheong I, Foss CA, Zhang X, Peters BA, Agrawal N, Bettegowda C, Karim B, Liu G, Khan K, et al. Pharmacologic and toxicologic evaluation of C. Novyi-NT spores. Toxicol Sci. 2005;88(2):562–75.
5. Axiak-Bechtel S, Fowler B, Yu DH, Amorim J, Tsuruta K, DeClue A. Chemotherapy and remission status do not alter pre-existing innate immune dysfunction in dogs with lymphoma. Res Vet Sci. 2014;97(2):230–7.
6. Fowler BL, Axiak SM, DeClue AE. Blunted pathogen-associated molecular pattern motif induced TNF, IL-6 and IL-10 production from whole blood in dogs with lymphoma. Vet Immunol Immunopathol. 2011;144(1-2):167–71.
7. LeBlanc CJ, LeBlanc AK, Jones MM, Bartges JW, Kania SA. Evaluation of peripheral blood neutrophil function in tumor-bearing dogs. Vet Clin Pathol. 2010;39(2):157–63.
8. Zhang Y, Axiak-Bechtel S, Friedman Cowan C, Amorim J, Tsuruta K, DeClue AE. Evaluation of immunomodulatory effect of recombinant human granulocyte-macrophage colony-stimulating factor on polymorphonuclear cell from dogs with cancer in vitro. Vet Comp Oncol. 2016;15(3):968–79.
9. Floras AN, Holowaychuk MK, Bienzle D, Bersenas AM, Sharif S, Harvey T, Nordone SK, Wood GA. N-terminal pro-C-natriuretic peptide and cytokine kinetics in dogs with endotoxemia. J Vet Intern Med. 2014;28(5):1447–53.
10. Karlsson I, Wernersson S, Ambrosen A, Kindahl H, Södersten F, Wang L, Hagman R. Increased concentrations of C-reactive protein but not high-mobility group box 1 in dogs with naturally occurring sepsis. Veterinary Immunology and Immunopathology. 2013;156(1–2):64–72.
11. Filiz Ibraimi, Björn Ekberg, Dario Kriz, Gertrud Danielsson, Leif Bülow. Preparation of a portable point-of-care in vitro diagnostic system, for quantification of canine C-reactive protein, based on a magnetic two-site immunoassay. Analytical and Bioanalytical Chemistry, 2013;405(18):6001–6007.
12. Deitschel SJ, Kerl ME, Chang CH, DeClue AE. Age-associated changes to pathogen-associated molecular pattern-induced inflammatory mediator production in dogs. J Vet Emerg Crit Care (San Antonio). 2010;20(5):494–502.
13. Yu D, Kim J, Park C, Park J. Serial changes of CD4+CD25+FoxP3+ regulatory T cell in canine model of sepsis induced by endotoxin. J Vet Med Sci. 2014; 76(5):777–80.
14. Maletzki C, Gock M, Klier U, Klar E, Linnebacher M. Bacteriolytic therapy of experimental pancreatic carcinoma. World J Gastroenterol. 2010;16(28): 3546–52.
15. Van Andel RA, Hook RR Jr, Franklin CL, Besch-Williford CL, van Rooijen N, Riley LK. Effects of neutrophil, natural killer cell, and macrophage depletion on murine Clostridium piliforme infection. Infect Immun. 1997;65(7):2725–31.

13

Ultrasonographic features of adrenal gland lesions in dogs can aid in diagnosis

Elena Pagani[1*], Massimiliano Tursi[1], Chiara Lorenzi[1], Alberto Tarducci[1], Barbara Bruno[1], Enrico Corrado Borgogno Mondino[2] and Renato Zanatta[1]

Abstract

Background: Ultrasonography to visualize adrenal gland lesions and evaluate incidentally discovered adrenal masses in dogs has become more reliable with advances in imaging techniques. However, correlations between sonographic and histopathological changes have been elusive. The goal of our study was to investigate which ultrasound features of adrenal gland abnormalities could aid in discriminating between benign and malignant lesions. To this end, we compared diagnosis based on ultrasound appearance and histological findings and evaluated ultrasound criteria for predicting malignancy.

Results: Clinical records of 119 dogs that had undergone ultrasound adrenal gland and histological examination were reviewed. Of these, 50 dogs had normal adrenal glands whereas 69 showed pathological ones. Lesions based on histology were classified as cortical adrenal hyperplasia ($n = 67$), adenocarcinoma ($n = 17$), pheochromocytoma ($n = 10$), metastases ($n = 7$), adrenal adenoma ($n = 4$), and adrenalitis ($n = 4$). Ultrasonographic examination showed high specificity (100%) but low sensitivity (63.7%) for identifying the adrenal lesions, which improved with increasing lesion size. Analysis of ultrasonographic predictive parameters showed a significant association between lesion size and malignant tumors. All adrenal gland lesions >20 mm in diameter were histologically confirmed as malignant neoplasms (pheochromocytoma and adenocarcinoma). Vascular invasion was a specific but not sensitive predictor of malignancy. As nodular shape was associated with benign lesions and irregular enlargement with malignant ones, this parameter could be used as diagnostic tool. Bilaterality of adrenal lesions was a useful ultrasonographic criterion for predicting benign lesions, as cortical hyperplasia.

Conclusions: Abnormal appearance of structural features on ultrasound images (e.g., adrenal gland lesion size, shape, laterality, and echotexture) may aid in diagnosis, but these features alone were not pathognomic. Lesion size was the most direct ultrasound predictive criterion. Large and irregular masses seemed to be better predictors of malignant neoplasia and lesions <20 mm in diameter and nodular in shape were often identified as cortical hyperplastic nodules or adenomas.

Keywords: Adrenal gland, Ultrasonography, Dogs, Lesion, Tumor

Background

In human medicine, the use of advanced imaging techniques (e.g., ultrasound, computed tomography, scintigraphy, and magnetic resonance imaging) has resulted in the increasing identification of incidental adrenal gland lesions [1]. Among the methods of diagnostic imaging, ultrasound is considered a relatively rapid, non-invasive, inexpensive and reliable modality to evaluate suspected

adrenal masses [2]. Beginning in the mid-1990s, ultrasound imaging has become a widely used diagnostic tool in veterinary medicine. Its application in small animal practice has yielded extensive information on normal adrenal gland appearance in the dog [3–10], but it has also led to an increase in the incidental discovery of adrenal masses. Though a common occurrence in diagnostic imaging, adrenal masses can constitute a significant clinical dilemma in the dog [11]. They may be benign (e.g., hyperplasia, myelolipoma, cortical adenoma) or malignant (e.g., pheochromocytoma, cortical carcinoma, and metastases) [12]. Adrenal gland lesions (nodules and masses)

* Correspondence: elena.pagani@unito.it
[1]Department of Veterinary Sciences, University of Turin, Largo Paolo Braccini 2-5, 10095 Grugliasco, TO, Italy
Full list of author information is available at the end of the article

commonly develop in older dogs, but surgery is indicated in only a small fraction of such cases, usually in malignant and hormone-secreting tumors [13]. While ultrasonography is an effective method for localizing adrenal lesions, standardized ultrasound criteria to distinguish benign from malignant lesions or functional cortisol-secreting from non-functional tumors are lacking [12]. In large-scale studies involving human patients, ultrasound morphological and dimensional criteria have proven reliable in differentiating adrenal lesions: tumor malignancy potential estimated on the basis of its dimensions alone showed that about 90% of malignant tumors were >40 mm in diameter [1, 14]. In the dog, only one study to date has compared the ultrasonographic appearance of adrenal lesions with their histopathological characteristics. The study was unable to establish definitive ultrasound criteria to differentiate benign from malignant lesions owing in part to the small sample size [12]. In the present study involving a large sample of dogs, we asked which ultrasound characteristics of adrenal lesions could predict for malignancy and how accurate ultrasound diagnosis (specificity and sensitivity) was as compared with histopathological diagnosis.

Methods

For this retrospective study, we reviewed the clinical records of dogs presented to the Veterinary Teaching Hospital, University of Turin (Italy), between 2009 and 2015. Dogs for which a definitive histopathological diagnosis was available and that had undergone adrenal gland ultrasonography were included whether or not the manifestation of clinical signs was related to adrenal disease. Adrenal glands were removed and collected during adrenal glandectomy or at necropsy if the dog was euthanized. The glands were placed in 10% buffered formalin and stained with hematoxylin and eosin, Grimelius argyrophil, and Gomori trichrome stains for histopathological examination. An experienced veterinary pathologist (M.T.), unaware of the ultrasonographic findings, reviewed the macroscopic and histopathology sections of all adrenal glands.

Ultrasonography was performed using a B-mode ultrasonographic scanner (MyLab 70 X Vision machine, Esaote, Florence, Italy), with linear (7.5–12 MHz) and microconvex transducers (5.5–6.6MHz). An experienced examiner (R.Z.) carried out the ultrasonographic procedures. During abdominal ultrasonography, both adrenal glands were scanned; if lesions were detected, adrenal gland echostructure, echogenicity, dimension, laterality, number, and adjacent vascular invasion were recorded and evaluated. Lesions were classified as follows: A) homogeneous enlargement defined as normal adrenal gland shape with rounded contour; B) irregular enlargement defined as total loss of normal adrenal shape,

echostructure, and dimension, with a mass aspect; C) nodular lesion defined as a round, well-defined focal parenchymal lesion, without loss of global shape; and D) multiple nodules defined as multiple, well-defined focal parenchymal lesions, without loss of adrenal global shape. Lesion size was determined by measuring the greatest dorsoventral and craniocaudal dimension in a longitudinal plane, as described by Hoerauf et al. (1999) [15]. Conventional gray-scale and color Doppler ultrasound were used to assess the adjacent vascular structures.

Statistical analysis to compare the ultrasonographic predictive parameters among benign and malignant lesions was performed by R software (version 3.1.2, R Core Team 2015). The Shapiro-Wilk normality test was used to assess normality of the data. Since data were not normally distributed, they were reported as medians and ranges. Categorical parameters (side and shape) were analysed using $\chi 2$ test and Fisher's exact test, while numerical parameter (size) by Kruskal–Wallis test and Wilcoxon signed-rank test was used as post hoc test. Significance was set at $P < 0.05$. Ultrasound sensitivity and specificity in detecting adrenal lesions were calculated using 2x2 contingency tables.

Ultrasound characteristics of each lesion were compared with their corresponding histopathological characteristics. The processing concerning the description of the statistic distributions of observations was achieved by a self-developed routine implemented in the IDL 8.0 programming language (ITT Visual Information Solutions).

Results

The clinical records of 119 dogs that had undergone ultrasound adrenal gland and histological examination were reviewed. Unilateral adrenal glandectomy was performed in 9 dogs and necropsy in 110. Histology was performed on 229 adrenal glands. Histopathological changes were noted in adrenal glands obtained from 69/119 dogs, with bilateral lesions in 36 dogs and unilateral in 33. Adrenal glands were histologically normal in 50/119 dogs.

Dogs with adrenal gland lesions, based on histopathological exam, were generally older (median age 10.5 years, range 1–17; median body weight 17.5 kg, range 2.3–52) than those with normal adrenal glands (median age 5.8 years, range 1.5–12; median body weight 23.1 kg, range 3.5–65) and equally distributed between sexes, 47.5% were male and 52.5% female. Forty-seven different breeds were included. The most commonly represented breeds were mixed breed (32), German Shepherd Dog (7), Labrador Retriever (5), Beagle (5), Boxer (5), Pit bull (4), French Bulldog (3), Bull Terrier (3), Yorkshire Terrier (3), Golden Retriever (3), Doberman Pincher (3), Schnauzer (3), Border Collie (2), Dogue de Bordeaux (2), Dachshund (2), Cocker Spaniel (2), Dalmatian (2), and Doberman (2).

Other less represented breeds (31) were found. Age, sex, weight and breed were not significantly different between dogs with normal adrenal glands and pathological ones and between malignant and benign lesions.

Histological diagnosis revealed cortical hyperplasia ($n = 67$), adenocarcinoma ($n = 17$), pheochromocytoma ($n = 10$), metastases ($n = 7$), adenoma ($n = 4$), and other minor lesions (adrenalitis) ($n = 4$). The prevalence of adrenal neoplasms was 18%, of which 82.2% were primary adrenal tumors and 17.8% metastatic lesions. Ultrasound imaging to detect adrenal lesions had high specificity (100%) but low sensitivity (63.7%). Adrenal lesions were not displayed in 56.8% (62/109) of cases: 67.7% (47/62) as cortical hyperplasia, 9.6% (6/62) as cortical adenocarcinoma, 6.4% (4/62) as metastasis, 4.8% (3/62) as cortical adenoma, 1.6% (1/62) as pheochromocytoma, and 1.6% (1/62) as adrenalitis.

Table 1 presents the number, type, and characteristics of adrenal lesions identified at ultrasonography and histopathology.

Adrenal carcinoma was the most common type of adrenal primary neoplasia (17/31), and it was generally unilateral, affecting the left and right adrenal gland in 8 (47%) and 9 (53%) dogs, respectively. Adrenal glandectomy was performed in 9 dogs with histopathologically confirmed unilateral adrenal carcinoma while necroscopy was performed in the other 8 cases, in 4 of which the contralateral gland was found atrophic. The adrenal gland usually maintained its normal shape. In 82.3% (14/17) of cases the tumor presented a nodular shape (single or multiple nodules) (Fig. 1), of which 76.4% (13/17) showed a lesion >10 mm. Of note, in 2 cases ultrasound overestimated the actual lesion size. The median diameter was 15 mm (range 3-37). The echotexture was generally heterogeneous, with several small areas of inner calcification

producing acoustic shadowing. In the patients with adrenocortical carcinoma, echogenicity ranged from hypo- to hyperechoic, compared to the renal cortex, and it was associated with microscopic findings of focal areas of necrosis and hemorrhage. Evidence of vascular invasion of the phrenicoabdominal vessels was noted in 23.5% (4/17) of dogs with a right-sided tumor. No invasion of the caudal vena cava or abdominal aorta was noted. Ultrasonography failed to detect lesions in 6 cases: lesions were <3 mm in 4 cases and <20 mm in 2 cases.

Pheochromocytoma was the second most frequent primary adrenal neoplasia (10/31). In 5 cases a large, amorphous encapsulated mass, with irregular margins and loss of normal shape and parenchymal structure, was visualized (Fig. 2). The remaining lesions were solitary or multiple nodules with normal adrenal shape. In 6/10 cases, pheochromocytoma was >10 mm in diameter and in 3 cases ultrasound overestimated the actual lesion size. The median diameter was 13 mm (range 7–62). No specificity in echogenicity was noted. Tumor thrombus extending into the phrenicoabdominal vein and caudal vena cava was visualized in 40% (4/10) of cases. In 1 case, both adrenal glands were affected by a pheochromocytoma caudally displacing the kidneys, with distortion of normal renal shape. No distant metastases were found in any of these 10 dogs. Ultrasound failed to detect pheochromocytoma in only 1 case and no gross lesions were detected at necroscopy.

Cortical adenoma was a rare adrenal primary neoplasia (4/31), presenting as solitary or multiple nodular lesions affecting both adrenal glands (median diameter 5.5 mm, range 4–15). The only one visualized on ultrasound appeared as heterogeneous multifocal nodules throughout the parenchymal tissue, with several small areas of inner calcification (Fig. 3).

Table 1 Ultrasonographic and histopathological features of adrenal gland lesions

Histopathological diagnosis		No. of lesions	Adrenal side			Lesion shape				Lesion size (mm)			
			L	R	Bi	A	B	C	D	<3	3.1-10	10.1-20	>20.1
Cortical Hyperplasia	US	20	6	4	10	3		17				15	5	
	AP	67	1	2	64	1	1	23	42	34	31	2	
Cortical Adenoma	US	1	1						1			1	
	AP	4	2	2				2	2		3	1	
Cortical Carcinoma	US	11	5	6		1	3	6	1			5	6
	AP	17	8	9		1	2	12	2		4	9	4
Pheochromocytoma	US	9	2	5	2		5	2	2			3	6
	AP	10	3	5	2		5	2	3		4	2	4
Metastasis	US	3		1	2			1	2	2	1		
	AP	7		1	6				7	6	1		

US Ultrasonographic findings, *AP* histopathological findings, *L* left side, *R* right side, *Bi* bilateral side. *A* Homogeneous enlargement, *B* Irregular enlargement, *C* Nodular lesion, *D* Multiple nodular lesions. Minor lesions (4 adrenalitis) were not express in the table because not detect by both ultrasonographic and macroscopical evaluations

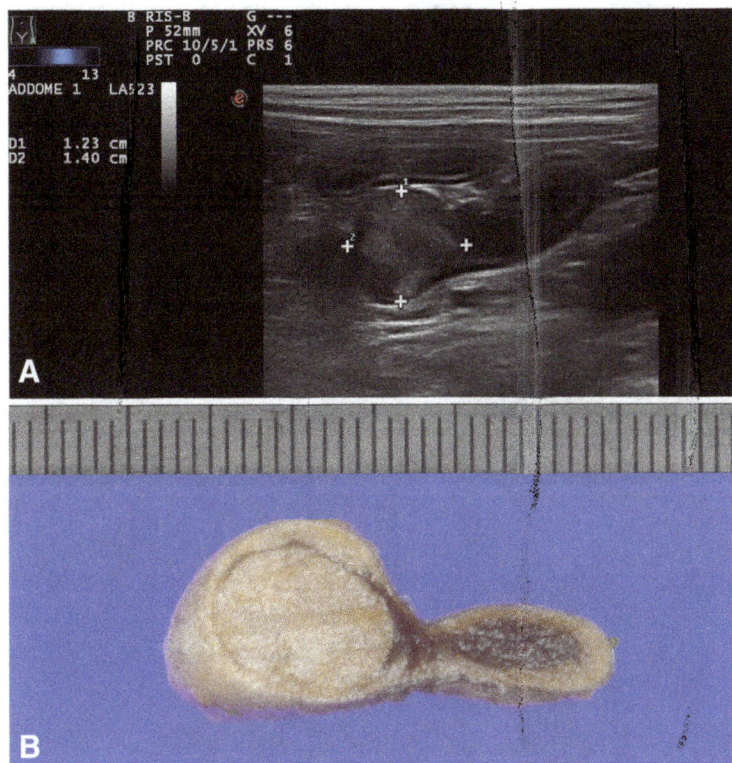

Fig. 1 CORTICAL CARCINOMA: **a**) ultrasonographic and **b**) macroscopical images of left adrenal cortical carcinoma nodular lesion of, illustrating a left adrenal nodular lesion, 12 x14 mm size, middle uniform echogenicity, and well defined margins

Compared with adrenocortical adenomas, the nodules in cortical hyperplasia were smaller and more numerous. Adrenocortical hyperplasia (67 cases) affected both adrenal glands in 32/35 (91%) cases. All adrenal glands affected by cortical hyperplasia maintained their normal shape. In 97% of the cases they were <10 mm and in 55% of them they had a multinodular aspect affecting the entire glandular parenchyma. Ultrasound detected cortical hyperplasia in 30% of cases; hyperplasia was characterized by focal nodules ranging from 3.1 to 10 mm in diameter (Fig. 4).

Adrenal metastasis was usually bilateral and presented as multifocal and heterogeneous nodules with irregular margins (Fig. 5). The adrenal metastases stemmed from 2 primary neoplasms: splenic hemangiosarcoma with bilateral lesions in 3 dogs and lung carcinoma in 1 dog. All metastatic lesions were <10 mm in diameter.

A comparison between the ultrasonographic predictive parameters for the diagnosis of benign (cortical hyperplasia and cortical adenoma) and malignant (cortical carcinoma, pheochromocytoma, metastasis) lesions showed significant statistical differences ($P < 0.05$) for all the parameters evaluated (lesion side, shape and size) (Table 2). Furthermore, a statistically significant association was noted between ultrasonographic nodular shape and the presence of benign lesions, such as cortical hyperplasia

and cortical adenoma ($P = 0.006$), whereas an irregular enlargement of the adrenal glands was significantly associated with malignant neoplasia, such as pheochromocytoma and cortical carcinoma ($P = 0.004$). Bilaterality of adrenal lesions was significantly associated with benign lesions, such as cortical hyperplasia ($P = 0.04$) and right adrenal lesions with malignant lesions ($P = 0.03$).

Discussion

The prevalence of adrenal gland neoplasia in our study was 18.1%, of which 81.7% were primary adrenal neoplasia and 18.3% metastatic lesions. The most frequent neoplastic type was adrenocortical carcinoma (44.7%), followed by pheochromocytoma (26.3%), metastases (18.4%), and adrenocortical adenoma (10.5%). A high prevalence (32%) of adrenal cortical hyperplasia was also noted. As reported in humans, the majority of histologically diagnosed adrenal lesions were benign, such as cortical hyperplasia (65.1% of cases in our series) rather than neoplastic [1]. Our results are in agreement with data reported by a previous study in dogs based on histological examination showing a prevalence of 19% of adrenal neoplasia and 41.5% cortical hyperplasia [16].

Adrenal lesions are more likely to be found in older dogs [11] with a median age of 10.5 years for dogs with adrenal gland lesions and 5.8 years for those with

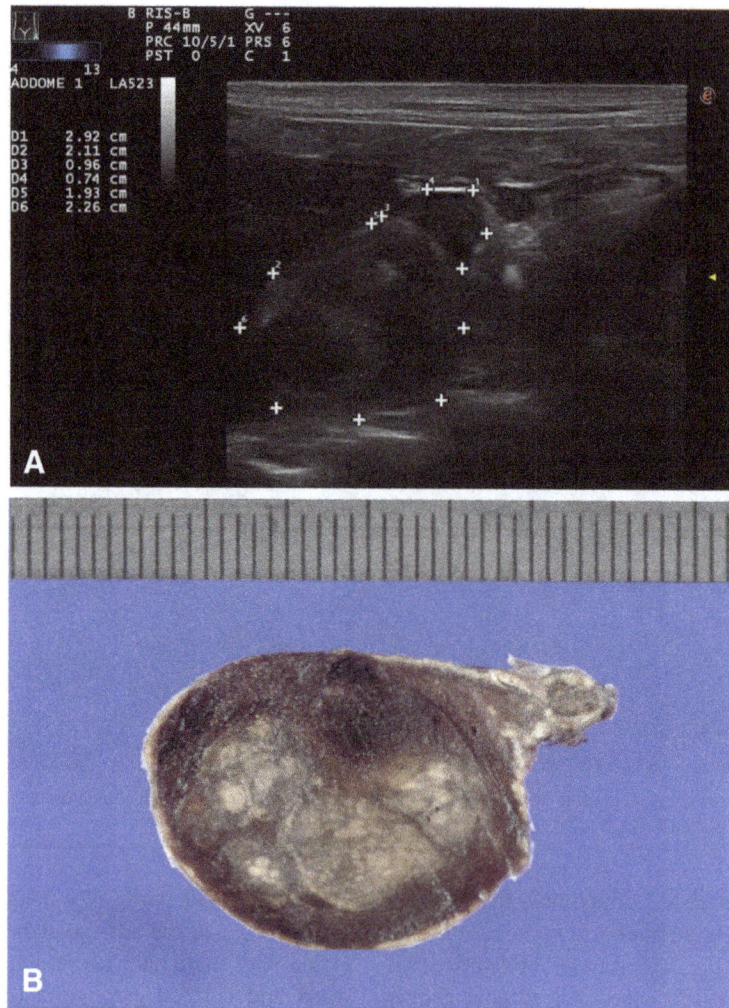

Fig. 2 PHEOCHROMOCYTOMA: **a**) ultrasonographic and **b**) macroscopical images of right adrenal mass pheochromocytoma of, 19 x 22 mm size, heterogenic echotexture and irregular margins

normal adrenal glands. Although no statistically significant differences between age and type of adrenal lesions were found ($P = 0.20$), the incidence of cortical hyperplasia seemed to increase with advancing age, with 67% of the dogs showing cortical hyperplasia being ≥ 8 years old. Chronic or severe illness in old dogs may reflect an increase in adrenocortical demand in response to stress and cause adrenocortical hyperplasia. Adrenocortical hyperplasia is also described to be more frequent in small dogs, but in this study there was no significant correlation between adrenal lesion type and body weight [11].

In terms of diagnostic tools, ultrasound imaging had high specificity (100%) but low sensitivity (63.7%) in the detection of lesions. However, sensitivity seemed to improve with increasing lesion dimension. Ultrasonography failed to detect lesions <3 mm in diameter in 95% of the cases and lesions between 3 and 10 mm in 46.8% of the cases. Ultrasound failed to detect 67.7% (47/62) of

cortical hyperplasia lesions and 5/7 of the metastatic lesions. In contrast, nearly all lesions (20/22) >10 mm were correctly detected.

Lesions that appear benign on ultrasound images can be confused with other types of abnormalities, including malignancy. Our data indicate that although structural features, such as lesion size, shape, laterality, and echotexture, may provide helpful diagnostic ultrasound criteria, such features alone are not necessarily pathognomonic. Of the parameters evaluated, lesion size seemed to be a distinguishing feature, as smaller adrenal lesions associated with a benign outcome whereas larger ones were more likely malignant ($P = 0.001$). Adrenal gland lesion dimension may be a useful ultrasonographic indicator to predict malignancy. Seventy percent (19/27) of adrenal primary tumors were in fact >10 mm, 30% >20 mm, and all adrenal lesions >20 mm in diameter were malignant tumors (pheochromocytoma and carcinoma both in 4 cases each).

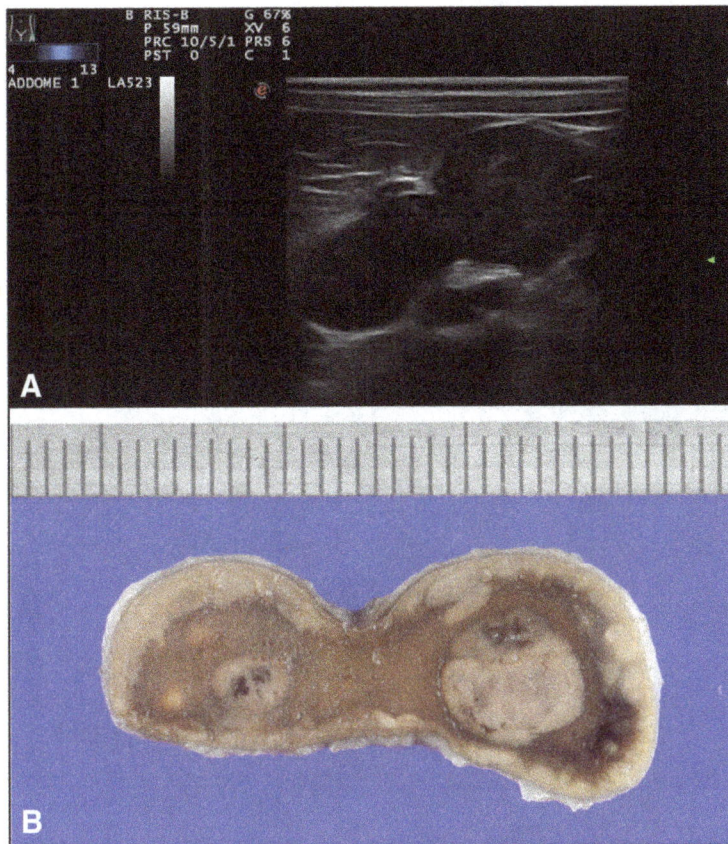

Fig. 3 CORTICAL ADENOMA: **a)** ultrasonographic and **b)** macroscopical images of left adrenal gland cortical adenoma showing with heterogeneous multifocal nodules with small areas of necrosis, calcification, and hemorrhaging

This finding is consistent with previous reports describing malignant adrenal tumors as lesions >20 mm in diameter [17–19] or 75% between 20 and 40 mm and 100% >40 mm in maximum diameter [12]. In agreement with this Cook et al. (2014) recently showed that malignancy should be strongly suspected in adrenal masses measuring >20 mm in diameter. In in such cases adrenal glandectomy seem highly recommended [11]. Similar data were reported also in human studies, where larger lesions (>40 mm) were more likely associated with malignant tumors [20]. In our study, adrenal lesions <3 mm were usually benign, with 85% (34/40) of the cases histologically diagnosed as cortical hyperplasia. However, small size can still be misleading because other small lesions may be malignant, as seen in the 6 cases of metastases. No data are available on adrenal gland lesions measuring <10 mm because this is the accepted cut-off value of adrenal gland maximum diameter set as an exclusion criterion [11].

Among the other ultrasonographic lesion features, abnormal adrenal gland shape may be a useful tool in diagnosis. Nodular shape was significantly associated with cortical hyperplasia, which was highly represented (67/119); however, all the metastatic lesions, the majority of which were cortical carcinoma (14/17), and approximately half of pheochromocytoma, showed a nodular or multinodular ultrasonographic aspects. In contrast, irregular adrenal gland enlargement was seen only in the presence of primary malignant tumors, as previously reported [12].

Adrenal laterality (right or left sides) was not found to be a useful predictor for adrenal gland abnormality, whereas bilateral lesions were significantly associated with cortical hyperplasia. As described in previous studies, however, this morphological feature could be confused with malignant metastatic lesions and with rare cases of pheochromocytoma [11, 19].

According to human and veterinary literature, vascular invasion may be a useful indicator of malignancy. Indeed, all 8 cases (4/17 cortical carcinoma and 4/10 pheochromocytoma) were diagnosed as vascular infiltration of malignant neoplastic cells, but it was not specific for the type of primary adrenal neoplasia [1, 12, 21]. In our sample, vascular invasion was a specific, but not sensitive ultrasonographic parameter. However, a possible but uncommon association between adrenal hyperplasia and vascular invasion of the distal aorta consequent to the

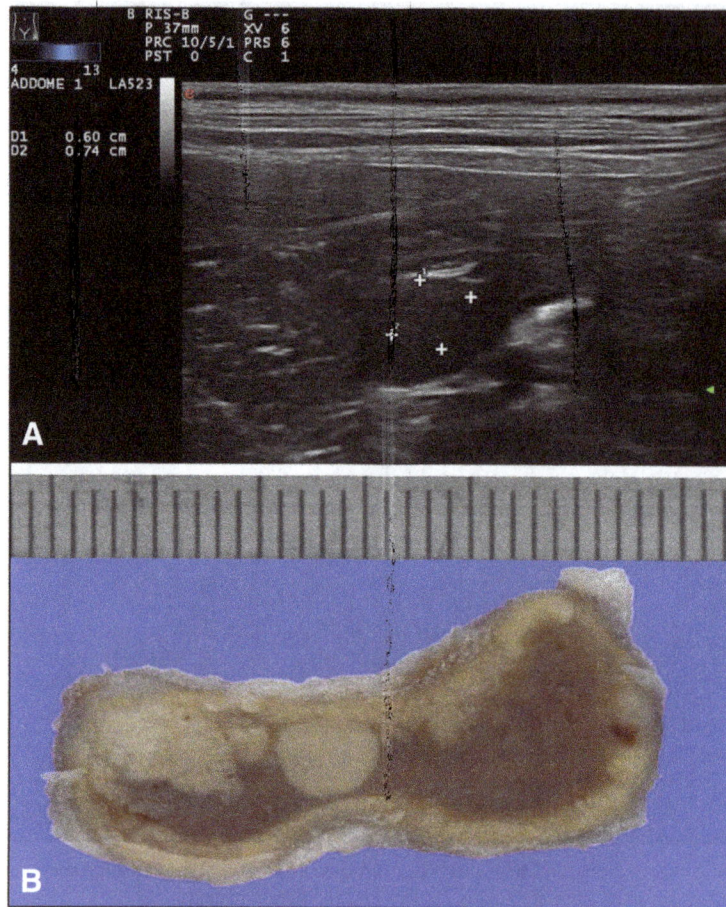

Fig. 4 CORTICAL HYPERPLASIA: **a**) ultrasonographic and **b**) macroscopical images of left adrenal gland cortical hyperplasia with multinodular aggregated lesions

hypercoagulability state often accompanied hyperadrenocorticism has been described [12].

Consistent with previous findings, adrenocortical carcinomas were generally unilateral, with an equal distribution between sides [22], with atrophy of the contralateral gland in 4 cases, suggesting a hormone-dependent neoplasia, as described elsewhere [2]. In agreement with previous studies [12] cortical adenomas were macroscopically characterized by a nodular pattern. In humans, they usually present as homogeneous hypoechogenic and solid focal or multifocal nodules with well-defined borders [1]. The only adenoma identified by ultrasound in our study appeared as heterogeneous multifocal nodules with several small areas of inner calcification producing acoustic shadowing. Calcification, necrosis, and hemorrhage are not microscopic features typical of adenoma but they are usually found in large lesions [12, 21]. Differentiation between cortical adenoma and adenocarcinoma based on shape, parenchymal structure, and mineralization was not possible, since 50% of adenoma and carcinoma show calcium parenchymal deposition [22].

In half of the cases of pheochromocytoma, the tumor was visualized as a large, amorphous encapsulated mass, with irregular margins and loss of normal shape and parenchymal structure. The remaining lesions presented as solitary or multiple nodules maintaining normal global shape. This pattern of pheochromocytoma has rarely been described [11, 12] and could be confused with other neoplastic lesions. Echogenicity was not specific for malignancy. The mixed echopatterns seemed to correlate with the microscopic evidence of hemorrhagic necrotic areas, as described by Poffenbarger et al. [18]. Larger pheochromocytoma seemed to be more heterogeneous, with predominant cystic-necrotic areas. Vascular tumor thrombus was present in 40% of cases, but without distant metastases, consistent with observations by Rosenstein [23]. In humans, pheochromocytoma is usually a benign tumor and as such is not expected to invade adjacent tissues [1]. In our study, all 10 cases of histologically diagnosed pheochromocytoma were malignant with vascular invasion, confirming its association with malignancy in dogs [12, 15].

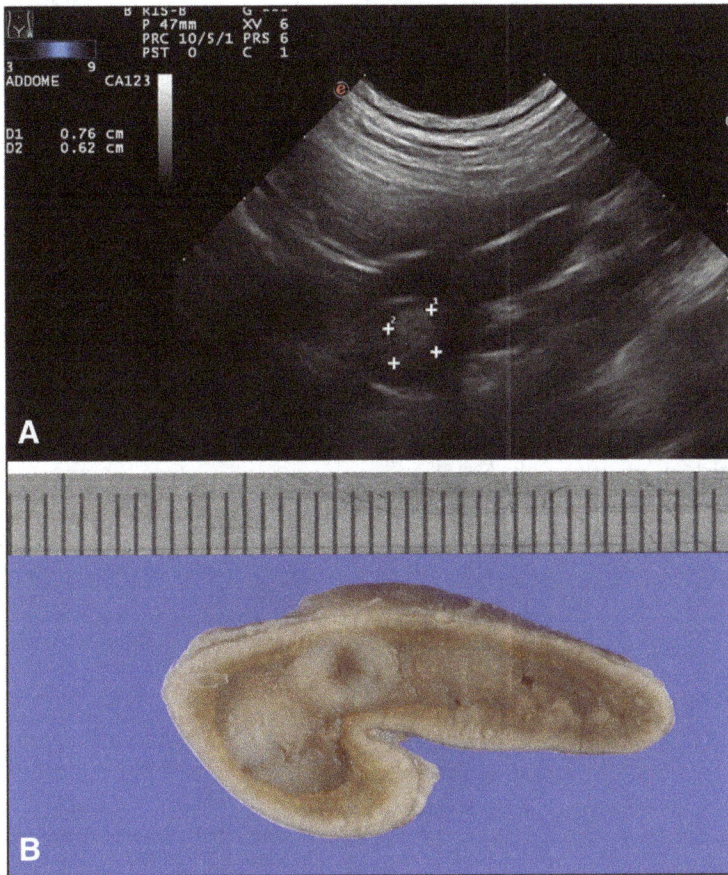

Fig. 5 METASTASES: **a**) ultrasonographic and **b**) macroscopical images showing a right adrenal gland lung carcinoma metastases with multifocal and heterogenic nodular lesions with irregular margins

Adrenal metastasis was frequently bilateral, presenting as multifocal and heterogeneous nodules with irregular margins. In humans, adrenal metastases vary considerably in size and infiltration pattern depending on the type of primary neoplasia from which they originate and are usually described as bilateral lesions [1]. In our series, the metastatic lesions showed similar characteristics, which could have been due to the high prevalence (85.7%) of the same primary neoplasia.

The present study has some limitations. Uncommon lesions of canine adrenal glands, such as myelolipomas, which might have led to different conclusions about ultrasound accuracy [24], were not included,. Furthermore, a high number of dogs that underwent necropsy were affected by the presence of terminal illness, which might bias the population enrolled.

Conclusions

As the use of ultrasonography as a diagnostic screening tool continues to increase, we can expect to recognize and diagnose more cases of occult or preclinical adrenal disease. Advances in diagnostic imaging technologies will also improve the identification of small lesions (<10 mm). Although most of them were benign, such as hyperplastic

Table 2 Ultrasonographic predictive parameters for the diagnosis of benign and malignant adrenal lesions

Histopathological diagnosis	No. of lesions	Adrenal side			Lesion shape				Lesion size
		n (%)			n (%)				Median (Range) mm
		L	R	Bi	A	B	C	D	
Benign Lesions	21	7 (50)	4 (25)	10 (71.4)	3 (75)	0 (0)	17 (65.4)	1 (16.7)	7.05 (3-16.1)
Malignant Lesions	23	7 (50)	12 (75)	4 (28.6)	1 (25)	8 (100)	9 (34.9)	5 (83.3)	10.8 (3-70.5)
p-value		1	0.03*	0.04*	0.33	0.004*	0.006*	0.18	0.0001*

L left side, R right side, Bi bilateral side. A Homogeneous enlargement, B Irregular enlargement, C Nodular lesion, D Multiple nodular lesions. *P <0.05

nodules, they could still constitute a challenging clinical issue. Large masses or nodules (>20 mm), associated or not with vascular invasion, seemed to be a direct parameter to predict malignant adrenal gland neoplasia, while vascular invasion was a specific but not sensitive predictor of malignancy. Lesions <20 mm in diameter and with nodular shape were usually cortical hyperplastic nodules or adenomas. Other criteria, such as adrenal gland laterality, were not specific for predicting malignancy, because only the right side was significantly associated with malignant lesions and bilateral lesions, such as cortical hyperplasia, were more likely to be benign. Clinical signs and laboratory findings of hormonal hypersecretion in the differential diagnosis and workup of adrenal gland lesions require close cooperation between radiologist and endocrinologist, given that only 5–15% of adrenocortical tumors are functional and clinical signs of pheochromocytoma are often unspecific [18, 19].

Abbreviations
A: Homogeneous enlargement; AP: Histopathological findings; B: Irregular enlargement; Bi: Bilateral side; C: Nodular lesion; D: Multiple nodular lesions; L: Left side; R: Right side; US: Ultrasonographic findings

Acknowledgements
The authors thank the technical staff of the pathological anatomy laboratory for their assistance.

Funding
This research had not funding sources.

Authors' contributions
EP and RZ carried out the studies and drafted the manuscript. CL participated in the design of the study. EB performed the statistical analysis. MT carried out the interpretation of the histological examinations. BB and AT conceived of the study, and participated in its design and coordination and helped to draft the manuscript. All authors read and approved the final manuscript.

Competing interests
The authors declare that they have no competing interests.

Consent to publish
Not applicable.

Author details
[1]Department of Veterinary Sciences, University of Turin, Largo Paolo Braccini 2-5, 10095 Grugliasco, TO, Italy. [2]Department of Agriculture, Forest and Food Sciences, University of Turin, L. Paolo Braccini, 2, 10095 Grugliasco, TO, Italy.

References
1. Fan J, Tang J, Fang J, Li Q, He E, Li J, Wang Y. Ultrasound Imaging in the Diagnosis of Benign and Suspicious Adrenal Lesions. Med Sci Monit. 2014;20:2132–41.
2. Benchekroun G, de Fornel-Thibaud P, Rodriguez Pineiro MI, Rault D, Besso J, Cohen A, et al. Ultrasonography criteria for differentiating ACTH dependency from ACTH independency in 47 dogs with hyperadrenocorticism and equivocal adrenal asymmetry. J Vet Intern Med. 2010;24:1077–85.
3. Shelling CG. Ultrasonography of the adrenal gland. Probl Vet Med. 1991;3:604–17.
4. Grooters AM, Biller DS, Merryman J. Ultrasonographic parameters of normal canine adrenal glands: comparison to necropsy findings. Vet Radiol Ultrasound. 1995;36:126–30.
5. Douglass JP, Berry CR, James S. Ultrasonographic adrenal gland measurements in dogs without evidence of adrenal disease. Vet Radiol Ultrasound. 1997;38:124–30.
6. Barberet V, Pey P, Duchateau L, Combes A, Daminet S, Saunders JH. Intra- and interobserver variability of ultrasonographic measurements of the adrenal glands in healthy Beagles. Vet Radiol Ultrasound. 2010;51:656–60.
7. Choi J, Kim H, Yoon J. Ultrasonographic adrenal gland measurements in clinically normal small breed dogs and comparison with pituitary-dependent hyperadrenocorticism. J Vet Med Sci. 2011;73(8):985–9.
8. Mogicato G, Layssol-Lamour C, Conchou F, Diquelou A, Raharison F, Sautet J, et al. Ultrasonographic evaluation of the adrenal glands in healthy dogs: repeatability, reproducibility, observer-dependent variability, and the effect of bodyweight, age and sex. Vet Rec. 2011;168(5):130.
9. de Chalus T, Combes A, Bedu AS, Pey P, Daminet S, Duchateau L, et al. Ultrasonographic adrenal gland measurements in healthy Yorkshire Terriers and Labrador Retrievers. Anat Histol Embryol. 2013;42:57–64.
10. Soulsby SN, Holland M, Hudson JA, Behrend EN. Ultrasonographic evaluation of adrenal gland size compared to body weight in normal dogs. Vet Radiol Ultrasound. 2014;56:317–26.
11. Cook AK, Spaulding KA, Edwards JF. Clinical findings in dogs with incidental adrenal gland lesions determined by ultrasonography: 151 cases (2007-2010). J Am Vet Med Assoc. 2014;244:1181–5.
12. Besso JG, Penninck DG, Gliatto JM. Retrospective ultrasonographic evaluation of adrenal lesions in 26 dogs. Vet Radiol Ultrasound. 1997;38:448–55.
13. Massari F, Nicoli S, Romanelli G, Buracco P, Zini E. Adrenalectomy in dogs with adrenal gland tumors: 52 cases (2002-2008). J Am Vet Med Assoc. 2011;239:216–21.
14. Papierska L, Cichocki A, Sankowski AJ, Cwikła JB. Adrenal incidentaloma imaging - the first steps in therapeutic management. Pol J Radiol. 2013;78:47–55.
15. Hoerauf A, Reusch C. Ultrasonographic Characteristics of both adrenal glands in 15 dogs with functional adrenocortical tumors. J Am Anim Hosp Assoc. 1999;35:193–9.
16. Myers NC. Adrenal incidentalomas. Diagnostic workup of the incidentally discovered adrenal mass. Vet Clin North Am Small Anim Pract. 1997;27:381–99.
17. Kantrowitz BM, Nyland TG, Feldman EC. Adrenal ultrasonography in the dog. Vet Radiol. 1986;27:91–6.
18. Poffenbarger EM, Feeney DA, Hayden DW. Gray-scale ultrasonography in the diagnosis of adrenal neoplasia in dogs: 6 cases (1981-1986). J Am Vet Med Assoc. 1988;192:228–32.
19. Bondyad H, Feeney DA, Caywood DD, Hayden DW. Pheochromocytoma in dogs: 13 cases (1980-1985). J Am Vet Med Assoc. 1987;191(12):1610–5.
20. Kasperlik-Zeluska AA, Rosłonowska E, Słowinska-Srzednicka J, et al. Incidentally discovered adrenal gland mass (incidentaloma): investigation and management of 208 patients. Clin Endocrinol. 1997;46:29–37.
21. Lyon SM, Lee MJ. Imaging the non-hyperfunctioning adrenal mass. Imaging. 2002;14:137–46.
22. Reusch C, Feldman EC. Canine hyperadrenococrticism due to adrenocortical neoplasia: pretreatment evaluation of 41 dogs. J Vet Int Med. 1991;5:3–10.
23. Rosenstein DS. Diagnostic imaging in canine pheochromocytoma. Vet Radiol Ultrasound. 2000;41(6):499–506.
24. Tursi M, Iussich S, Prunotto M, Buracco P. Adrenal Myelolipoma in a Dog. Vet Pathol. 2005;42:232–5.

14

Release kinetics of tumor necrosis factor-α and interleukin-1 receptor antagonist in the equine whole blood

Simon Rütten[1], Gerald F. Schusser[2], Getu Abraham[1*] and Wieland Schrödl[3]

Abstract

Background: Horses are much predisposed and susceptible to excessive and acute inflammatory responses that cause the recruitment and stimulation of polymorphnuclear granulocytes (PMN) together with peripheral blood mononuclear cells (PBMC) and the release of cytokines. The aim of the study is to develop easy, quick, cheap and reproducible methods for measuring tumor necrosis factor alpha (TNF-α) and interleukin-1 receptor antagonist (IL-1Ra) in the equine whole blood cultures ex-vivo time- and concentration-dependently.

Results: Horse whole blood diluted to 10, 20 and 50 % was stimulated with lipopolysaccharide (LPS), PCPwL (a combination of phytohemagglutinin E, concanavalin A and pokeweed mitogen) or equine recombinant TNF-α (erTNF-α). TNF-α and IL-1Ra were analyzed in culture supernatants, which were collected at different time points using specific enzyme-linked immunosorbent assays (ELISA). Both cytokines could be detected optimal in stimulated 20 % whole blood cultures. TNF-α and IL-1Ra releases were time-dependent but the kinetic was different between them. PCPwL-induced TNF-α and IL-1Ra release was enhanced continuously over 24–48 h, respectively. Similarly, LPS-stimulated TNF-α was at maximum at time points between 8–12 h and started to decrease thereafter, whereas IL-1Ra peaked later between 12–24 h and rather continued to accumulate over 48 h. The equine recombinant TNF-α could induce also the IL-1Ra release.

Conclusions: Our results demonstrate that similar to PCPwL, LPS stimulated TNF-α and IL-1Ra production time-dependently in whole blood cultures, suggesting the suitability of whole blood cultures to assess the release of a variety of cytokines in health and diseases of horse.

Keywords: Horse, TNF-α, IL-1receptor antagonist, ELISA, Whole blood culture, Inflammation

Background

Tumor necrosis factor α (TNF-α), in addition to being cytotoxic for certain tumor cells [1, 2], has turned out to be a pro-inflammatory cytokine that is involved in the regulation of immunity and several inflammatory diseases in humans [3, 4] and animals including horses [5, 6]. These animals are much predisposed and susceptible to excessive and acute inflammatory responses that cause the recruitment and stimulation of polymorphnuclear granulocytes (PMN) and peripheral blood mononuclear cells (PBMC) as frequently observed in gastrointestinal diseases [7], laminitis [8], recurrent airway obstruction [9, 10] and

endometritis [11]. In horses as well as in humans, the systemic release of TNF-α appears to be an essential early mediator in inflammatory and immunologic reactions during host defense [12–14]. Also, several studies have shown a direct correlation between disease severity/lethality and TNF-α concentration [7, 15, 16].

Moreover, it has been described that TNF-α can orchestrate the production of other cytokines such as interleukin (IL)-1, IL-6 and IL-8 to promote inflammation including increased leukocyte extravasation [17, 18], cellular and tissue damage in multiple organs and clinical features of sepsis [19, 20], both in experimental animal disease models and in human diseases. Evidence exists that excessive production of the cytokines TNF-α and IL-1 significantly contributes to the development of multiple organ damage in endotoxemia and sepsis in

* Correspondence: gabraham@rz.uni-leipzig.de
[1]Institute of Pharmacology, Pharmacy and Toxicology, Faculty of Veterinary Medicine, Leipzig University, An den Tierkliniken 15, 04103 Leipzig, Germany
Full list of author information is available at the end of the article

humans [21], in the equine endometritis [22], equine asthma [5, 23] and colic [7].

The elevated TNF-α and IL-1 levels trigger often high production of the interleukin-1 receptor antagonist (IL-1Ra), the first described naturally occurring cytokine or hormone-like molecule that functions as a specific IL-1 receptor antagonist and produced by various cell types, including mononuclear cells and neutrophils [24, 25]. IL-1Ra is elevated in plasma of human patients with a variety of inflammatory, infectious, and post-surgical conditions, indicating the importance of hepatic production of this anti-inflammatory protein (for review see reference [26]). Also, administered LPS increased the plasma concentration of IL-1 and concomitantly of IL-1Ra [27], suggesting highly likely that IL-1Ra diffuses from the circulation into tissues and influences the local ratio of IL-1Ra to IL-1 to suppress competitively the IL-1, subsequently to attenuate IL-1-induced TNF-α and IL-6 production [25, 28]. In vitro, it has been also shown that TNF is capable of inducing the production of IL-1Ra [29, 30]. TNF-α has been described to be associated with the human endotoxemia and several inflammatory disorders, and blocking of this cytokine seems to inhibit endotoxin-induced IL-1Ra release [21]; indeed, this relationship to TNF-α has not been examined in horses.

Generally, in the horse, cytokine production can be influenced by several factors including various nutritional, physiological and pathological factors as well as drugs; thus, there is still much interest in measuring the concentrations of different cytokines. In man, successful ex-vivo ELISA-based method of TNF-α measurement has been well established in whole blood system [17, 31] which is quick, less expensive than the analysis in isolated cell systems and can be adapted to field use. In contrast, in horses, current literature review indicates that different matrices have been used to assess TNF-α production ex vivo which did not warrant the generation of uniform data; for example, in bronchoalveolar lavage fluid (BALF) [32], serum [15], plasma [33] or isolated and cultured leukocytes [34–36]. Indeed, different protocols showed culturing PMN influences cell functions and presumably cytokine release [37]. Despite the fact that there are also some studies that used equine whole blood to assess cytokine releases, little was attempted to assess systematically the kinetics of TNF-α production in relation to IL-1Ra production and in different volumes of the whole blood as specialized circulating connective tissue by retaining all blood components.

Thus, we have used the equine whole blood cultures to investigate: first, the relationship between cultures of equine whole blood dilutions and stimulated TNF-α and IL-1Ra release; second, to characterize time-concentration-responses of TNF-α and IL-1Ra production within individuals and different blood dilutions; third, effects of lipopolysaccharide (LPS), a combination of phytohem-agglutinin E, concanavalin A and pokeweed mitogen (PCPwL) and equine recombinant TNF-α (erTNF-α) on TNF-α and IL-1Ra in whole blood cultures. Finally, we wished to evaluate, to our knowledge the first time, whether elevated TNF-α can enhance the IL-Ra activity in the equine whole blood cultures. Our results indicate that TNF is involved not only in the secretion of agonistic members of the cytokine network in endotoxemia but also in that of an important antagonistic member (i.e., IL-1Ra), assuming that blockade of TNF-α results in a general down-regulation of the cytokine system.

Methods

Animals

For the kinetic time-course studies of TNF-α and IL-1Ra releases, blood samples were collected from three-five healthy horses of mixed breeds and 8–14 years of age. They were neither under treatment for the last three weeks before sampling nor were given immune-suppressing drugs. Animals were kept in an individual pen, fed with hey and concentrates three times a day, but had access to water ad libitum. Blood samples were collected from horses, which belong to the Large Animal Clinic of the Leipzig University.

Reagent and antibody dilutions

TNF-α antibodies[1] were reconstituted to final stock concentrations of 1 mg/ml (capture) and 0.25 mg/ml (detection) in ultra-pure water.[2] Complete RPMI 1640 medium contained basal RPMI 1640 medium[2], Penicillin G[2] (100 U/ml), Streptomycin[2] (100 µg/ml) and heparin[2] (10 U/ml). The TNF-α-capture antibody was diluted in 0.1 M NaHCO₃ solution with ultra-pure water to a working concentration of 3 µg/ml. The detection antibody was diluted to a working concentration of 250 ng/ml in PBST-buffer, containing 2 % heat inactivated (56 °C, 30 min) and sterile-filtered rabbit serum.[3] Streptavidin-horseradish-peroxidase[4] (HRP) was diluted 1:50000 in PBST containing Dulbecco's phosphate buffered saline (PBS) solution[5] and 0.1 % Tween 20.[6] With regard to IL-1Ra, antibodies and reagents were processed in accordance with the manufacturer's instructions (Equine IL-1ra/IL-1 F3 DuoSet ELISA).[7]

Blood sampling, whole blood cell culture and stimulation

Blood samples were collected via jugular venipuncture into 9 mL vacutainer tubes with Li-Heparin (16 U × mL⁻¹) (S-Monovette).[8] Blood dilutions, culturing and whole blood stimulations were carried out under sterile conditions. Within 30 min after sampling, whole blood was diluted at a ratio of 1:2 (50 %), 1:5 (20 %) and 1:10 (10 %) in a complete RPMI 1640 medium, respectively.

For the stimulation of TNF-α and IL-1Ra releases, diluted blood was incubated in 24-well culture plates (total volume 2 ml/well). Samples were stimulated with either LPS[9] (1000 ng/ml; Escherichia coli O111:B4) or with PCPwL (100 ng/ml) (a combination of phytohemagglutinin E,[10] concanavalin A[10] and pokeweed mitogen[10]) (as positive control) or with medium alone. Moreover, whole blood cultures were treated with the equine recombinant TNF-α[11] (erTNF-α; 20 ng/ml) to stimulate IL-1Ra antagonist release. Each culture plate was then incubated for 72 h at 37 °C under 5 % CO_2 atmosphere. To assess the time course of cytokine releases, aliquots of the supernatant/well were collected at time points of 0, 1, 2, 4, 6, 8, 12, 16, 24, 48 and 72 h. These aliquots were centrifuged (10000 rpm) at 4 °C for 3 min and the supernatant was separated from the cell debris and frozen at −20 °C until analysis of the cell-associated cytokines.

Detection of TNF-α and IL-1Ra production

Concentrations of cytokines in whole blood cell culture supernatants were determined by enzyme-linked immunosorbent assay (ELISA) system. All samples from each blood dilutions were analyzed in one ELISA.

Measurement of TNF-α

The TNF-α protein level was measured using the equine TNF-α sandwich ELISA that was established in our laboratory. For this purpose, 96-microtiter well plates[12] were coated with 100 μl/well of a polyclonal antibody specific for equine TNF-α and incubated overnight at 4–6 °C. Thereafter, samples were allowed to reach room temperature. Plates were then washed twice with 400 μl/well washing buffer (distilled water containing 0.9 % NaCl and 0.05 % Tween 20) using an automated 8-channel washer.[13]

Assay conditions were optimized by adding a series of calibrators on every assay plate that consisted of 7-point serial dilutions of equine recombinant TNF-α starting from 24.3 ng/ml to 0.033 ng/ml in duplicates in complete RPMI 1640 cell culture medium containing PBST in the presence of 10, 20 or 50 % horse serum. Also, duplicate wells of each plate contained only medium. For each ELISA plate, the optical density (OD) at 450 nm was measured, and the standard curves were established by plotting mean absorbance for each standard concentration against the target protein concentration with OD 450 nm as the Y-axis using GraphPad Prism Software program. These curves were used to determine protein expression levels.

Basal and stimulated levels of TNF-α and IL-1Ra in whole blood culture supernatant samples were measured using ELISA. In brief, for each point of assay, 50 μl of pure cell culture supernatant were pipetted into each well of 96-microtiter well plates and diluted 1:2 by adding 50 μl PBST-buffer. Samples were then incubated for 1 h at room temperature. After three times rinsing the plates with washing buffer, 100 μl of the polyclonal biotin-labeled detecting antibody were added to each sample and incubated for further 2 h at room temperature. After three washing steps, plates were incubated with 100 μl horseradish peroxidase-conjugated streptavidin for 1 h at room temperature. After four washing steps, 100 μl of freshly prepared substrate solution (containing 3 mM H_2O_2 and 1 mM tetramethylbenzidine[14] (TMB) in 0.2 M citrate buffer, pH 4.0) were added to each well. The chromogenic substrate was converted from colorless to blue by streptavidin-HRP conjugate. The reaction was stopped after 15 min at room temperature by adding 50 μl of 1 M sulfuric acid solution, and the optical density (OD) was read at 450 and 620 nm with a spectrophotometer (Tecan Plate reader[15]). The levels of TNF-α in whole blood supernatant samples were interpolated from the erTNF-α standard calibration curves calculated as described above.

Measurement of IL-1Ra

IL-1Ra concentrations were measured in whole blood culture supernatants according to the manufacturers' guidelines with slight modifications. Briefly, 96-microtiter well plates were coated with polyclonal equine anti-IL-1Ra antibody and incubated overnight at room temperature, followed by washing and blocking steps. Freshly thawed whole blood supernatant samples and the equine IL-1Ra standard (at different concentrations starting from 40 ng/ml to 0.16 ng/ml) were diluted at a ratio of 1:10 and incubated. Following several washing steps, biotinylated secondary IL-1Ra antibody, streptavidin-HRP conjugate and enzyme substrate were added at different time points as given in the guidelines. Further procedures were performed analogous to the TNF-α ELISA.

Data calculation and statistical analysis

Results are presented as means ± SEM. The levels of TNF-α and IL-1Ra in whole blood supernatants were interpolated from the erTNF-α and IL-1Ra standard calibration curves which were established using Graph-Pad Prism 6.01[16]. Variations in cytokine productions in the different whole blood cultures and time courses of incubation as well as different cytokine stimulants were assessed by two-way analysis of variance (ANOVA) using SigmaPlot 12.5[17] with Holm-Sidak post-hoc test. Cytokine productions in different culture conditions were plotted and statistical significance was calculated. Differences giving P value < 0.05 were considered significant.

Results

Relationship between whole blood dilutions and cytokine releases

The ex vivo production of TNF-α and IL-1Ra was determined in horses using heparin-displaced whole blood

Table 1 Maximal TNF-α concentration after stimulation with LPS or PCPwL

BC (%)	LPS	PCPwL	
	8 h	24 h	72 h
10 %	296 ± 153	103 ± 103	345 ± 106
20 %	538 ± 219	304 ± 164	517 ± 163
50 %	1104 ± 279	865 ± 187	661 ± 316

Supernatant TNF-α level (pg/ml) was compared between different whole blood volumes after stimulation with LPS or PCPwL. Maximal concentrations were obtained after the start of stimulation at various time points until 72 h. Data represent means ± SEM of three different horses. BC, blood concentration

samples collected in a single draw. Samples were diluted 1:2 (50 %), 1:5 (20 %) and 1:10 (10 %) with complete RPMI 1640 medium. The PCPwL- but also LPS-stimulated TNF-α and IL-1Ra production was linear with different concentrations of the equine whole blood, whereby the highest cytokine concentration was achieved at whole blood dilution of 50 %. In all whole blood dilutions, PCPwL stimulated continuously TNF-α release over 24 h to the maximum and similarly but within 12 h of stimulation, LPS activated TNF-α production (Table 1). The stimulation with these both stimulating agents and additionally with erTNF-α yielded on average a maximum IL-1Ra production in all whole blood dilutions over 48 h of stimulation (Table 2). Despite the linearity of ELISA signals for TNF-α and IL-1Ra as a function of whole blood dilution, there were high background signals and strong adherence of diluted blood in the pipette tips at a volume of 50 % (with large variation in cytokine concentration). These errors were considered significant; thus, in all subsequent experiments, 20 % equine whole blood dilution, which provided low data variation of cytokine concentration, was routinely used, since also 10 % dilution tended not to result in reliable data.

Time-course kinetics of TNF-α release in whole blood cell culture

In the next step, the relationship between equine whole blood dilutions and time-course of LPS-stimulated TNF-α production in comparison to PCPwL was examined. As depicted in Figs. 1 and 2, the mean production of TNF-α in relation to whole blood dilution was affected by time. One hour after LPS addition, the level of TNF-α started to increase and maximum levels were achieved

at the incubation time between 8–12 h. Thereafter, TNF-α concentration started to decrease continuously up to 72 h (Fig. 1a). In whole blood cultures of both 10 and 20 % dilutions, PCPwL stimulated the TNF-α production to a similar extent as LPS, but the concentration of TNF-α increased gradually and peaked until up to 72 h while in 50 % diluted whole blood cultures TNF-α level declined continuously after 24 h of incubation (Fig. 1b). Comparing both stimulating agents, LPS seems to stimulate TNF-α production more than PCPwL, and this was also dependent on whole blood dilutions (Fig. 2). Together, due to the data fluctuation of TNF-α releases, which were obtained at whole blood dilutions of 10 or 50 % and the variable peak time courses obtained after PCPwL and also after LPS stimulation, 12-h incubation is assumed to be an optimal condition to measure TNF-α in 20 % whole blood cultures.

Time-course kinetics of IL-1Ra activation

Strong and significant activation of IL-1Ra release was obtained in 50 % diluted equine whole blood cultures regardless of the used stimulating agents (LPS, PCPwL or erTNF-α) (Fig. 3a-c). Interestingly, it was able to detect IL-1Ra release first after about 4 h of stimulation of the whole blood cultures of 20 and 50 % dilutions and the maximum response was obtained after 48 h and declined after 72 h. Similar data of IL-1Ra release were obtained when 10 % whole blood cultures were stimulated but maximum response was obtained here after about 72 h of incubation. As shown in Fig. 4, there were little significant differences between IL-1Ra levels obtained from three whole blood dilutions stimulated by all three stimulating agents (LPS, PCPwL or erTNF-α) over 72 h.

Discussion

The present study dissects equine whole blood dilution-dependent and time-course secretion of TNF-α and IL-1Ra after stimulation by PCPwL, LPS as well as erTNF-α (only IL-1Ra was stimulated) ex vivo. The decisive results were: PCPwL and also LPS triggered TNF-α and IL-1Ra releases in a blood volume-dependent manner (50 % > 20 % >10 %). In whole blood cultures, TNF-α exhibited a kinetic profile similar to that of IL-1Ra, but peaked explicitly prior to IL-1Ra activity. TNF-α peaked 8–12 h after LPS addition while the IL-1Ra level was at

Table 2 Maximal IL-1Ra production after stimulation with LPS, PCPwL or erTNF- α

BC (%)	LPS		PCPwL	erTNF-α	
	48 h	72 h	48 h	48 h	72 h
10 %	5643 ± 1520	5809 ± 1426	8045 ± 2965	5083 ± 2364	5120 ± 2323
20 %	11368 ± 1713	8502 ± 1667	11451 ± 1620	11167 ± 994	8829 ± 178
50 %	26375 ± 4842	21260 ± 7332	25982	>40000	27529 ± 4010

Supernatant IL-1Ra production (pg/ml) was compared between different whole blood volumes after stimulation with LPS, PCPwL or erTNF-α. Maximal concentrations were obtained after the start of stimulation at various time points until 72 h. Data represent means ± SEM of three different horses. BC, blood concentration

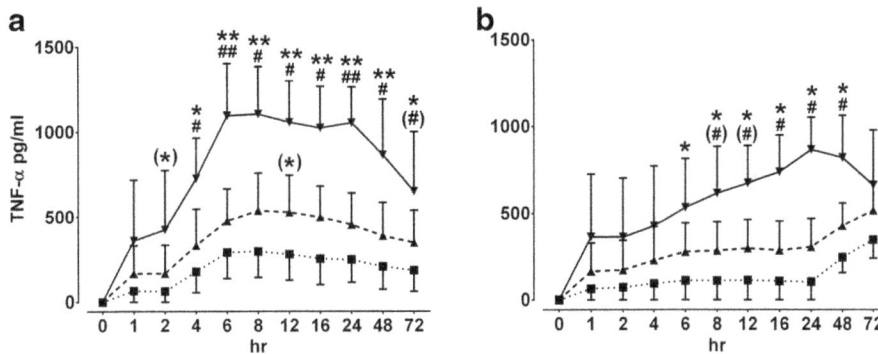

Fig. 1 Effect of time and blood dilution on TNF-α production in whole blood culture. Time-dependent TNF-α production was measured in equine whole blood cell culture supernatants obtained from different blood volume dilutions after stimulation by LPS (1000 ng/ml) (a) and PCPwL (100 ng/ml) (b). 10 % (■), 20 % (▲), and 50 % (▼) whole blood volumes were used to assess TNF-α over 72 h (hr). Data represent means ± SEM of three different horses. ** $p < 0.001$/* $p < 0.05$/(*) $0.05 \geq p < 0.1$ versus 10 % BC, ## $p < 0.001$/# $p < 0.05$/(#) $0.05 \geq p < 0.1$ versus 20 % BC. BC, blood concentration

maximum 24 h later and remained at that level for further 24 h. The effect of several stimuli on cytokine releases was often investigated in isolated leukocytes of horses [34–36] and humans [38, 39]. Also, cytokines could be assessed in human whole blood cultures [31, 37–39], but to our knowledge, very rarely or even not analyzed the time-dependent kinetics of TNF-α release in relation to IL-1Ra production in an equine whole blood-volume-dependent manner.

For reasons that the optimal stimulation conditions to assess cytokine releases in the equine whole blood cultures were not well known, the aim of the current study was to first find out which blood volumes can provide a reproducible signal-to-noise ratio of cytokine standard and sample concentration curves. In the whole blood medium, which resembles closely the physiological milieu, it was observed that the PCPwL- or LPS-stimulated TNF-α and IL-1Ra release was reduced in whole blood cultures with increasing dilutions (cf. Tables 1 and 2). Indeed, the data obtained from whole blood cultures of

1:2-diltution (50 %-vol.) were subjected fluctuations, presumably due to more background signals as a result of strong adherence of the blood to the pipette tips when compared to the data obtained from equine whole blood cultures of the 20 and 10 % dilutions. Even if 10 % whole blood samples would require smaller starting blood samples to assess cytokines, signals obtained here were weak. On the other hand, the 1:5-dilution (20 %-vol.) of the whole blood delivered consistently high reproducible cytokine data. This validated novel, cheap, optimized and straightforward approach was further used to quantify TNF-α and IL-1Ra in whole blood cultures of the horse, and can be suggested for the use in field conditions. Our data are in agreement with data from earlier studies that demonstrated stable cytokine production in diluted human whole blood cultures (dilution ranged: 1:4 to 1:10) [31, 38, 39]. These authors compared whole blood cultures with isolated monocytes or PBMC and showed constant cytokine reproducibility in whole blood cultures than in isolated cells, thus, suggested that whole

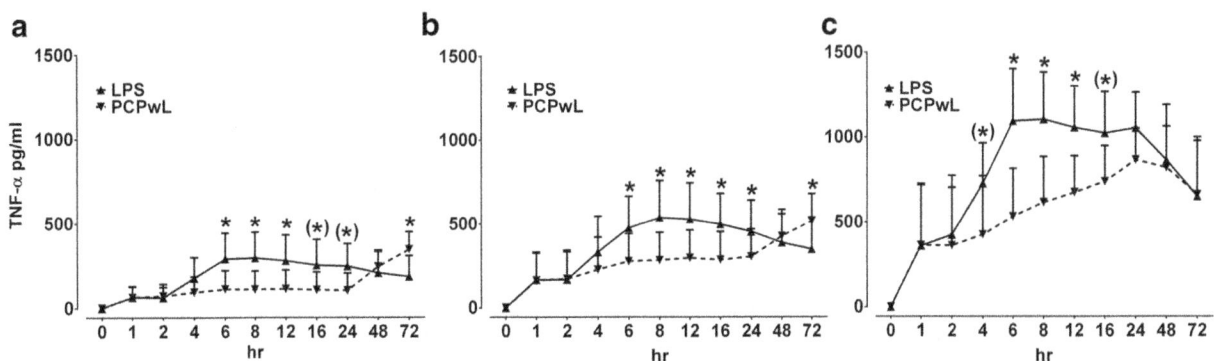

Fig. 2 Comparison of LPS- and PCPwL-stimulated TNF-α production. LPS- and PCPwL-stimulated TNF-α production was measured in 10 % (a), 20 % (b) and 50 % (c) whole blood cultures over time. Data represent means ± SEM of three different horses. ** $p < 0.001$/* $p < 0.05$/(*) $0.05 \geq p < 0.1$. BC, blood concentration

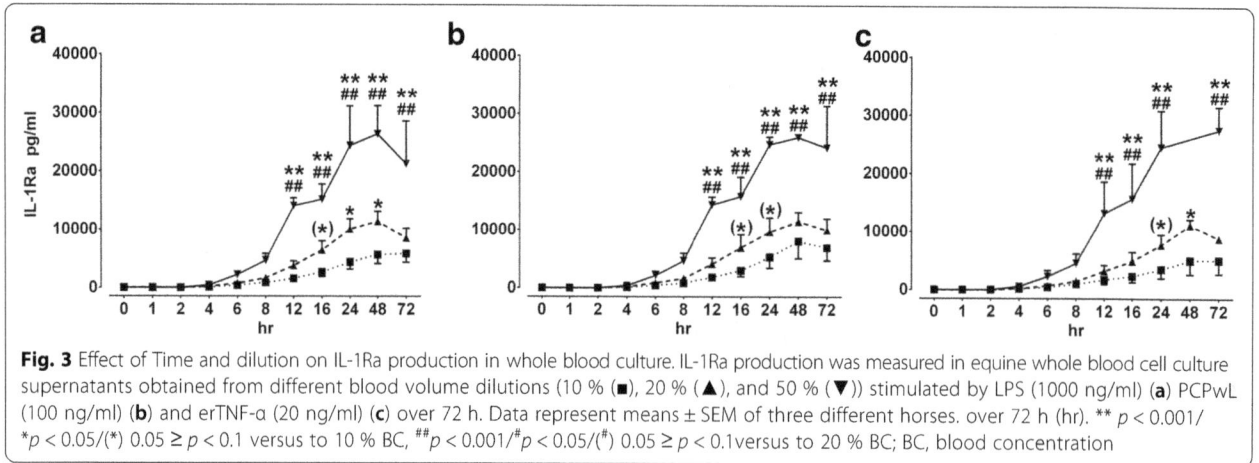

Fig. 3 Effect of Time and dilution on IL-1Ra production in whole blood culture. IL-1Ra production was measured in equine whole blood cell culture supernatants obtained from different blood volume dilutions (10 % (■), 20 % (▲), and 50 % (▼)) stimulated by LPS (1000 ng/ml) (**a**) PCPwL (100 ng/ml) (**b**) and erTNF-α (20 ng/ml) (**c**) over 72 h. Data represent means ± SEM of three different horses. over 72 h (hr). ** $p < 0.001$/ *$p < 0.05$/(*) $0.05 \geq p < 0.1$ versus to 10 % BC, ##$p < 0.001$/#$p < 0.05$/(#) $0.05 \geq p < 0.1$versus to 20 % BC; BC, blood concentration

blood is a better suited medium than isolated blood cell cultures for cytokine studies in humans. Even though in the current study leukocytes were not isolated, it can be suggested that large-scale ex vivo cytokine assessment can be undertaken with equine whole blood cultures.

Similar to the effect of whole blood dilution on equine TNF-α and IL-1Ra production, there was an effect of time on the release of both cytokines ex vivo after stimulation with PCPwL or LPS. With regard to TNF-α, the release kinetics in whole blood stimulation ex vivo were similar to those reported in vivo after LPS-challenge of horses [40–42]. In these in vivo models of endotoxemia, the low-dose LPS challenge of horses resulted in a predictable effect on increasing plasma TNF-α activity that peaked between 1–4 h (average 1.5–2.5 h). In our study, cytokine levels increased after 1-h stimulation of the equine whole blood cultures with LPS and peaked between 8–12 h. This time was considered as an optimal incubation condition for further experiments, since stimulation of blood cultures for longer times resulted in decreased TNF-α production e.g. until 72 h.

Interestingly, we could also demonstrate the first time that IL-1Ra can be detected in relation to TNF-α production in the equine whole blood cultures and can be also affected with time. Both PCPwL and LPS could induce a continuous production of IL-1Ra over 48 h, indicating that the elevated TNF-α may contribute to the high level of IL-1Ra even beyond the peak time points, which were observed for the former cytokine. The activated IL-1Ra levels were much higher than the levels of TNF-α, presumably, to block the biological effects of IL-1 [25, 27] which is concomitantly released during inflammatory processes in several tissue and organ systems. Furthermore, in the current study, stimulation of the equine whole blood cultures with the equine recombinant TNF-α (erTNF-α) resulted in enhanced activity of IL-1Ra, in agreement with the data obtained from human studies [43–45]. In man, this relationship has been shown during endotoxemia [21] and high level of acute-phase protein [46, 47] and could be linked to the involvement of TNF-α in the course of several diseases. However, in horses, excessive IL-1Ra production in relation to TNF-α release has not yet been associated with disease pathogenesis and severity. In the first place, IL-1Ra

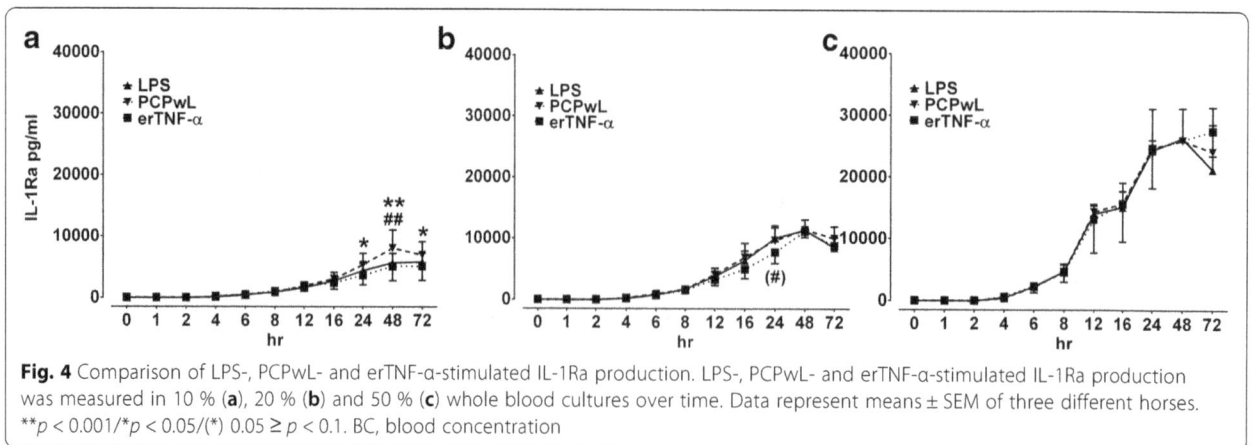

Fig. 4 Comparison of LPS-, PCPwL- and erTNF-α-stimulated IL-1Ra production. LPS-, PCPwL- and erTNF-α-stimulated IL-1Ra production was measured in 10 % (**a**), 20 % (**b**) and 50 % (**c**) whole blood cultures over time. Data represent means ± SEM of three different horses. **$p < 0.001$/*$p < 0.05$/(*) $0.05 \geq p < 0.1$. BC, blood concentration

is claimed to attenuate the IL-1-dependent activities [25] which are necessary in tissue remodeling which often occur in several fibrotic equine diseases such as in the recurrent airway obstruction (RAO).

Conclusions

Together, this study indicates the suitability of whole blood cultures to assess ex vivo or in vivo the production of a variety of cytokines of healthy or diseased horses (e.g. inflammatory disorders of the airways, gastro-intestinal tract, uterus, liver etc.), presumably, more than isolated PMN or PBMC cultures. The equine whole blood assay system is additionally an efficient tool to elucidate interactions of cytokines within the inflammatory responses and may provide equine veterinarians with new therapeutic approaches. Dilution of the whole blood to a ratio of 1:5 (20 %) and an incubation time of 12 h can be considered as optimal conditions to assess stimulated cytokines.

Endnotes

[1]ThermoFisher Scientific, Rockford, Illinois, USA
[2]Biochrom, Berlin, Germany
[3]Biowest, Nuaille', France
[4]ThermoFisher Scientific, Rockford, Illinois, USA
[5]Biochrom, Berlin, Germany
[6]Roth, Karlsruhe, Germany
[7]R&D Systems, Wiesbaden, Germany
[8]Sarstedt, Nümbrecht, Germany
[9]Sigma-Aldrich, Taufkirchen, Germany
[10]Biochrom, Berlin, Germany
[11]Perbio science, Rockford, Illinois, USA
[12]BD Bioscience, Heidelberg, Germany
[13]Nunc, Roskilde, Denmark
[14]Sigma-Aldrich, Taufkirchen, Germany
[15]Tecan, Crailsheim, Germany
[16]Graphpad Software Inc., La Jolla, California, USA
[17]Systat Software Inc., San Jose, California, USA

Abbreviations

BALF, Bronchoalveolar lavage fluid; ELISA, Enzyme-linked immunosorbent assay; erTNF-α, Equine recombinant tumor necrosis factor alpha; HRP, Horseradish-peroxidase; IL, Interleukin; IL-1Ra, Interleukin-1 receptor antagonist; LPS, Lipopolysaccharide; PBMC, Peripheral blood mononuclear cells; PBST, Solution containing phosphate buffered saline and Tween 20; PCPwL, Combination of phytohemagglutinin E, concanavalin A and pokeweed mitogen; PMN, Polymorphnuclear granulocytes; TMB, Tetramethylbenzidine; TNF-α, Tumor necrosis factor alpha

Acknowledgments
We thank Rita Diehl for thoughtful comments and helping in statistical analysis.

Funding
Research reported in this work was supported by the Federal Ministry for Economic Affairs and Energy.

Authors' contributions
SR, GFS, GA and WS designed the research and wrote the paper. SR and WS performed the experiment. SR, GFS, GA and WS analyzed the data and wrote the paper. GA corrected the English language. All authors gave their final approval of the manuscript.

Competing interests
The authors declare that they have no competing interests.

Consent for publication
Not applicable.

Author details
[1]Institute of Pharmacology, Pharmacy and Toxicology, Faculty of Veterinary Medicine, Leipzig University, An den Tierkliniken 15, 04103 Leipzig, Germany. [2]Department of Large Animal Medicine, Faculty of Veterinary Medicine, Leipzig University, An den Tierkliniken 11, 04103 Leipzig, Germany. [3]Institute of Bacteriology and Mycology, Faculty of Veterinary Medicine, Leipzig University, An den Tierkliniken 29, 04103 Leipzig, Germany.

References
1. Männel DN, Moore RN, Mergenhagen SE. Macrophages as a source of tumoricidal activity (tumor-necrotizing factor). Infect Immun. 1980;30:523–30.
2. Ruff MR, Gifford GE. Rabbit tumor necrosis factor: mechanism of action. Infect Immun. 1981;31:380–5.
3. Broide DH, Lotz M, Cuomo AJ, Coburn DA, Federman EC, Wasserman SI. Cytokines in symptomatic asthma airways. J Allergy Clin Immunol. 1992;89:958–67.
4. Chung KF, Barnes PJ. Cytokines in asthma. Thorax. 1999;54:825–57.
5. Giguère S, Viel L, Lee E, MacKay RJ, Hernandez J, Franchini M. Cytokine induction in pulmonary airways of horses with heaves and effect of therapy with inhaled fluticasone propionate. Vet Immunol Immunopathol. 2002;85:147–58.
6. Franchini M, Gill U, von Fellenberg R, Bracher VD. Interleukin-8 concentration and neutrophil chemotactic activity in bronchoalveolar lavage fluid of horses with chronic obstructive pulmonary disease following exposure to hay. Am J Vet Res. 2000;61:1369–74.
7. Morris DD, Moore JN, Crowe N. Serum tumor necrosis factor activity in horses with colic attributable to gastrointestinal tract disease. Am J Vet Res. 1991;52:1565–9.
8. De la Rebière de Pouyade G, Serteyn D. The role of activated neutrophils in the early stage of equine laminitis. Vet J. 2011;189:27–33.
9. Pirie RS. Recurrent airway obstruction: a review. Equine Vet J. 2014;46:276–88.
10. Laan TT, Bull S, Pirie R, Fink-Gremmels J. The role of alveolar macrophages in the pathogenesis of recurrent airway obstruction in horses. J Vet Intern Med. 2006;20:167–74.
11. Woodward EM. Troedsson, M H T. Inflammatory mechanisms of endometritis. Equine Vet J. 2015;47:384–9.
12. Werners AH, Bull S, Fink-Gremmels J. Endotoxaemia: a review with implications for the horse. Equine Vet J. 2005;37:371–83.
13. Beutler B, Cerami A. The biology of cachectin/TNF–a primary mediator of the host response. Annu Rev Immunol. 1989;7:625–55.
14. MacKay RJ. Inflammation in horses. Vet Clin North Am Equine Pract. 2000;16:15–27.
15. Lavoie-Lamoureux A, Beauchamp G, Quessy S, Martin JG, Lavoie JP. Systemic inflammation and priming of peripheral blood leukocytes persist during clinical remission in horses with heaves. Vet Immunol Immunopathol. 2012;146:35–45.
16. Morris DD, Moore JN. Tumor necrosis factor activity in serum from neonatal foals with presumed septicemia. J Am Vet Med Assoc. 1991;199:1584–9.

17. DeForge LE, Remick DG. Kinetics of TNF, IL-6, and IL-8 gene expression in LPS-stimulated human whole blood. Biochem Biophys Res Commun. 1991;174:18–24.

18. Fiers W. Tumor necrosis factor. Characterization at the molecular, cellular and in vivo level. FEBS Lett. 1991;285:199–212.

19. Sheron N, Lau J, Daniels H, Goka J, Eddleston A, Alexander GJ, et al. Increased production of tumour necrosis factor alpha in chronic hepatitis B virus infection. J Hepatol. 1991;12:241–5.

20. Bradham CA, Plümpe J, Manns MP, Brenner DA, Trautwein C. Mechanisms of hepatic toxicity. I. TNF-induced liver injury. Am J Physiol. 1998;275:387–92.

21. van der Poll T, van Deventer SJ, ten Cate H, Levi M, ten Cate JW. Tumor necrosis factor is involved in the appearance of interleukin-1 receptor antagonist in endotoxemia. J Infect Dis. 1994;169:665–7.

22. Christoffersen M, Woodward E, Bojesen AM, Jacobsen S, Petersen MR, Troedsson MH, Lehn-Jensen H. Inflammatory responses to induced infectious endometritis in mares resistant or susceptible to persistent endometritis. BMC Vet Res. 2012;29:8:41.

23. Bullone M, Lavoie JP. Asthma "of horses and men"–how can equine heaves help us better understand human asthma immunopathology and its functional consequeces? Mol Immunol. 2015;66:97–105.

24. Dinarello CA. Interleukin-1 and interleukin-1 antagonism. Blood. 1991;77:1627–52.

25. Dinarello CA, Thompson RC. Blocking IL-1: interleukin 1 receptor antagonist in vivo and in vitro. Immunol Today. 1991;12:404–10.

26. Arend WP. The balance between IL-1 and IL-1Ra in disease. Cytokine Growth Factor Rev. 2002;13:323–40.

27. Granowitz EV, Santos AA, Poutsiaka DD, Cannon JG, Wilmore DW, Wolff SM, et al. Production of interleukin-1-receptor antagonist during experimental endotoxaemia. Lancet. 1991;338:1423–4.

28. Arend WP, Malyak M, Guthridge CJ, Gabay C. Interleukin-1 receptor antagonist: role in biology. Annu Rev Immunol. 1998;16:27–55.

29. McColl SR, Paquin R, Menard C, Beaulieu AD. Human neutrophils produce high levels of the interleukin I receptor antagonist in response to granulocyte/macrophage colony-stimulating factor and tumor necrosis factor-a. J Exp Med. 1992;176:593–8.

30. Martel-Pelletier J, McCollum R, Pelletier JP. The synthesis of IL-I receptor antagonist (IL-I ra) by synovial fibroblasts is markedly increased by the cytokines TNF-a and IL-I. Biochim Biophys Acta. 1993;1175:302–5.

31. Damsgaard CT, Lauritzen L, Calder PC, Kjaer TM, Frøkiaer H. Whole-blood culture is a valid low-cost method to measure monocytic cytokines - a comparison of cytokine production in cultures of human whole-blood, mononuclear cells and monocytes. J Immunol Methods. 2009;340:95–101.

32. Richard EA, Depecker M, Defontis M, Leleu C, Fortier G, Pitel P, et al. Cytokine concentrations in bronchoalveolar lavage fluid from horses with neutrophilic inflammatory airway disease. J Vet Intern Med. 2014;28:1838–44.

33. McFarlane D, Holbrook TC. Cytokine dysregulation in aged horses and horses with pituitary pars intermedia dysfunction. J Vet Intern Med. 2008;22:436–42.

34. MacKay RJ, King RR, Dankert JR, Reis KJ, Skelley LA. Cytotoxic tumor necrosis factor activity produced by equine alveolar macrophages: preliminary characterization. Vet Immunol Immunopathol. 1991;29:15–30.

35. Morris DD, Moore JN, Fischer K, Tarleton RL. Endotoxin-induced tumor necrosis factor activity production by equine peritoneal macrophages. Circ Shock. 1990;30:229–36.

36. Karagianni AE, Kapetanovic R, McGorum BC, Hume DA, Pirie SR. The equine alveolar macrophage: functional and phenotypic comparisons with peritoneal macrophages. Vet Immunol Immunopathol. 2013;155:219–28.

37. Strieter RM, Remick DG, Ham JM, Colletti LM, Lynch 3rd JP, Kunkel SL. Tumor necrosis factor-alpha gene expression in human whole blood. J Leukoc Biol. 1990;47:366–70.

38. Yaqoob P, Newsholme EA, Calder PC. Comparison of cytokine production in cultures of whole human blood and purified mononuclear cells. Cytokine. 1999;11:600–5.

39. De Groote D, Zangerle PF, Gevaert Y, Fassotte MF, Beguin Y, Noizat-Pirenne F, et al. Direct stimulation of cytokines (IL-1 beta, TNF-alpha, IL-6, IL-2, IFN-gamma and GM-CSF) in whole blood. I Comparison with isolated PBMC stimulation. Cytokine. 1992;4:239–48.

40. Morris DD, Crowe N, Moore JN. Correlation of clinical and laboratory data with serum tumor necrosis factor activity in horses with experimentally induced endotoxemia. Am J Vet Res. 1990;51:1935–40.

41. Cudmore LA, Muurlink T, Whittem T, Bailey SR. Effects of oral clenbuterol on the clinical and inflammatory response to endotoxaemia in the horse. Res Vet Sci. 2013;94:682–6.

42. Alcott CJ, Sponseller BA, Wong DM, Davis JL, Soliman AM, Wang C, et al. Clinical and immunomodulating effects of ketamine in horses with experimental endotoxemia. J Vet Intern Med. 2011;25:934–43.

43. Langereis JD, Oudijk ED, Schweizer RC, Lammers JJ, Koenderman L, Ulfman LH. Steroids induce a disequilibrium of secreted interleukin-1 receptor antagonist and interleukin-1β synthesis by human neutrophils. Eur Respir J. 2011;37:406–15.

44. Marie C, Pitton C, Fitting C, Cavaillon JM. IL-10 and IL-4 synergize with TNF-alpha to induce IL-1ra production by human neutrophils. Cytokine. 1996;8:147–51.

45. Marsh CB, Wewers MD. Cytokine-induced interleukin-1 receptor antagonist release in mononuclear phagocytes. Am J Respir Cell Mol Biol. 1994;10:521–5.

46. Gabay C, Smith MF, Eidlen D, Arend WP. Interleukin 1 receptor antagonist (IL-1Ra) is an acute-phase protein. J Clin Invest. 1997;99:2930–40.

47. Gabay C, Gigley J, Sipe J, Arend WP, Fantuzzi G. Production of IL-1 receptor antagonist by hepatocytes is regulated as an acute-phase protein in vivo. Eur J Immunol. 2001;31:490–9.

15

Estimating canine cancer incidence: findings from a population-based tumour registry in northwestern Italy

Elisa Baioni[1]* [iD], Eugenio Scanziani[2], Maria Claudia Vincenti[3], Mauro Leschiera[4], Elena Bozzetta[5], Marzia Pezzolato[5], Rosanna Desiato[1], Silvia Bertolini[1], Cristiana Maurella[1] and Giuseppe Ru[1]

Abstract

Background: Canine cancer registry data can be put to good use in epidemiological studies. Quantitative comparison of tumour types may reveal unusual cancer frequencies, providing directions for research and generation of hypotheses of cancer causation in a specific area, and suggest leads for identifying risk factors. Here we report canine cancer incidence rates calculated from a population-based registry in an area without any known specific environmental hazard.

Results: In its 90 months of operation from 2001 to 2008 (the observation period in this study), the population-based Piedmont Canine Cancer Registry collected data on 1175 tumours confirmed by histopathological diagnosis. The incidence rate was 804 per 100,000 dog-years for malignant tumours and 897 per 100,000 dog-years for benign tumours. Higher rates for all cancers were observed in purebred dogs, particularly in Yorkshire terrier and Boxer. The most prevalent malignant neoplasms were cutaneous mastocytoma and hemangiopericytoma, and mammary gland complex carcinoma and simplex carcinoma.

Conclusions: The Piedmont canine cancer registry is one of few of its kind whose operations have been consistently supported by long-term public funding. The registry-based cancer incidence rates were estimated with particular attention to the validity of data collection, thus minimizing the potential for bias. The findings on cancer incidence rates may provide a reliable reference for comparison studies. Researches conducted on dogs, used as sentinels for community exposure to environmental carcinogens, can be useful to detect excess risks in the incidence of malignant tumours in the human population.

Keywords: Population-based cancer registry, Dog, Incidence, Tumours, Cancer epidemiology, Sentinel animal

Background

Canine cancer registry data can be put to good use in epidemiological studies. Quantitative comparison of tumour types may reveal unusual cancer frequencies, providing direction for research and generation of hypotheses of cancer causation in a specific area, and suggest leads for identifying risk factors.

The pivotal role of the sentinel animal some species play at a low level in the trophic chain, e.g., to show the effect of endocrine disruptors, [1] could also be assumed

by dogs. The existence of a tumour registry in this species can pinpoint variations in cancer incidence in target organs. One task of such registries is to determine whether potential correlations exist between an increase or decrease in cancer incidence and environmental hazards. In a study conducted 25 years ago on companion animals as a sentinel for environmentally related human diseases, a correlation was found whereby changes in the canine proportionate incidence ratios preceded human incidence rates by 2 years, suggesting that fluctuations in proportionate incidence ratios of tumours in dogs may be useful for predicting changes in cancer patterns in humans [2]. Because these variations can only be discerned when the size of an observed population is

* Correspondence: elisa.baioni@izsto.it
[1]Biostatistics, Epidemiology and Risk Analysis Unit, Istituto Zooprofilattico Sperimentale del Piemonte, Liguria e Valle d'Aosta, Via Bologna 148, 10154 Torino, Italy
Full list of author information is available at the end of the article

known, and knowledge of the animal population size of a specific area is required for estimating the incidence of zoonotic diseases [3], veterinary epidemiologists face numerous hurdles to arriving at a correct estimate of an animal population at risk.

To get around this problem, some registries have obtained the denominator from pet insurance company databases [4, 5], but with the risk of having an incomplete denominator and introducing a systematic error. Insured dogs likely represent a selected subset of the real composition of an area's dog population. [6]. Recognizing this limitation, veterinary studies have underscored the importance of selecting a delimited geographic area as referential for case collection when establishing animal population-based tumour registries. After an area has been selected, a distinction is made between cases belonging to the area and those not belonging to it. Cases belonging to the area but diagnosed outside of it then need to be identified and retrieved, and cases of animals living outside of it need to be excluded. It is acknowledged that the owners of dogs with cancer will often use veterinary services whereby cases are detected and reported, ultimately restricting the denominator to dogs receiving veterinary care.

The first population-based canine tumour registry was set up by the California State Department of Public Health to estimate the cancer incidence in dogs and cats resident in two counties in California, and to measure the effects of age, sex and breed on cancer development [7]. Over a 3-year period, malignant neoplasm cases in dogs and cats were reported to the registry through the collaboration of county veterinarians. The cases were categorized by their primary tumour site according to the International Classification of Diseases, Revision 7 (ICD-7). The estimated annual incidence rates for malignant cancers of all anatomic sites were 381.2/100,000 dogs and 155.8/100,000 cats.

Ten years later, MacVean et al. [8] investigated the denominator for the cancer incidence rate for dogs seen by veterinarians in one year in two counties. Histopathological diagnosis was offered free to the practitioners participating in the registry. The annual incidence rate for malignant neoplasms was 507/100,000 dogs, or double that of the Californian registry. Other European studies, using as denominator the cynological organization databases, reported incidence rates for some specific breeds [9–11].

The results of two cancer registration projects in Italy have recently been published. The Animal Tumour Registry of Genoa estimated an incidence rate for malignant cancers of 185.7/100,000 dogs [12]. The Animal Tumour Registry of Venice and Vicenza counties was set up in 2005 and provides free histopathological testing to veterinary practices in its catchment area. The

estimated incidence rate for malignant neoplasms was 142.8/100,000 dogs [13].

Here we report canine cancer incidence data collected between 2001 and 2008 for a small, well-delimited geographical area in northwestern Italy. As the data were obtained from a population-based registry, the Piedmont Canine Cancer Registry, for an area without any known specific environmental hazard, they may be considered a reliable estimate of reference incidence rates and so may serve as comparison data for other registries.

Methods
Denominator
The catchment area was selected according to the following criteria: 1) a population of less than 20,000 dog units with an annually expected number of suspected cases bearable by the histopathological laboratory (the bearable burden of diagnostic testing was calculated using as "expected incidence" the figures reported in Dorn et al. [7] in their population-based registry in California); 2) both urban and rural environments to allow internal comparisons within the dataset; 3) a geographically well-delimited area.

Based on the above criteria, an area (Fig. 1) comprising 46 municipalities in northernwestern Piedmont was selected, where 17,770 dogs were recorded in the canine identification and registration system, which at the time (2001) was still in hard copy format. The area is under the administration of a single local health unit. It is bordered to the west and north by geographical barriers (Alps); on its southern and eastern borders it is surrounded by municipalities within the same local health unit that acted as a buffer area for data collection. The 22 veterinary practitioners in the catchment area and the buffer area were involved in the collection and identification of suspected tumours. The ArcGIS version 9.2 (ESRI, Redlands, CA, USA) was used to create the thematic map.

Surveys were carried out to estimate the real size of the dog population, removing the deceased subjects and including the unregistered dogs within the local canine identification and registration systems.

A capture-recapture (CR) method (Lincoln Petersen) [14] - normally used in ecology - was adopted and applied to the canine population of the catchment area. The CR method has been already applied to define the reference animal population in cancer registries [13] and is routinely used in epidemiological studies. The first stage of the method is the capture of a number of individuals (M), marked, and subsequently released within the general population.

In a second stage, a new random sample (n) is captured, out of which (m) is found to be already marked. If the marked subjects perfectly merge with the unmarked

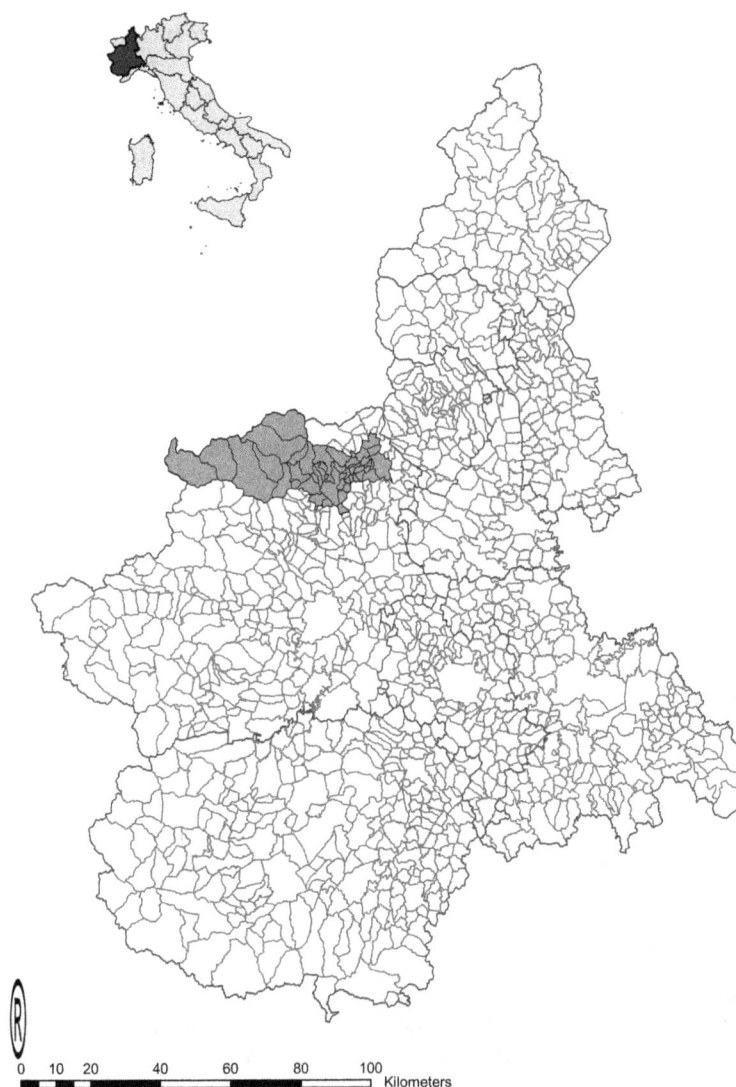

Fig. 1 The catchment area of the canine tumour registry. *Left angle*: map of Italy and Piedmont; *Right angle*: map of Piedmont and the catchment area

animals, the proportion of the marked individuals within the unknown overall population N and within the second sample n remains constant: $m / n = M / N$.

In this study, the first 'capture' is represented by the data from the regional canine identification and registration system, corrected after excluding the deceased subjects. This preliminary correction was carried out on the basis of a pilot telephone survey of the dog owners. The sample size of the survey (n = 545) was calculated on the basis of an expected prevalence rate of 15% of deceased dogs, an error of 3%, a 95% confidence interval (CI), and an expected response rate of 80%. The sample was stratified according to the number of dogs registered per municipality. The second random sample (recapture) was obtained by means of an anonymous questionnaire survey to estimate the proportion of unregistered dogs

and, therefore, the overall population; the sample size was calculated using the same parameters (expected prevalence 15%, accepted error 3%, 95% CI). Moreover, the second survey was also used to estimate the structure of the canine population by age, sex, and breed and to estimate the proportion of owned dogs receiving veterinary care. The latter data were needed to estimate the proportion of the dog population that was actually seen in veterinary practices and could provide the incident cases to the laboratory. In urban areas the questionnaires were distributed in public offices (exam reservation centres), whereas in rural areas through the collaboration of the post office services which served also as questionnaire collection sites: 2000 hard copies of the questionnaire were printed out and distributed.

Finally, a dog population census based on 28,068 questionnaires sent to each household and covering most (44 out of 46) of the involved municipalities was conducted in 2005, four years after the start of the registration, by the local official veterinary service and used to validate and update the capture-recapture estimates.

Numerator

A parallel public awareness campaign was launched through announcements in local print and media channels to inform dog owners about the canine tumour registry and its services. The tumour samples collected by biopsy, post-mortem or surgical removal were sent to the two diagnostic laboratories participating in the project and analysed free of charge. In addition, a dissection room was set up by the official veterinary service of the area for post-mortem examination and cancer detection if the owner decided to have the dog euthanised.

All veterinary practices were provided with a standardised case report form specifically designed for the collection of canine cancer cases. Because very few dogs had a subcutaneous microchip carrying their identification number, the animal's name, breed, date of birth, sex, and the owner's surname and address of the place of residence were recorded to identify each animal. Where the breed was not clearly indicated or two breeds were reported as indication of a mixed breed, this was included in the category "crossbreed". Tumour data included anatomic site, lesion size, date of excision, and any related historical and clinical information (e.g., ovariohysterectomy or castration status). The participating practitioners were also provided with a form to report cases in which cancer diagnosis had been obtained from laboratories other than the two project laboratories.

Formalin-fixed samples were routinely processed, paraffin-embedded and stained with haematoxylin and eosin for histological examination. Immunohistochemical analysis was performed to characterise poorly differentiated neoplasms. Tumours were classified and coded according to the Classification of tumours of domestic animals, World Health Organization Tumor Fascicles and the International Classification of Diseases for Oncology, 3rd edition (ICD-0) [15–17].

Based on the histopathological diagnosis, each type of neoplasm of a multiple primary tumours was classified as a separate cancer and added to the numerator

Cancer incidence calculation

A database (Microsoft Access) was created for collecting all cancer cases: information about sex, age, place of residence, veterinarian, number of tumours in the same dog, tumour classification, and tumour behaviour were entered into the database.

Incidence rates were calculated for histologically assessed malignant and benign tumours. In particular, specific rates by age, breed and sex were estimated with 95% confidence intervals. The incidence rates were expressed as the number of cases per 100,000 dog-years. A rate ratio was calculated to compare two subsequent registration period and its 95% confidence level was calculated to detect an eventual statistical significant difference (i.e. in case the 95% confidence interval would not include a value of 1). Statistical data analysis was performed using STATA software SE 11 (Stata Corp., College Station, TX, USA).

Results

Dog population size and structure

When the registration activity started in 2001, the reference canine population was estimated through a capture-recapture approach that yielded an overall population of 10,095 dogs (95% confidence interval (CI) 9705–10,485). As the first capture was based on dogs registered with the local identification and registration systems, 590 telephone interviews with dog owners were conducted (87% response rate) to preliminarily estimate the proportion of deceased dogs still registered. About half (55%) of the registered dogs had already died; therefore, the number of dogs registered and still alive (first capture) was estimated to be 8005. The second capture was obtained through an anonymous questionnaire survey (31.35% response rate) that yielded the identification of 627 dogs, 497 of which (79.3%) were recaptured as already registered with the canine registry office (95% CI 75.8–82.3). A 2005 midterm census of the municipalities in the catchment area (44 out of 46) confirmed the previous population estimates: the canine population was 9987 dogs as compared to the 9097 dogs estimated in the same 44 municipalities with the capture-recapture method (with a potential underestimation of 9.6%). Owing to the incompleteness of the census data (one of the two municipalities excluded was the largest town in the area), only the capture-recapture estimates were used as denominators for computing the incidence rates.

In the second survey, 91% of dog owners reported that they regularly used veterinary services for their dog's health care (95% CI 88–93), suggesting that the veterinary practitioners were able to find tumours in 9182 dogs out of the 10,095 calculated. Based on the population size and the observation period (90 months), the total dog-years of observation to calculate the incidence rates were 68,865. In all, 55% of the dogs were male (95% CI 51–59%) and 48% were purebred (95% CI 44–52%), with 23 pure breeds (mainly German shepherd dog, Boxer, Yorkshire terrier, English setter and Siberian husky). Figure 2 shows the population structure by age.

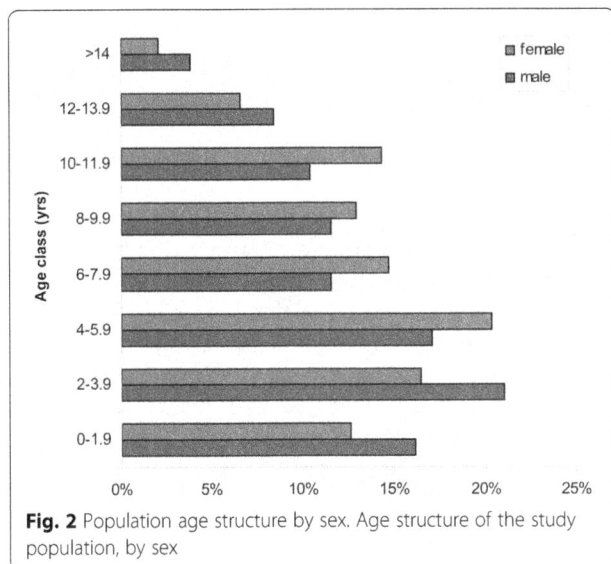

Fig. 2 Population age structure by sex. Age structure of the study population, by sex

Numerators and incidence rates

In its 90 months of operation, the Piedmont Canine Cancer Registry collected data on 1172 tumours, of which 618 benign and 554 malignant tumours were confirmed by histopathological diagnosis. Figure 3 presents the distribution of cases by most frequent tumour site.

The crude incidence rate was 804 per 100,000 dog-years for malignant tumours and 897 per 100,000 dog-years for benign tumours. As there was a decreasing trend for cancer cases at the end of 2002, we also calculated the incidence rates after splitting the registration period into two parts, before and after 01 June 2003 (period 1 vs. period 2); no statistically significant difference in the rates of malignant tumours was found (rate ratio [RR] 1.09, 95% CI 0.89–1.31) (Table 1).

Overall, the higher cancer incidence rates in the female dogs were largely due to the high number of mammary tumours.

Higher incidence rates for all cancers were observed in purebreds. The incidence rates by breed are presented in Table 2. The most common breeds in the study population were the German shepherd dog (7785 dog-years),

the Italian segugio (2003 dog-years), the English setter (1335 dog-years), and the Maremma sheepdog (1335 dog-years).

The cancer rates by age class in male and female dogs were similar up to the biennial class of 4–5.9 years, after which the rates started to diverge, with an increase noted for the females and a decrease for the males after the 10–11.9 age class (Fig. 4). The distribution of malignant tumours by sex and tumour site is shown in Fig. 5.

The most commonly affected organs were the mammary gland (n = 585), skin (n = 229), and ovaries (n = 40) in the female dogs and the skin (n = 242), testicles (n = 112), and spleen in the male dogs.

Table 3 reports the incidence rates of tumours by histological type and organ of origin (cases per 100,000 dog-years at risk) in the most frequently affected sites.

Discussion

Here we present the findings obtained from a canine population-based cancer registry that we conducted in northwestern Italy for a 90-month period from 2001 to 2008. The Piedmont canine cancer registry is one of few of its kind whose operations have been consistently supported by long-term public funding. The incidence rate of malignant and benign tumours was about 800 and 900 cases per 100,000 dog-years at risk, respectively, with the largest impact on females and purebred dogs. The highest incidence rates by sex and tumour site were observed for mammary and cutaneous tissues in females and cutaneous tissues and testicles in males. These results were obtained by paying particular attention to the validity of the data collection process, thus minimizing the potential for bias.

Given the constraints derived from working with a canine population, considerable effort was expended to estimate the relevant denominators in terms of population size and structure. Moreover, we were able to obtain detailed reports of cases of incidental tumours by selecting a small-medium size catchment area and through public awareness campaigns coupled with enhanced participation of veterinary practices offered scientific support and histological examinations free of charge.

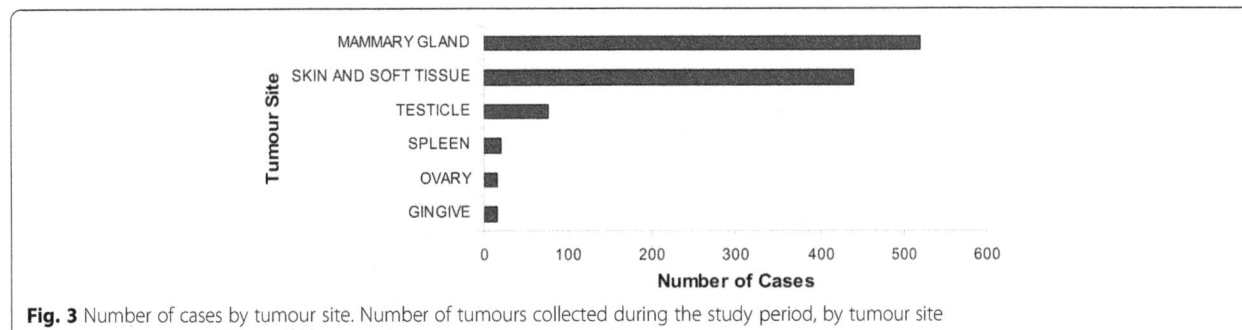

Fig. 3 Number of cases by tumour site. Number of tumours collected during the study period, by tumour site

Table 1 Crude incidence rates

	Number of cases	Dog-years	IR	95% CI
Crude	554	68,865	804	739–874
Female	344	31,113	1106	992–1229
Male	209	37,748	554	481–634
Purebred	311	32,820	948	845–1059
Crossbreed	233	36,045	646	566–735
Period 1	151	17,599	858	727–1006
Period 2	403	51,266	786	711–867

Malignant tumour incidence rates by sex, breed, and calendar period (cases per 100,000 dog-years at risk). *CI* denotes confidence interval, *IR* incidence rate

Though our study may have limitations, they do not necessarily compromise its internal or external validity. By mobilizing the available human and economic resources and restricting the cancer registration to a relatively small area (canine population of about 10,000 units), we were able to maintain the activities for a 90-month period, with a total of about 70,000 dog-years at risk which were then used as the overall denominator. The resulting overall incidence rates were found to be stable; however, less precise estimates could also have been obtained by looking at subgroups (e.g., municipality, breed, age class). For this reason, we carried out few subgroups analyses within our dataset.

As mentioned, there remains the potential for some residual bias in the quantification of the denominators and the numerators. Selection bias is less likely to be a problem with population-based registries than, for example, hospital-based registries [18, 19] or canine

Table 2 Breeds

Breed	Number of cases	Dog-years	IR	95% CI
Yorkshire terrier	19	555	3423	2061–5346
Boxer	34	1223	2781	1925–3885
Alaskan malamute	3	113	2667	548–7759
Chow chow	3	113	2667	548–7759
Pinscher	7	443	1582	635–3256
Dalmatian	5	338	1481	480–3452
English cocker spaniel	9	668	1348	616–2558
Italian pointer	3	225	1333	275–3897
Siberian husky	14	1223	1145	626–1921
Rottweiler	10	893	1120	537–2059
English setter	13	1335	974	519–1665
German shepherd dog	71	7785	912	712–1150

Malignant tumour incidence rates in the most common breeds in the study population (cases per 100,000 dog-years at risk). *CI* denotes confidence interval, *IR* incidence rate. Breeds with incidence rates below 900 cases per 100,000 dog-years at risk not shown

registries using databases from pet insurance companies where cross-breed dogs or aged dogs are apt to be underrepresented [6, 20].

With regard to the capture-recapture strategy that was applied to estimate the unknown canine population size, some of the assumptions this approach [14] requires may not have been fully met, e.g., working on a closed population and using random samples (assumptions that are unlikely to be met in a field situation); however, there are no evident reasons that preclude that the recruited dogs were equally likely to be captured in each of the two samples. The midterm census of 44 of the 46 municipalities in the catchment area indicated no large deviation from the direct enumeration of the existent dogs.

Additionally the population structure by breed- or age-strata may not be as precise as the population size. The structure was obtained from our second capture (the anonymous questionnaire survey) only. Unfortunately, the data on the first capture (i.e., the canine identification and registration system) and the midterm census were available only in hard copy format, precluding any practical way to further analyse the data. Therefore, the incidence rates are likely to be more robust when the denominator was the entire population (e.g., crude malignant rate or site-specific rates) rather than when the denominators referred to individual breeds or age classes.

Finally, with regard to the cases of incidental tumours, a certain degree of underdetection may have occurred. In particular, a proportion of tumours may have gone undiagnosed (e.g., a deep organ tumour), or not reported as not requiring histological confirmation (e.g., osteosarcoma, lymphoma) or may have been diagnosed by laboratories other than ours and not reported by the collaborating veterinary practitioners. In an attempt to minimize these problems, the collaborating veterinary practitioners were given standardized case report forms and local laboratories were contacted.

Assuming an unbiased estimation of cancer occurrence, the incidence rates in our registry are higher than those reported by similar population-based registries in Italy [12, 13] where the crude incidence rates for all malignant cancer were less than 200 cases per 100,000 dog-years at risk. The differences, albeit evident, are smaller when the comparison is carried out with data from international population-based registries ([7, 8, 21]). Rates higher than ours were reported in a registry that used as a denominator for cancer incidence all dogs insured with a pet U.K. insurance company [4]. The higher cancer rates we found cannot be convincingly linked to exposure of the dogs to as yet undetected environmental risk factors in the catchment area. Instead, the excess incidence may more likely stem from the effect of a

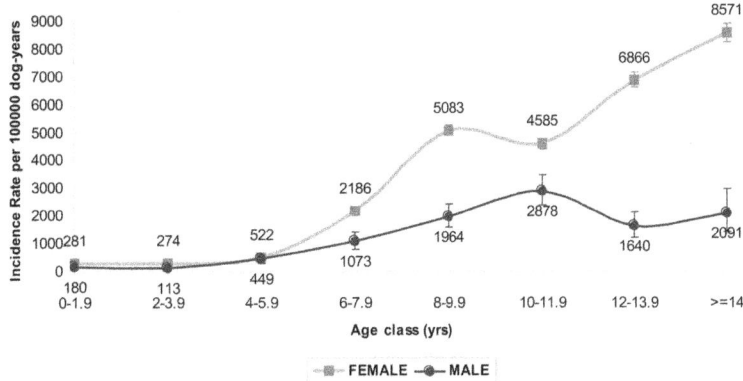

Fig. 4 Age and sex-specific incidence rates. Age and sex specific incidence rates: cases per 100,000 dog-years at risk

different distribution of confounding factors such as age and breed, which are known determinants of cancer in dogs [22–24]. Unfortunately, in most of the comparable studies, data on the population structure by age and breed were not available, preventing any appropriate comparison of rates. Moreover unlike other studies, in ours the denominators were reduced to take into account the real proportion of dogs under veterinary care, an adjustment not reported elsewhere.

Another explanation for the high cancer rates we found may be due to the way we managed the data on multiple primary tumours, which are a common finding in dogs [25–27]. Based on the histopathological diagnosis, each type of neoplasm was classified as a separate

cancer and added to the numerator. Other canine registries may not have done this. Finally, the potential risk of overestimation due to the inclusion of cases sourced from outside the registry catchment area was minimized by applying the preliminary case inclusion/exclusion criteria established in the registration protocol.

The distribution of cancer types in our registry is fairly consistent with the literature. As reported elsewhere [7–13, 21], the most prevalent malignant neoplasms were mammary carcinoma and cutaneous mastocytoma. The high prevalence of seminoma found in the Norwegian dog population [22] is analogous to the high incidence estimated in our registry. With regard to breed, the higher incidence rates in purebred rather than in cross-breed dogs were evident for Yorkshire terrier and Boxer, breeds known [5, 7, 27] to be particularly at risk of developing neoplasms, for which a genetic predisposition has been suggested. In the female dogs, the observed cancer trend by age matches those seen in other studies, with an exponential increase in elderly females for all tumours [9] or specifically for mammary tumours [5].

Comparison with the recent findings from two other Italian cancer registries [12, 13] shows that the distribution of tumours is substantially similar. In our registry, the ratio of malignant to benign tumours was 0.90:1, as compared to 0.96:1 in Genoa and 1:1 in the Veneto Region. The incidence of malignant cancer was higher in females than in males (2.5 times, 2.7 times, and 1.7 times in the study area, Genoa, and Veneto, respectively) and in purebred dogs than in cross-breed dogs (1.5 times in Piedmont and 2 times in Veneto where data were available). Finally, the distribution by tumour site (mammary and cutaneous/soft tissues tumours in females and cutaneous/soft tissues and genital tract tumours in males) was quite similar for all three registries. The exceptionally higher incidence of lymphoma in dogs of both sexes in the Genoa registry may have been due to

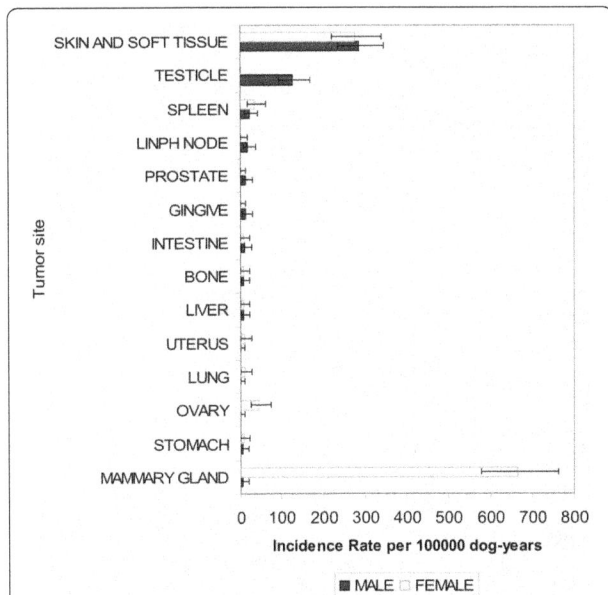

Fig. 5 Malignant tumours: site- and sex-specific incidence rates. Site and sex specific incidence rates for malignant tumours: cases per 100,000 dog-years at risk

Table 3 Tumour site and histological type

Site	Tumour	ICD-O code	Number of cases	Dog-years	IR	95% CI
Mammary gland	Complex Carcinoma	8010/3	60	31,113	193	147–248
	Carcinoma Simplex	8231/3	36	31,113	116	81–160
	Tubulopapillary Carcinoma	8263/3	18	31,113	58	34–91
	Carcinoma In Situ	8010/2	18	31,113	58	34–91
	Solid Carcinoma	8230/3	16	31,113	51	29–84
Skin	Mastocytoma	9740/3	73	68,865	106	83–133
	Hemangiopericytoma	9150/1	28	68,865	41	27–59
Genital tract	Seminoma	9061/3	25	37,748	66	43–98
	Sertoli Cell Tumour	8640/1	13	37,748	34	18–59
Spleen	Hemangiosarcoma	9120/3	13	68,865	19	10–32

Incidence rates of malignant tumours (cases per 100,000 dog-years at risk) by histological type and site (only the higher incidence rates are shown). *CI* denotes confidence interval, *IR* incidence rate *ICD-O* International Classification of Diseases for Oncology

the inclusion of cancers diagnosed by cytology or because of exposure to unknown risk factors present in a large city.

The Piedmont canine cancer registry is based on a large target population that combine rural and urban environments and on a population-based study design; for this reason our findings have the necessary external validity to be generalized, after adjustment for breed and age, to the canine population of northwestern Italy.

Assuming that the incidence rates from a population-based registry have external validity, national and international standards should be developed and shared to be able to make any meaningful comparison across studies. The adoption of an international classification and coding system, like the International Classification of Diseases for Oncology used in human cancer registries [28], would facilitate the exchange of comparable data and the possibility to carry out multicenter studies [29].

Finally, basic epidemiological methods (e.g., standardization techniques) to account for the confounding effect of age and breed should always be applied: data on population structure should be collected and made available in each study and, as proposed by Thrusfield [30], an international normal dog population should be established and shared as an external standard.

Conclusions

As highlighted by Kelsey et al. [19], the data from population-based canine cancer registries may facilitate the identification of a less select group of cases for case-control studies and allow examination of trends over time and geographic differences in cancer incidence. The findings from the current study provide data on the incidence of canine tumours. The incidence rates may be useful for assessing the impact of neoplastic diseases

in the canine population in northwestern Italy and may serve as a reference when setting up studies to detect excess risks in the incidence of malignant tumours in dogs used as sentinels for community exposure to environmental carcinogens.

Acknowledgments
This work was supported by Piedmont Region (Ricerca Sanitaria Finalizzata 2000 & 2002, Ricerca Scientifica Applicata 2003). The authors are grateful to the public veterinary service (ASL TO4) and the veterinary practitioners involved in the project.

Funding
This work was supported by Piedmont Region (Ricerca Sanitaria Finalizzata 2000 & 2002, Ricerca Scientifica Applicata 2003). The funders had no role in study design, data collection and analysis, decision to publish, or preparation of the manuscript.

Authors' contributions
EBA carried out the research project, analysed and interpreted the data, and drafted the manuscript; EBO and ES performed the histopathological analysis and revised the manuscript; MCV assisted in the design of the study; MP carried out all laboratory procedures and contributed to the histopathological diagnosis, ML was responsible for conception of the study and necropsy examinations; RD and SB carried out the statistical analysis to estimate the canine population denominators and contributed to the conception of the study, CM assisted in the conduct and reporting of the study, GR supervised the project and contributed to the manuscript. All authors read, revised and approved the final manuscript.

Consent for publication
Not applicable.

Competing interests
The authors declare that they have no competing interests.

Author details
[1]Biostatistics, Epidemiology and Risk Analysis Unit, Istituto Zooprofilattico Sperimentale del Piemonte, Liguria e Valle d'Aosta, Via Bologna 148, 10154

Torino, Italy. [2]Department of Veterinary Science and Veterinary Public Health, Università degli Studi di Milano, Milan, Italy. [3]Azienda Sanitaria Locale Valle d'Aosta, Aosta, Italy. [4]Azienda Sanitaria Locale TO4, Ivrea, Turin, Italy. [5]Histopathology Unit, Istituto Zooprofillattico Sperimentale del Piemonte, Liguria e Valle d'Aosta, Torino, Italy.

References

1. Ottinger MA, Dean KM. Neuroendocrine impacts of endocrine-disrupting chemicals in birds: life stage and species sensitivities. J Toxicol Environ Health B Crit Rev. 2011;14(5–7):413–22.

2. Garbe PL. The companion animal as a sentinel for environmentally related human diseases. Acta Vet Scand Suppl. 1988;84:290–2.

3. Patronek GJ, Beck AM, Glickman LT. Dynamics of dog and cat populations in a community. J Am Vet Med Assoc. 1997;210(5):637–42.

4. Dobson JM, Samuel S, Milstein H, Rogers K, Wood JL. Canine neoplasia in the UK: estimates of incidence rates from a population of insured dogs. J Small Anim Pract. 2002;43(6):240–6.

5. Egenvall A, Bonnett BN, Ohagen P, Olson P, Hedhammar A, von Euler H. Incidence of and survival after mammary tumors in a population of over 80,000 insured female dogs in Sweden from 1995 to 2002. Prev Vet Med. 2005;69(1–2):109–27.

6. Egenvall A, Nodtvedt A, Penell J, Gunnarsson L, Bonnett BN. Insurance data for research in companion animals: benefits and limitations. Acta Vet Scand. 2009;51:42.

7. Dorn CR, Taylor DO, Schneider R, Hibbard HH, Klauber MR. Survey of animal neoplasms in alameda and contra costa counties, California. II. Cancer morbidity in dogs and cats from Alameda County. J Natl Cancer Inst. 1968;40(2):307–18.

8. MacVean DW, Monlux AW, Anderson PS Jr, Silberg SL, Roszel JF. Frequency of canine and feline tumors in a defined population. Vet Pathol. 1978;15(6):700–15.

9. Moe L. Population-based incidence of mammary tumours in some dog breeds. Journal of Reproduction & Fertility - Supplement. 2001;57:439–43.

10. Anfinsen KP, Grotmol T, Bruland OS, Jonasdottir TJ. Breed-specific incidence rates of canine primary bone tumors–a population based survey of dogs in Norway. Can J Vet Res. 2011;75(3):209–15.

11. Boerkamp KM, Teske E, Boon LR, Grinwis GC, van den Bossche L, Rutteman GR: Estimated incidence rate and distribution of tumours in 4,653 cases of archival submissions derived from the Dutch golden retriever population. BMC Vet Res. 2014;10:34–6148–10-34.

12. Merlo DF, Rossi L, Pellegrino C, Ceppi M, Cardellino U, Capurro C, et al. Cancer incidence in pet dogs: findings of the animal tumor registry of Genoa, Italy. J Vet Intern Med. 2008;22(4):976–84.

13. Vascellari M, Baioni E, Ru G, Carminato A, Mutinelli F. Animal tumour registry of two provinces in northern Italy: incidence of spontaneous tumours in dogs and cats. BMC Vet Res. 2009;5:39.

14. Chao A, Tsay PK, Lin S, Shau W, Chao D. The applications of capture-recapture models to epidemiological data. Stat Med. 2001;20(20):3123–57.

15. Anonymous International histological classification of tumors of domestic animals. Bull World Health Organ. 1974;50(1–2):1–142.

16. Beveridge WI, Sobin LH. International histological classification of tumours of domestic animals: introduction. Bull World Health Organ. 1976;53(2–3):137–41.

17. Fritz A. ICD-O international classification of diseases for oncology: 3. ed ed. Geneva: World health organization; 2000.

18. Withrow SJ, Vail DM. Withrow & MacEwen's small animal clinical oncology 4th ed. Philadelphia: W.B. Saunders Company; 2007. p. 846.

19. Kelsey JL, Moore AS, Glickman LT. Epidemiologic studies of risk factors for cancer in pet dogs. Epidemiol Rev. 1998;20(2):204–17.

20. Wood JLN, Dobson J, Rogers K. An epidemiological study of cancer in British dogs based on insurance company data. Proceedings of the 9th symposium of the International Society for Veterinary Epidemiology and Economics. 2000;956-958.

21. Reid-Smith R, Bonnett B, Martin S, Kruth S, Abrams-Ogg A, Hazlett M. The incidence of neoplasia in the canine and feline patient populations of private veterinary practices in Ontario. Proceedings of the 9th Symposium of the International Society for Veterinary Epidemiology and Economics, Breckenridge, Colorado: International Symposia on Veterinary Epidemiology and Economics; 2000;460

22. Nodtvedt A, Gamlem H, Gunnes G, Grotmol T, Indrebo A, Moe L. Breed differences in the proportional morbidity of testicular tumours and distribution of histopathologic types in a population-based canine cancer registry. Vet Comp Oncol. 2011;9(1):45–54.

23. Dobson JM. Breed-predispositions to cancer in pedigree dogs. ISRN Vet Sci. 2013;2013:941275.

24. Priester WA, McKay FW. The occurrence of tumors in domestic animals. Natl Cancer Inst Monogr. 1980;54:1-210.

25. Mulligan RM. Multiple primary tumors in dogs. Cancer Res. 1944;4(8):505–9.

26. Dorn CR, Taylor DO, Chaulk LE, Hibbard HH. The prevalence of spontaneous neoplasms in a defined canine population. Am J Public Health Nations Health. 1966;56(2):254–65.

27. Bronden LB, Nielsen SS, Toft N, Kristensen AT. Data from the Danish veterinary cancer registry on the occurrence and distribution of neoplasms in dogs in Denmark. Vet Rec. 2010;166(19):586–90.

28. Dos Santos Silva I. Cancer epidemiology: principles and methods. Lyon: International Agency for Research on Cancer. 1999;442.

29. Nodtvedt A, Berke O, Bonnett BN, Bronden L. Current status of canine cancer registration - report from an international workshop. Vet Comp Oncol. 2012;10(2):95–101.

30. Thrusfield MV. Demographic characteristics of the canine and feline populations of the UK in 1986. J Small Anim Pract. 1989;30(2):76–80.

16

Identification of the two KIT isoforms and their expression status in canine hemangiosarcomas

Yi-Chen Chen[1,2], Jiunn-Wang Liao[2], Wei-Li Hsu[3]* and Shih-Chieh Chang[1,4]*

Abstract

Background: KIT is a tyrosine kinase growth factor receptor. High expression of KIT has been found in several tumors including canine hemangiosarcoma (HSA). This study investigated the correlation of KIT expression and *c-kit* sequence mutations in canine HSAs and benign hemangiomas (HAs).

Results: Immunohistochemistry (IHC) staining confirmed KIT expression in 94.4 % (34/36) of HSAs that was significantly higher than 0 % in HAs (0/16). Sequencing the entire *c-kit* coding region of HSAs and normal canine cerebellums (NCCs) revealed GNSK-deletion in exon 9. As for exon 9 genotyping by TA-cloning strategy, GNSK-deletion *c-kit* accounted for 48.6 % (68/140) colonies amplified from 12 KIT-positive HSAs, a significantly higher frequency than 14.1 % (9/64) of colonies amplified from six NCCs.

Conclusions: Due to the distinct expression pattern revealed by IHC, KIT might be used to distinguish benign or malignant vascular endothelial tumors. Moreover, the high incidence of GNSK-deletion *c-kit* in canine HSAs implicates KIT isoforms as possibly participating in the tumorigenesis of canine HSAs.

Keywords: Canine, Hemangiosarcoma, *c-kit*, GNSK-deletion, Isoform, KIT

Background

Hemangiosarcomas (HSAs) are highly malignant tumors of vascular endothelial origin, which occur more frequently in dogs than other domestic species and are characterized by a high fatality rate [1, 2]. Surgical excision remains the primary treatment for most dogs with HSAs [3]. However, owing to a poor outcome by surgery alone, adjuvant chemotherapy is suggested for canine HSAs [4].

KIT protein, encoded by proto-oncogene *c-kit*, is a tyrosine kinase growth factor receptor for stem cell factor (SCF). Generally, KIT is activated by autophosphorylation upon the binding of its ligand SCF [5]; however it is constitutively expressed in a number of cells including mast cells, and hematopoietic stem cells

[6]. In humans, KIT is often expressed in angiosarcomas, but it is not detected in most benign vascular tumors, and KIT positivity is more likely related to an immature phenotype [7]. As with human tissues, KIT is expressed in a large proportion of canine HSAs [8]. It has been demonstrated that activating mutations of *c-kit* typically confer constitutional KIT phosphorylation leading to downstream activation independent of ligand binding [9]. Among the 21 exons, the common activating mutations are located in exons 11 and 17, coding for juxtamembrane domain and tyrosine kinase domain of KIT, respectively [10–12]. Gain-of-function mutations have been proposed to contribute to neoplastic growth of several tumor mast cell lines [13]. Sequence analysis of canine mast cell tumors (MCTs) identified several mutations in exons 8, 9, 11, and 17 of *c-kit* RNA [14]. In contrast to MCTs, no mutation was found in these two exons (11 and 17) of *c-kit* gene in KIT-positive neoplasms of vascular cell origin [7].

Imatinib (Gleevec; Novartis), the tyrosine kinase inhibitor that targets activating mutations of *c-kit*, has been used in patients with gastrointestinal stromal

* Correspondence: wlhsu@dragon.nchu.edu.tw; scchang@dragon.nchu.edu.tw
[3]Graduate Institute of Microbiology and Public Health, College of Veterinary Medicine, National Chung Hsing University, 250 Kuo-Kuang Road, Taichung 40227, Taiwan
[1]Department of Veterinary Medicine, College of Veterinary Medicine, National Chung Hsing University, 250 Kuo-Kuang Road, Taichung 40227, Taiwan
Full list of author information is available at the end of the article

tumors (GIST) harboring a *c-kit* exon 11 mutation. Decreases in tumor mass and increases of survival time have been reported [15, 16].

At present, *c-kit* gene polymorphism was detected in various canine tumors [17], but information of mutations or the impact of the *c-kit* gene in canine HSAs was limited. Since *c-kit* gene mutations could influence the expression level of KIT, and also the sensitivity of kinase inhibitor (such as imatinib mesylate) treatment [18], a systemic investigation of the mutation status of *c-kit* would provide prognostic information for tumor pathogenesis and also for the clinical response of patients under imatinib therapy [19]. Hence, this study aimed to evaluate the contribution of KIT expression and also genetic variations in the malignancy of canine HSAs.

Methods

Samples

Dogs with cutaneous hemangiomas (HAs) or splenic/cutaneous HSAs presented to the Veterinary Medical Teaching Hospital from 2005 to 2012 were enrolled. Medical records included breed, age, sex, number of tumors, tumor size, anatomical location, clinical history, physical examination, complete blood count, serum biochemical profile, thoracic and abdominal radiographs, abdominal ultrasonography, fine-needle cytological examination and needle core biopsy or surgical excision for histological examination. All HSAs were staged according to the World Health Organization staging system for canine splenic HSAs [9] and cutaneous HSAs [20]. The protocol of study was approved by the Institutional Animal Care and Use Committee of National Chung Hsing University [IACUC Number: 102–70].

In total, 52 specimens (16 HAs by surgical excision, 24 HSAs by surgical excision and 12 cutaneous HSAs by needle core biopsy) were included in this study. For histologic examination, specimens were fixed in neutral-buffered 10 % formalin overnight, and then processed routinely. Sections were stained with haematoxylin and eosin. Histologic grading of HSAs was assigned by cumulative scores of differentiation, mitotic rate (the number of mitotic figures per 10 high magnification fields) and percentage of necrosis [21].

Immunohistochemistry (IHC) analysis

Serial sections of formalin-fixed and wax-embedded tissues were deparaffinized and rehydrated. Table 1 lists primary and secondary antibodies and antigen retrieval procedures used in immunohistochemical (IHC) analysis. Antigen retrieval was modified from a previous study [22]. Slides in buffer solution were cooled at room temperature for 20 min, and incubated with peroxidase-blocking reagent (S200389, Dako) for 30 min, and then treated with primary antibodies. In each interval of the following procedures, sections were rinsed with a mixture of Tris-Buffered Saline and Tween-20. Slides were then reacted with secondary antibody followed by incubation of DAB and chromogen (dilution 1 μL in 100 μL) from a commercial ChemMate EnVision detection kit (K5007, Dako). Finally, sections were counterstained with Mayer's hematoxylin for 2 min then rinsed with DDW, and incubated with 37 mM ammonia water for 5 s and rinsed with DDW.

For immunolabelingvon Willebrand factor (vWF), a canine subcutaneous granuloma acted as a positive control, and normal vessels in tissues surrounding the tumor served as an internal positive control [8]. For immunolabeling vimentin or KIT, normal adipose tissues [23] or a normal canine cerebellum (NCC) [24] was used as a positive control respectively. Replacement of primary antibody with antibody dilution buffer served as a negative control.

To score expression, this study followed an immunoreactive score (IRS) system from a previous study [25] in which IRS = SI (staining intensity) x PP (percentage of positive cells). SI was assigned as 0, negative; 1, weak; 2, moderate; and 3, strong. PP was defined as 1, <10 % positive cells; 2, 10–50 % positive cells; and 3, >50 % positive cells. Ten high magnification fields were randomly chosen for IRS evaluation. The expression level was classified as 'negative', 'weak', or 'strong', corresponding to IRS values of

Table 1 Primary and secondary antibodies and antigen retrieval procedures used in IHC analysis of this study

Antibody	pAb/mAb (clone)	Host	Source	Antigen retrieval (buffer, microwave, interval)	Time for incubation		
					Primary Ab	Secondary Ab	DAB+ Chromagen
von Willebrand factor	pAb	Rabbit anti human	Dako	Citrate buffer (0.01 M pH 6.0), 700 W-10 min and 300W-10 min	1:200, 30 min	10 min	1 min
vimentin	mAb (V9)	Mouse anti human	Dako	TE buffer (pH 9.0), 700 W-10 min and 400W-10 min	1:150, 1 h	10 min	10 min
KIT	pAb	Rabbit anti human	Dako	TE buffer (pH 9.0),700 W-10 min and 400W-10 min	1:400, 30 min	10 min	2 min

pAb polyclonal antibody, *mAb* monoclonal antibody, *TE buffer* Tris-EDTA buffer solution

0–1, 2–4 and 6–9, respectively. For KIT expression, three patterns were determined as pattern I, a membrane associated pattern with little to no cytoplasmic staining; pattern II, a focal (paranuclear or Golgi-like) cytoplasmic pattern with only occasional minor membrane staining, and pattern III, a diffuse cytoplasmic pattern [26].

Identification of *c-kit* coding sequences

Total RNA extracted with Trizol (Invitrogen) from 12HSAs with KIT-overexpression and from a NCC for amplifying wild-type open reading frame of *c-kit* gene were reverse transcribed into cDNA. A solution of 2 µg RNA, 2 µL of 5 µM random primers, 4 µL of 2.5 mM dNTP and 7 µL DDW were incubated at 65 °C for 5 min, then chilled on ice for 5 min. The mixture of reverse transcriptase solution, which included 1 µL of 0.1 M dithiothreitol, 1 µL reverse transcriptase (Superscript III, Invitrogen), 4 µL of 5× First Strand Buffer (Invitrogen) and 1 µL RNase inhibitor (Promega), was added and heated at 50 °C for 60 min, then inactivated at 70 °C for 15 min and chilled on ice.

Sequencing of the entire *c-kit* coding region was determined by PCR using several sets of primers followed by automated sequencing. Primers were designed according to a previously published canine *c-kit* cDNA sequence [27]. Sequences, as well as locations of primers, are listed in Table 2.

In general, PCR solution included 2.5 µL of 10× Taq buffer, 2.5 µL of 2.5 mM dNTP, 1 µL of 5 mM of both sense and anti-sense primer, 0.5 U DreamTaq DNA polymerase (EP0702, Fermentas), 2 µl of RT reaction mixture and 15.5 µL DDW. PCRwas performed by carrying outinitial denaturation for 5 min at 95 °C, followed by 40 thermocycles: 1 min at 95 °C, annealing for 45 s at 52 to 62 °C (Table 2) and then 1 min at 72 °C, and final polymerization for 7 min at 72 °C. Amplified products were electrophoresed with 1.5 % agarose gel and visualized with a UV illuminator.

The amplified fragments with expected size were purified by a commercial gel extraction kit (DF300, Qiagen), which was performed with an automated sequencing(Mission Biotech Co., Taipei, Taiwan). The sequences obtained from a NCC were initially compared with a canine *c-kit* sequence [GenBank: AF448148]. Sequences of HSAs were aligned with those of NCC using the BLAST program on the NCBI.

Cloning of PCR amplicon containing the exon 9 region of *c-kit*

To clarify sequences of the most 3′end of *c-kit* exon 9 of HSAs, DNA fragments containing exon 9 were amplified by PCR with primers set EX9F/R (Table 2) and were then purified. Ligation was conducted by a TOPO TA Cloning Kit (450641, Invitrogen) followed by transforming to TOP10 competent cells and plating onto an LB

Table 2 Sequences and locations of *c-kit* primers used in this study

Designation	Sequence (5'-3')	Primer location
1F	CGATGAGAGGCGCTCGC	27–34
1R	GGCGTAACACA TGAACACTCCAG	891–913
2F	GCTGGCATCATGGTGACTTC	819–838
2R	CATGGGTTTCTGTAGATACTTGTAGG	1668–1693
3F	CACACCTTTGCTGATTGGCT	1591–1610
3R	GATTCGACCATGAGTAAGGAGG	2419–2440
4F	GGGTATGGCATTCCTGGC	2359–2376
4R	GCTTCACACATCTTCGTGTACCA	2937–2959
AF	GCTCAGAGTCTATCGCAGCCACCG	3–26
AR	CTGCCTTCTCTGTGATCCATTCGTTG	271–296
BF	GCTGTCCAAGAAATTCACCCTG	619–640
BR	ATATTACTTTCATTGTCAGACTTGGG	1124–1149
CF	AAAACTCGTCTCTGTCACCGTCTG	1422–1445
CR	GATCTCCTCAACAACCTTCCACTG	1691–1714
DF	AAATCAGAGTTAATAGTCAGTGTCGG	133–158
DR	TTTATCCACATCGAGTCCACG	729–749
EX9F	CAACAATGTAGGCAGGAGTTCTG	1495–1517
EX9R	CAGCAAAGGTGTGAACAGGG	1572–1591

F forward, *R* reverse

Annealing temperature dependent on combination of the primers: 55 °C for 1F and 1R, 56 °C for 2F and 2R, 52 °C for 3F and 3R, 61 °C for AF and AR, 54 °C for BF and BR, 57 °C for CF and CR, 54 °C for DF and DR, 57 °C for AF and BR, 55 °C for P2F and CR, 56 °C for CF and P3R, and 54 °C for EX9F and EX9R

plate containing ampicillin as well as X-gal and IPTG for the case of blue/white screening.

After 16 h of incubation, 10 to 14 white colonies randomly picked from each plate were cultured at 37 °C overnight and then the plasmid DNA was extracted via High-Speed Plasmid Mini Kit, (PD300, Geneaid). Plasmids with insertion of *c-kit* DNA were initially confirmed by the digestion pattern using are striction enzyme *Eco*RI (New England Biolabs Inc.) followed by automated sequencing (Mission Biotech Co.).

Statistical analysis

The statistical analysis was performed using Statistical Package for the Social Science (Version 19.0, SPSS Taiwan Corp). Univariate logistic regression was used to establish the correlation between variables and KIT immunolabeling patterns. P-value <0.05 indicated a statistically significant difference between categorized groups.

Results

Animals

As listed in Additional file 1: Table S1, of the 16 dogs with HAs, seven were male and nine were female. Dogs with HSAs included 24 males and 12 females. Pedigree dogs comprised eight breeds and accounted for 56.3 % (9/16) of dogs with HAs, and 58.3 % (21/36) of dogs with HSAs, which included Maltese ($n = 3$), Pomeranian ($n = 2$), and Golden Retriever ($n = 2$) with HAs, and Golden Retriever ($n = 8$), Miniature Schnauzer ($n = 5$), Beagle ($n = 2$), Maltese ($n = 2$), and Labrador Retriever ($n = 2$) with HSAs. Labrador retriever and Shetland sheepdog each accounted for 1/16 with HA; and Caucasian sheepdog and Welsh Corgi each accounted for 1/36 with HSA. The other 43.7 % (7/16) of HA and 41.7 % (15/36) of HSA occurred in mixed dogs. The median age in dogs with HA was 11.8 years (range 2–16 years), and 13.4 years (range 4–18 years) in dogs with HSA.

Clinical stages of HSA included stage III in 58.3 % (21/36), stage II in 22.2 % (8/36), and stage I in 19.5 % (7/36) of dogs. Histological grades were assigned as grade I in 5.6 % (2/36), grade II in 33.3 % (12/36), and graded III in 61.1 % (22/36) of dogs.

Detection of KIT expression by IHC

To study the correlation of KIT expression with *c-kit* sequence mutations in canine HSAs, initially, KIT expression in canine HSAs and KIT expression in HAs were detected by IHC analysis, of which, KIT staining was optimized using NCC as a positive control (Fig. 1a), and omitting KIT antibody as a negative control. As listed in Table 3, vWF expression was demonstrated in all HSAs (36/36, 100 %), vimentin expression was shown in 97.2 % of HSAs (35/36), and KIT expression was detected in 94.4 % of HSAs (34/36), whereas negative KIT expression was found in all HAs (16/16, 100 %, and Fig. 1b). All KIT-positive HSAs (34/34, 100 %) showed a diffuse cytoplasmic immunostaining pattern (Fig. 1 panels c-d).

Identification of *c-kit* gene sequences of HSA

In order to identify possible mutations of the *c-kit* gene in canine HSAs, amplicons covering the entire coding region of the *c-kit* gene were amplified by PCR using several sets of primers followed by automated sequencing. Initially, sequences representing wild type *c-kit* gene were amplified from a NCC. Compared with the *c-kit* coding sequences [GenBank: AF448148], a G to A transversion ($G^{1275}A$), a silent mutation at codon 425 of KIT, was identified in our NCC sample.

Next, the full length *c-kit* coding region of 12 HSAs with high KIT expression level (samples were indicated in Additional file 1: Table S1) was amplified for sequence identification. Compared with the wild-type *c-kit* sequences, the 1275 nucleotide (nt) was either A or G; 50 % (6/12) of HSAs harbored the $A^{1275}G$ substitution. In addition, 8.3 % (1/12) of HSA samples contained 3 other genetic variations at $C^{159}T$ (codon 53), $C^{414}T$ (codon 138), and $A^{507}G$ (codon 169) of *c-kit*. Overall, these four point mutations were silent mutations that did not alter amino acids.

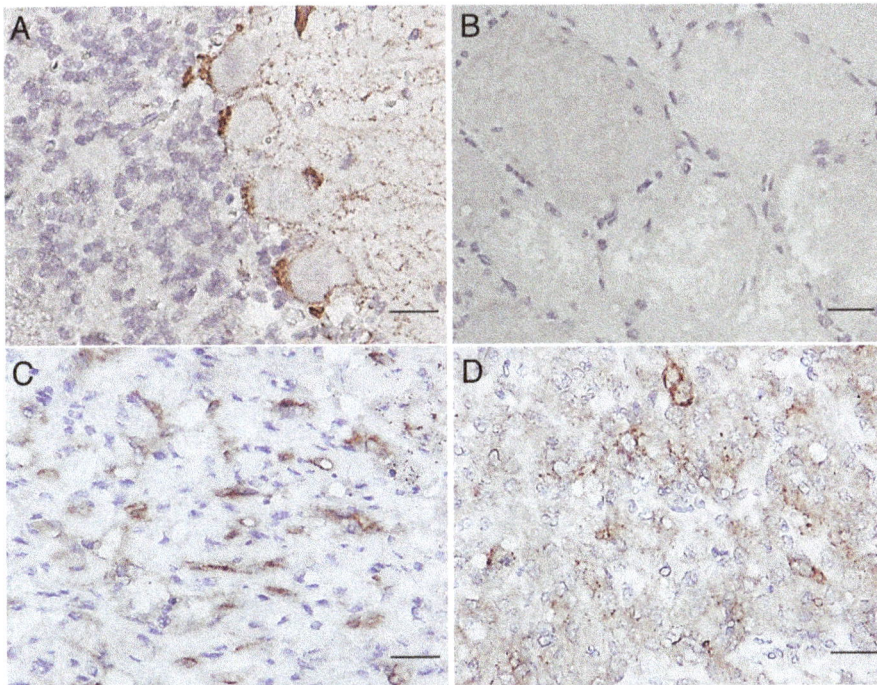

Fig. 1 Immunohistochemical staining for KIT. **a** Strong immunolabelling in the cytoplasm of Purkinje cells of a NCC was used as a positive control for KIT immunostaining. **b** Expression of KIT was not detected in a HA. **c** Strong immunoreactivies were observed inasplenic HSA with stage III and grade 3. **d** Positive immunoreactivities were observed ina cutaneous HSA with stage III and grade 2. Sections counterstained with hematoxylin. Bar = 50 μm

Table 3 IHC analysis of vWF, vimentin and KIT expression in canine hemangiomas and hemangiosarcomas

	Number	Intensity (%)			Positively tumor cells (%)			Immunoreactivity		Chi-square	P value
		Weak	Moderate	Strong	< 10 %	10-50 %	> 50 %	Positive	Negative		
vWF for HSAs	36	0 (0%)	8 (22.2%)	28 (77.8%)	5 (13.9%)	7 (19.4%)	24 (66.7%)	36 (100%)	0 (0%)	-	-
Vimentin for HSAs	36	1 (2.8%)	2 (5.6%)	33 (91.6%)	4 (11.1%)	9 (25%)	23 (63.9%)	35 (97.2%)	1 (2.8%)	-	-
KIT for HAs	16	16 (100%)	0 (0%)	0 (0%)	16 (100%)	0 (0%)	0 (0%)	0 (0%)	16 (100%)	43.654	< 0.0001
KIT for HSAs	36	2 (5.6%)	9 (25%)	25 (69.4%)	6 (16.7%)	10 (27.8%)	20 (55.5%)	34 (94.4%)	2 (5.6%)		

vWF von Willebrand factor, HSAs hemangiosarcomas, HAs hemangiomas, Weak staining much weaker than positive control or negative, Moderate staining slightly weaker than positive control, Strong staining equal to positive control. -, not done. P values <0.05 indicate significant difference

Interestingly, as judged by sequencing chromatogram, overlapping noise signals starting from codon 513 to 516 (the most 3′ end) of the c-kit exon 9 were found in all DNA fragments amplified from HSAs (12/12, 100 %) (Fig. 2a, left panel), indicating the presence of sequence polymorphisms. This phenomenon was not found in those amplified from NCCs (Fig. 2a, right panel). Isolation of the PCR amplicons containing this region revealed two distinct products (Fig. 2b, indicated as arrowheads). Sequence alignment indicated that 12 nucleotides, coding for residues 513–516 (GNSK), were deleted from the exon 9 variant, as compared with that of wild type (Fig. 2c).

Investigation of sequence variations in exon 9 of c-kit

Based on the migration pattern of gel electrophoresis, two types of exon 9 amplicons were present in all HSA samples (12/12), and in 83.3 % (5/6) of NCCs (Fig. 3a). It is worthy of noting that the 12 nt deletion variant, designated GNSK-deletion herein, was the major product in HSAs samples that is distinct from normal canine tissues, which is consistent with sequencing chromatogram as indicated in Fig. 2a. Next, we investigated the correlation of the c-kit GNSK-deletion variant with canine HSAs.

To this end, we determined the approximate frequency of these two genotypes of c-kit exon 9 by cloning strategies [28]. DNA amplicons were cloned into TA vector following PCR, and more than ten bacterial colonies with c-kit exon 9 insertion randomly picked from individual cases were sequenced. In total, sequences of 140 clones containing exon 9, amplified from 12 HSA patients and 64 clones from 6 healthy canine cerebellums, were determined. The frequency of two c-kit exon

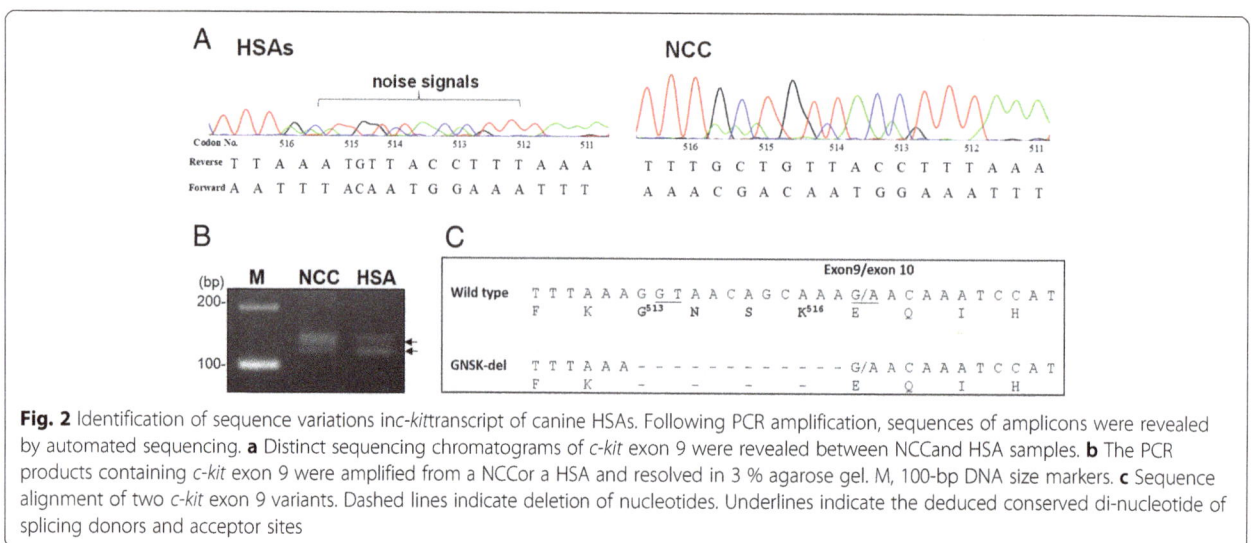

Fig. 2 Identification of sequence variations in c-kit transcript of canine HSAs. Following PCR amplification, sequences of amplicons were revealed by automated sequencing. **a** Distinct sequencing chromatograms of c-kit exon 9 were revealed between NCC and HSA samples. **b** The PCR products containing c-kit exon 9 were amplified from a NCC or a HSA and resolved in 3 % agarose gel. M, 100-bp DNA size markers. **c** Sequence alignment of two c-kit exon 9 variants. Dashed lines indicate deletion of nucleotides. Underlines indicate the deduced conserved di-nucleotide of splicing donors and acceptor sites

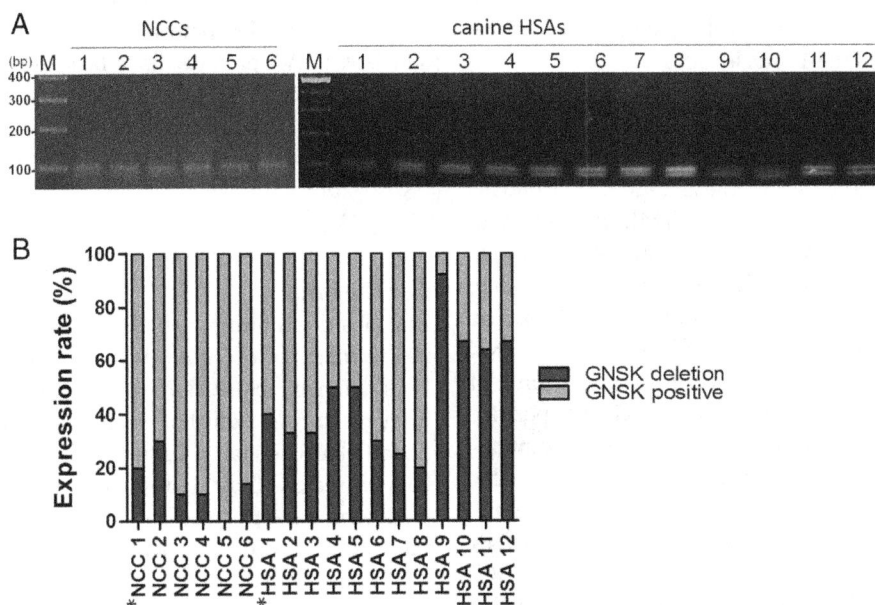

Fig. 3 The frequency of *c-kit* exon 9 variants in canine tissues. **a** PCR products containing the exon 9 region amplified from 6 healthy canine cerebellums (*left* panel) or 12 canine HSAs (*right* panel) were electrophoresed with 3 % agarose gel. **b** The approximate frequency of the *c-kit* exon 9 variants was determined by cloning strategy. Numbers of colonies containing genotype representing wild type (*grey bar*), or 12-nt del (*black bar*) of exon 9 were summarized

9 genotypes in each sample are shown in Fig. 3b. Overall, 72 colonies from HSAs and 55 colonies from NCCs resembled wild-type *c-kit* exon 9 sequences, whereas 68 clones from HSAs and 9 clones from NCCs were the GNSK-deletion. Overall, frequency of this *c-kit* RNA variant in HSAs was 48.6 % (68/140), significantly higher than 14.1 % (9/64) of NCCs (*P* = 0.004).

Discussion

The expression profile and the mutation status of KIT have been intensively studied in human tumors, in particular, GISTs and MCTs [29]. Mutational hot spots in different regions of the *c-kit* gene have been found in human tumors. However, little is known about the *c-kit* mutation status of canine tumors. In the present study, the frequency and location of *c-kit* gene mutations of canine HSA was investigated. We analyzed the entire coding region of the *c-kit* transcript and revealed a variant with a 12-nt deletion in exon 9. Previously, the GNSK deletion was detected in C2 canine malignant mast cell line, but not in NCC [30]. In addition, while preparing this manuscript, *c-kit* sequences of canine HSA was revealed [17]. In that study, Gramer et al., referred GNSK insertion (the full length *c-kit*) was not amplified in canine HSA, indicating GNSK-deletion allele possibly is the major transcript that is consistent with our findings. We further demonstrated, in fact, both wild type (full length) and GNSK-deletion genotypes were present in canine tumor samples.

Interestingly, GNSK- deletion was present in a significantly higher level in canine HSAs as compared with NCCs.

It is worthy of noting that previously identified high frequency mutations were not present in canine HSAs; for instance, mutations in exon 11 [31], and alterations in exon 9 of *c-kit* including SNPs and duplication in human GISTs [32, 33], and SNPs (missense mutations; $S^{479}I$, $N^{508}I$ substitution) in canine MCTs [7]. Interestingly, the GNSK-deletion presents not only in HSAs, but also in NCCs (to a much lower frequency); this variation was regarded as a *c-kit* isoform. Deletion of 12-nt (GGTAACAGCAAA, coding for $G^{513}NSK^{516}$ residues) has not been reported in previous studies on canine GISTs and MCTs [31, 34]. Based on the signal intensity of sequence chromatography and also the frequency estimated from TA cloning strategy, we suspect the two genotypes (wild type and GNSK-deletion) of KIT were expressed at similar levels in canine HSAs.

Furthermore, as GNSK-del mutation of exon 9 was not detected in genomic DNA of all samples, the presence of two *c-kit* RNAs is very likely due to alternative splicing during processes of pre-mRNA. Indeed, the deleted sequences (5′-GGTAACAGCAAAG-3′) in exon 9 comprised consensus splicing signals [35], i.e. the two nucleotides in italic font, of which the GT di-nucleotide at the 5′ end, and AG at the 3′ end (G residue is the first nucleotide in the adjacent exon 10) serves as a donor site and acceptor site of the splicing event, respectively.

Therefore, the presence of GT and AG di-nucleotides in the end of exon 9 would act as an alternative splicing signal leading to deletion of the 12 nucleotides.

In previous studies, the isoform with deletion of a tetrapeptide sequence (GNNK) in the extracellular juxtamembrane region of KIT has been demonstrated in mice and humans [36, 37]. While these two KIT isoforms share similar affinity to ligand SCF [24], expression of KIT with GNNK deletion induced stronger transformation effects in NIH3T3 cells and was more tumorigenic in nude mice, as compared with wild type KIT [38]. The underlying mechanism has been proposed; the GNNK negative isoform can be phosphorylated (on tyrosine) at a higher level and more rapidly than the GNNK-positive isoform upon SCF ligand binding that leads to stimulating a stronger downstream signaling [39]. Additionally, the GNNK negative isoform was more resistant to tyrosine kinase inhibitor when compared with the GNNK positive isoform in the absence of human SCF [40]. Moreover, it is worthy of noting that genotyping in this study revealed the presence of GNSK-deletion in NCCs, although to a lesser extent than in canine HSAs. This is in line with the results of IHC, in which malignant HSAs and NCCs expressed high levels of KIT. Expression of KIT in the cerebellum implicates the importance of KIT in maintenance of cerebellar functionality. Indeed, embryonic knockdown expression of KIT in the rat cortex indicates KIT participates in radial migration of cortical neurons and also in the correct formation of callosal projection neurons [41]. In addition, as seen in Fig. 3, the ratio of GNSK-deletion of *c-kit* transcripts in HSAs was significantly higher than that in NCCs, indicating the role that the GNSK-deletion isoform plays in the development of HSAs, possibly due to activating downstream signaling of KIT.

The results of IHC demonstrated that KIT is predominantly expressed in malignant canine HSAs while it is absent in benign HAs. This finding is consistent with one previous study [8]. In addition, expression of KIT in all canine HSAs displayed diffuse cytoplasmic staining, even in HSAs with various histologic grades. According to the definition of a previous report, the immunostaining pattern of KIT in canine HSAs was classified into pattern III [42]. It has been reported that pattern III is significantly associated with a high histologic grade, poor differentiation [43], local recurrence, and metastasis [42].

Although most HSAs expressed high levels of KIT, the downstream signal transduction pathways activated by KIT in canine HSAs remain unclear. The active and dysregulated dimeric KIT may result in neoplastic transformation of normal cells overexpressing KIT [13]. The constitutional phosphorylation of KIT

and activations of the downstream signaling pathways including the MAPK pathway, PI3K/AKT/mTOR pathway and JAK/STAT pathway have been reported [41, 44, 45]. Therefore, the role of GNSK-deletion KIT in the activation of downstream signaling pathways in canine HSAs or in the pathogenesis of canine HSAs warrants further investigation.

Conclusions

The positive immunoactivity of KIT was demonstrated in the majority of HSAs, while it was not detectable in HAs. Hence, expression of KIT might be used as a marker to distinguish benign or malignant vascular endothelial originated tumors. Sequencing of the entire coding region indicated previously reported sequence variations were not present in canine HSAs analyzed in this study. Instead, a KIT isoform with deletion of GNSK, generated by alternative splicing, was detected in all canine HSAs tested. Moreover, a significantly higher proportion of this GNSK-deletion isoform in canine HSAs than in normal cerebellum was demonstrated for the first time.

Abbreviations
GIST, gastrointestinal stromal tumors; HA, hemangioma; HSA, hemangiosarcoma; IHC, immunohistochemistry; IRS, immunoreactive score; MCT, mast cell tumor; NCC, normal canine cerebellum; PP, percentage of positive cell; SCF, stem cell factor; SI, staining intensity; vWF, von Willebrand factor

Acknowledgements
All authors wish to thank Yi-Ping Yang for assisting in histopathological examination of all canine HAs and HSAs. Shin-Hung Huang for normal canine cerebellums collection.

Funding
No funding was obtained for this study.

Authors' contributions
YCC conducted the experiments, analyzed the data, and prepared the manuscript. JWL evaluated the results of histopathological examinations and immunohistochemistry stains. WLH and SCC designed this research and revised the manuscript. All authors read and approved the final manuscript.

Competing interests
None of the authors of this paper has a financial or personal relationship with other people or organisations that could inappropriately influence or bias the paper content.

Consent for publication
Not applicable.

Author details

[1]Department of Veterinary Medicine, College of Veterinary Medicine, National Chung Hsing University, 250 Kuo-Kuang Road, Taichung 40227, Taiwan. [2]Graduate Institute of Veterinary Pathobiology, College of Veterinary Medicine, National Chung Hsing University, 250 Kuo-Kuang Road, Taichung 40227, Taiwan. [3]Graduate Institute of Microbiology and Public Health, College of Veterinary Medicine, National Chung Hsing University, 250 Kuo-Kuang Road, Taichung 40227, Taiwan. [4]Veterinary Medical Teaching Hospital, College of Veterinary Medicine, National Chung Hsing University, 250 Kuo-Kuang Road, Taichung 40227, Taiwan.

References

1. Brown NO, Patnaik AK, MacEwen EG. Canine hemangiosarcoma: retrospective analysis of 104 cases. J Am Vet Med Assoc. 1985;186(1):56–8.
2. Spangler WL, Culbertson MR. Prevalence, type, and importance of splenic diseases in dogs: 1,480 cases (1985–1989). J Am Vet Med Assoc. 1992;200(6): 829–34.
3. Dernell WS, Withrow SJ, Kuntz CA, et al. Principles of treatment for soft tissue sarcoma. Clin Tech Small Anim Pract. 1998;13(1):59–64.
4. Ogilvie GK, Powers BE, Mallinckrodt CK, et al. Surgery and doxorubicin in dogs with hemangiosarcoma. J Vet Intern Med. 1996;10(6):379–84.
5. Galli SJ, Zsebo KM, Geissler EN. The kit ligand, stem cell factor. Adv Immunol. 1994;55:1–96.
6. Vliagoftis H, Worobec AS, Metcalfe DD. The protooncogene c-kit and c-kit ligand in human disease. J Allergy Clin Immunol. 1997;100(4):435–40.
7. Miettinen M, Sarlomo-Rikala M, Lasota J. KIT expression in angiosarcomas and fetal endothelial cells: lack of mutations of exon 11 and exon 17 of C-kit. Mod Pathol. 2000;13(5):536–41.
8. Sabattini S, Bettini G. An immunohistochemical analysis of canine haemangioma and haemangiosarcoma. J Comp Pathol. 2009;140(2–3):158–68.
9. Kessler M, Maurus Y, Kostlin R. Hemangiosarcoma of the spleen: clinical aspects in 52 dogs. Tierarztl Prax Ausg K Kleintiere Heimtiere. 1997;25(6):651–6.
10. Hirota S, Isozaki K, Moriyama Y, et al. Gain-of-function mutations of c-kit in human gastrointestinal stromal tumors. Science. 1998;279(5350):577–80.
11. Moskaluk CR, Tian Q, Marshall CR, et al. Mutations of c-kit JM domain are found in a minority of human gastrointestinal stromal tumors. Oncogene. 1999;18(10):1897–902.
12. Nakahara M, Isozaki K, Hirota S, et al. A novel gain-of-function mutation of c-kit gene in gastrointestinal stromal tumors. Gastroenterology. 1998;115(5):1090–5.
13. Kitamura Y, Tsujimura T, Jippo T, et al. Regulation of development, survival and neoplastic growth of mast cells through the c-kit receptor. Int Arch Allergy Immunol. 1995;107(1–3):54–6.
14. Roskoski Jr R. Structure and regulation of Kit protein-tyrosine kinase–the stem cell factor receptor. Biochem Biophys Res Commun. 2005;338(3):1307–15.
15. Debiec-Rychter M, Dumez H, Judson I, et al. Use of c-KIT/PDGFRA mutational analysis to predict the clinical response to imatinib in patients with advanced gastrointestinal stromal tumours entered on phase I and II studies of the EORTC Soft Tissue and Bone Sarcoma Group. Eur J Cancer. 2004;40(5):689–95.
16. Kobayashi M, Kuroki S, Ito K, et al. Imatinib-associated tumour response in a dog with a non-resectable gastrointestinal stromal tumour harbouring a c-kit exon 11 deletion mutation. Vet J. 2013;198(1):271–4.
17. Gramer I, Kessler M, Geyer J. Detection of novel polymorphisms in the ckit gene of canine patients with lymphoma, melanoma, haemangiosarcoma, and osteosarcoma. Vet Res Commun. 2016. [Epub ahead of print].
18. Frost MJ, Ferrao PT, Hughes TP, et al. Juxtamembrane mutant V560GKit is more sensitive to Imatinib (STI571) compared with wild-type c-kit whereas the kinase domain mutant D816VKit is resistant. Mol Cancer Ther. 2002;1(12):1115–24.
19. Miettinen M, Lasota J. KIT (CD117): a review on expression in normal and neoplastic tissues, and mutations and their clinicopathologic correlation. Appl Immunohistochem Mol Morphol. 2005;13(3):205–20.
20. Wood CA, Moore AS, Gliatto JM, et al. Prognosis for dogs with stage I or II splenic hemangiosarcoma treated by splenectomy alone: 32 cases (1991–1993). J Am Anim Hosp Assoc. 1998;34(5):417–21.
21. Kuntz CA, Dernell WS, Powers BE, et al. Prognostic factors for surgical treatment of soft-tissue sarcomas in dogs: 75 cases (1986–1996). J Am Vet Med Assoc. 1997;211(9):1147–51.
22. Hellstrom S, Tengblad A, Johansson C, et al. An improved technique for hyaluronan histochemistry using microwave irradiation. Histochem J. 1990; 22(12):677–82.
23. Meis JM, Enzinger FM. Chondroid lipoma. A unique tumor simulating liposarcoma and myxoid chondrosarcoma. Am J Surg Pathol. 1993;17(11):1103–12.
24. London CA, Kisseberth WC, Galli SJ, et al. Expression of stem cell factor receptor (c-kit) by the malignant mast cells from spontaneous canine mast cell tumours. J Comp Pathol. 1996;115(4):399–414.
25. Shyu RY, Jiang SY, Chou JM, et al. RARRES3 expression positively correlated to tumour differentiation in tissues of colorectal adenocarcinoma. Br J Cancer. 2003;89(1):146–51.
26. Reguera MJ, Rabanal RM, Puigdemont A, et al. Canine mast cell tumors express stem cell factor receptor. Am J Dermatopathol. 2000;22(1):49–54.
27. Ma Y, Longley BJ, Wang X, et al. Clustering of activating mutations in c-KIT's juxtamembrane coding region in canine mast cell neoplasms. J Invest Dermatol. 1999;112(2):165–70.
28. Lacey EA. Microsatellite variation in solitary and social tuco-tucos: molecular properties and population dynamics. Heredity. 2001;86(Pt5):628–37.
29. Cruse G, Metcalfe DD, Olivera A. Functional deregulation of KIT: link to mast cell proliferative diseases and other neoplasms. Immunol Allergy Clin North Am. 2014;34(2):219–37.
30. London CA, Galli SJ, Yuuki T, et al. Spontaneous canine mast cell tumors express tandem duplications in the proto-oncogene c-kit. Exp Hematol. 1999;27(4):689–97.
31. Letard S, Yang Y, Hanssens K, et al. Gain-of-function mutations in the extracellular domain of KIT are common in canine mast cell tumors. Mol Cancer Res. 2008;6(7):1137–45.
32. Lux ML, Rubin BP, Biase TL, et al. KIT extracellular and kinase domain mutations in gastrointestinal stromal tumors. Am J Pathol. 2000;156(3):791–5.
33. Martin J, Poveda A, Llombart-Bosch A, et al. Deletions affecting codons 557–558 of the c-KIT gene indicate a poor prognosis in patients with completely resected gastrointestinal stromal tumors: a study by the Spanish Group for Sarcoma Research (GEIS). J Clin Oncol. 2005;23(25):6190–8.
34. Gregory-Bryson E, Bartlett E, Kiupel M, et al. Canine and human gastrointestinal stromal tumors display similar mutations in c-KIT exon 11. BMC Cancer. 2010;10:559.
35. Mount SM. A catalogue of splice junction sequences. Nucleic Acids Res. 1982;10(2):459–72.
36. Crosier PS, Ricciardi ST, Hall LR, et al. Expression of isoforms of the human receptor tyrosine kinase c-kit in leukemic cell lines and acute myeloid leukemia. Blood. 1993;82(4):1151–8.
37. Hayashi S, Kunisada T, Ogawa M, et al. Exon skipping by mutation of an authentic splice site of c-kit gene in W/W mouse. Nucleic Acids Res. 1991; 19(6):1267–71.
38. Caruana G, Cambareri AC, Ashman LK. Isoforms of c-KIT differ in activation of signalling pathways and transformation of NIH3T3 fibroblasts. Oncogene. 1999;18(40):5573–81.
39. Voytyuk O, Lennartsson J, Mogi A, et al. Src family kinases are involved in the differential signaling from two splice forms of c-Kit. J Biol Chem. 2003; 278(11):9159–66.
40. Chan EC, Bai Y, Bandara G, et al. KIT GNNK splice variants: expression in systemic mastocytosis and influence on the activating potential of the D816V mutation in mast cells. Exp Hematol. 2013;41(10):870–81.
41. Guijarro P, Wang Y, Ying Y, et al. In vivo knockdown of cKit impairs neuronal migration and axonal extension in the cerebral cortex. Dev Neurobiol. 2013; 73(12):871–87.
42. Thompson JJ, Yager JA, Best SJ, et al. Canine subcutaneous mast cell tumors: cellular proliferation and KIT expression as prognostic indices. Vet Pathol. 2011;48(1):169–81.
43. Gil da Costa RM, Matos E, Rema A, et al. CD117 immunoexpression in canine mast cell tumours: correlations with pathological variables and proliferation markers. BMC Vet Res. 2007;3:19.
44. Ronnstrand L. Signal transduction via the stem cell factor receptor/c-Kit. Cell Mol Life Sci. 2004;61(19–20):2535–48.
45. Adachi M, Hoshino Y, Izumi Y, et al. Immunohistochemical detection of a potential molecular therapeutic target for canine hemangiosarcoma. J Vet Med Sci. 2016;78(4):649–56.

17

Splenic malignant fibrous histiocytoma with concurrent hypertension and epistaxis in an Alaskan malamute dog

Jung-Hyun Kim[1], Hee-Jin Kim[1], Sung-Jun Lee[2] and Hun-Young Yoon[2*] (iD)

Abstract

Background: Malignant fibrous histiocytoma has been uncommonly described in dogs. Several extranasal neoplasias have been reported to result hypertensive epistaxis. There are, however, no published case reports of extranasal malignant fibrous histiocytoma with concurrent hypertension and epistaxis in dogs.

Case presentation: A 10-year-old dog presented with a spontaneous massive epistaxis persisting for 5 days. The dog exhibited unstable hypertension, which was considered as a cause of epistaxis. The complete blood count, prothrombin time, and activated partial thromboplastin time were within the reference limits, and other systemic examination showed no abnormalities except for a splenic mass occupying more than one third of the abdomen. Histologic examination of the resected spleen revealed the characteristic features of a malignant fibrous histiocytoma. One week after splenectomy, the hypertension and epistaxis resolved clinically and did not recur on the 5-month follow-up.

Conclusions: The dog's blood pressure and epistaxis normalized after malignant fibrous histiocytoma resection suggesting that hypertensive epistaxis may be a rare manifestation of canine malignant fibrous histiocytoma.

Keywords: Dog, Epistaxis, Hypertension, Malignant fibrous histiocytoma

Background

Malignant fibrous histiocytoma (MFH) is a soft tissue sarcoma characterized by the presence of variably fibroblastic to less obviously histiocytic cells and variable numbers of associated non-neoplastic inflammatory cells [1, 2]. MFH most frequently affects the lung, hilar lymph nodes, mesenteric lymph nodes, liver, and spleen [3], and various reported clinical signs of MFH depend on the tumor location. MFH is associated with a rapid clinical progression, grave prognosis, and usually fatal outcome [4]. Although MFH is the most common type soft tissue sarcoma reported in humans, it has been uncommonly described in veterinary medicine [5]. A previous survey of the types of tumors occurring in dogs found that MFH comprised only 0.34% of all reported tumors [6]. Generally, MFH is reported in older dogs [2], although one report describes a case involving a puppy [7].

Epistaxis is a common and potentially severe or fatal otolaryngologic emergency in dogs that may be caused by either local disease within the nasal cavity or systemic illness [8, 9]. Canine epistaxis may be caused by various disorders, including hemostatic abnormalities, neoplasia, infection, foreign bodies, nasal parasites, hyperviscosity syndrome, and vasculitis [9]. In veterinary medicine, systemic hypertension has also been considered as a potential cause of epistaxis, although the direct mechanism remains unclear [8]. Notably, several cases of epistaxis resulting from hypertension or bleeding disorder caused by an extranasal neoplasia have been reported in human and veterinary medicine [8, 10, 11]. However, a link between extranasal MFH with concurrent hypertension and epistaxis has not been reported previously in dogs [3, 4]. In this report, we present the first description of concurrent hypertension and epistaxis in a dog with a splenic MFH, and the subsequent return of blood pressure values to within reference ranges after splenectomy. Therefore, we review the veterinary literature and suggest the possibility regarding hypertension and epistaxis in a dog with splenic MFH.

* Correspondence: yoonh@konkuk.ac.kr
[2]Department of Veterinary Surgery, College of Veterinary Medicine, Konkuk University, #120 Neungdong-ro, Gwangjin-gu, Seoul 143-701, Korea
Full list of author information is available at the end of the article

Case presentation

Medical history and clinical sign

A 10-year-old spayed female Alaskan malamute (body weight 38 kg) was admitted to the Konkuk University Veterinary Medical Teaching Hospital with persistent intermittent bilateral epistaxis of 5 days' duration. Per the owner's report, once initiated, the epistaxis did not stop for 2 h despite nasal plugging. During the initial physical examination, the dog was bright and alert, with no nasal bleeding. No purpuric spots were observed throughout the body, and an oral examination revealed no remarkable findings. Thoracic auscultation revealed no abnormal sounds in the lung and cardiac fields, and an automated oscillometric blood pressure measurement revealed mild hypertension (systolic blood pressure 148 mmHg). However, abdominal palpation revealed a large, round, firm, painful mass on the upper-middle abdomen.

Hematology and biochemistry

Complete blood count, serum biochemistry profile, prothrombin time, and activated partial thromboplastin time analyses were performed to rule out coagulapathies, polycythemia, and thrombocytopenia as causes of epistaxis (Table 1). The complete blood count revealed neutrophilic leukocytosis (white blood cells 42.97×10^9 cells/L; reference range $6-17 \times 10^9$ cells/L) and anemia (hematocrit 30%; reference range 37–55%, hemoglobin 8.7 g/dL; RI 12–18 g/dL). Serum chemistry revealed mildly elevated alkaline phosphatase activity (378 U/L; reference range 15–127 U/L) and hypoalbuminemia (2.6 g/dL; reference range 2.9–4.2 g/dL). The results of coagulation tests were within reference limits (activated partial thromboplastin time 9.6 s; reference range 14–18 s, prothrombin time 8.2 s; reference range 6.2–8.2 s).

Diagnostic imaging

Thoracic radiography revealed a mild broncho-interstitial pattern in the overall lung field and a normal cardiac size.

Table 1 The results of coagulation tests, complete blood count, and serum biochemistry profile in a dog presenting with epistaxis

Variable	Result	Reference Interval
PT (seconds)	8.2	6.2–8.2
APTT (seconds)	9.6	14–18
WBC ($\times 10^9$ cells/L)	42.97	6–17
Haematocrit (%)	30	37–55
Platelet ($\times 10^9$ cells/L)	239	200–500
Alkaline phosphatase (U/L)	378	15–127
Total protein (g/dL)	6.8	5.4–7.4

APTT activated partial thromboplastin time, *PT* prothrombin time, *WBC* white blood cell

An abdominal ultrasound examination revealed a splenic mass with a heterogeneous appearance and irregular but encapsulated borders.

The dog's owner elected to pursue a rhinoscopy and computed tomography (CT) of entire body. Following anesthetization of the dog, the rhinoscopy was performed using flexible endoscopes (Fig. 1a and b). A retroflexed view of the bilateral nasal choana revealed no remarkable findings except an engorged vessel (Fig. 1c and d), and CT images revealed a normal nasal passage and intact cribriform plate. However, an abdominal CT scan detected a massive, continuous splenic mass measuring 13.2 cm × 13.5 cm × 8.4 cm in the mid-abdomen, as well as diffuse contrast-enhancement of the heterogeneous splenic parenchyma and an irregular margin (Fig. 2a). A thoracic CT scan indicated well-circumscribed, contrast-enhanced miliary nodules on the left cranial lung lobe, consistent with lung metastasis (Fig. 2b). The patient was hospitalized, during which time an episode of intractable and pulsatile epistaxis occurred without cessation for more than 1 h, despite nasal plugging. This episode caused the dog to become slightly agitated, with a temporary severe increase in blood pressure (systolic blood pressure 180–250 mmHg).

Surgery and histopathology

The owner consented to a surgical excision of the splenic tumor, and the dog underwent a surgical exploration of the abdominal cavity while in the dorsal recumbent position. A large (16 cm × 14 cm × 10 cm) mass at the tail of the spleen was found to attach to the greater omentum. The involved section of the greater omentum was resected, and a total splenectomy was performed. The abdomen was lavaged with warmed sterile saline and closed routinely. The dog recovered uneventfully with routine postoperative antibiotics. Histopathologically, the resected spleen comprised pleomorphic neoplastic cells; these included both round histiocyte-like cells and spindle cells with occasional multinucleate cells and mitotic activities ranging from one to four mitoses per high-power field (Fig. 3a). An immunohistochemistry stain for vimentin yielded a positive result (Fig. 3b), consistent with the mesenchymal origin, and the main differential diagnosis of spindle cell squamous carcinoma was excluded. A diagnosis of MFH was made based on the histologic and immunohistochemical findings.

Treatment and outcome

Butorphanol[1] (0.1 mg/kg intravenously every 8 h) was provided as postoperative analgesia for the first 24 h. Although intermittent minor episodes of epistaxis and transient hypertension occurred during the 7 days after splenectomy, the significant epistaxis had disappeared by the 5-month follow-up. Based on the histopathological findings, we recommended that the dog undergo adjuvant

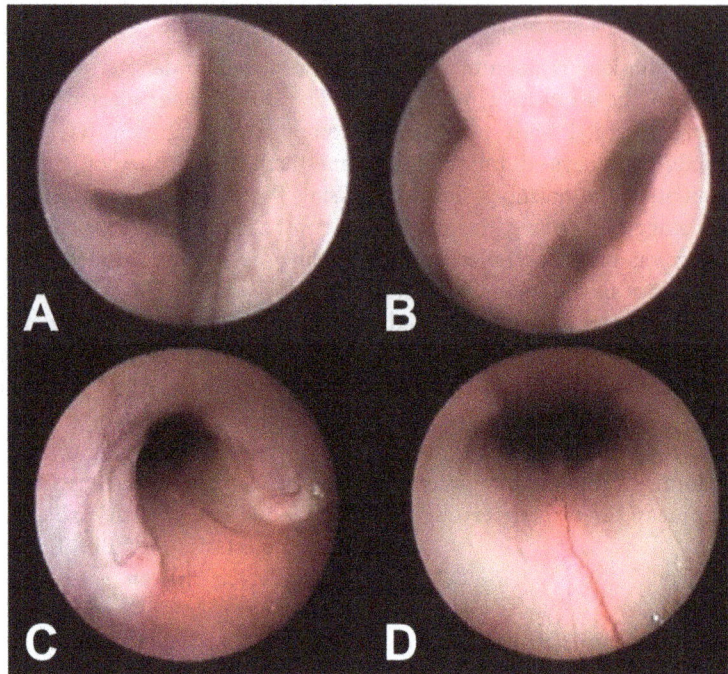

Fig. 1 Rhinoscopy and nasopharyngoscopy did not reveal a mass occupying the nasal and nasopharyngeal regions. Mild congestion was observed in the left (**a**) and right (**b**) nasal cavities. Nasopharyngoscopy revealed congestion in the nasopharyngeal region (**c**) and engorged vessels in the nasal cavity (**d**)

chemotherapy, but the owners refused. Five months after the first visit, however, the patient presented with acute anorexia and abdominal pain. Although her blood pressure was within normal limits (systolic blood pressure 125 mmHg), a complete blood count revealed neutrophilic leukocytosis (66.7×10^9 cells/L), anemia (hematocrit 26%, hemoglobin 9.5 g/dL), and thrombocytopenia (platelets 136×10^9 cells/L; reference range $200–500 \times 10^9$ cells/L). A serum chemistry analysis detected elevated hepatic enzyme levels (aspartate aminotransferase 84 U/L, RI 0–50 U/L, alkaline phosphatase activity 1260 U/L, gamma glutamyl transferase 14 U/L; reference range 0–7 U/L) and mild hypertriglyceridemia (173 mg/dL; reference range 10–100 mg/dL). An abdominal ultrasound revealed multiple nodules and masses of various sizes, shapes, and echogenecities that were spread diffusely throughout all liver lobes, leading to the diagnosis of metastatic liver masses and nodules. However, the owner declined further examinations and therapy because of the poor prognosis, and the patient was discharged at the owner's request. The dog died 3 days later at home; however, the owner unfortunately refused a necropsy.

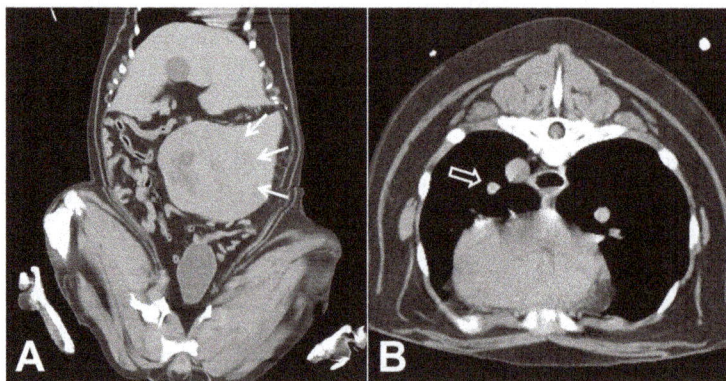

Fig. 2 Computed tomography of the (**a**) abdomen and (**b**) thorax. **a** A mass continuous with the splenic parenchyma was detected in the mid-abdomen. Note the diffuse heterogeneous contrast enhancement of the splenic parenchyma and irregular margin (mass size: 13.2 cm × 13.5 cm × 8.4 cm) (arrows). **b** Imaging of the thorax revealed a well-circumscribed, contrast-enhanced miliary nodule on the left cranial lung lobe (open arrow)

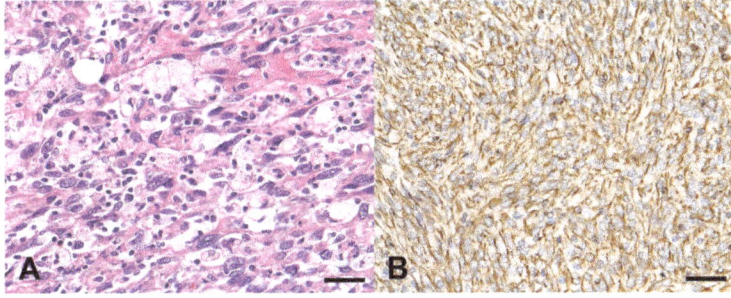

Fig. 3 Histopathology of a malignant fibrous histiocytoma resected from the spleen. **a** Note the plump, spindle-shaped fibroblasts and histiocyte-like cells and the storiform pattern. Oval or polygonal malignant spindle cells with anisokaryosis and coarse nuclei, as well as scattered inflammatory cells, are shown (hematoxylin and eosin, magnification × 400, scale bar = 35 μm). **b** Immunohistochemically, the tumor cells were strongly positive for vimentin (magnification × 400, scale bar = 35 μm)

Discussion

To the authors' knowledge, no previous report has described concurrent hypertension and epistaxis in the dog with MFH. In the present case, the hypertension and epistaxis resolved after the surgical resection of MFH. Accordingly, this the first report of concurrent systemic hypertension and epistaxis attributable to MFH in a dog, with resolution after splenectomy. The lack of clinical reports describing these concurrent diseases processes might be attributable either to the low prevalence of splenic MFH in dogs or the fact that blood pressure evaluations are not routinely performed when abdominal masses are detected.

Epistaxis may be caused by local disease within the nasal cavity or by systemic diseases that result in hemostatic disorders [9]. In a retrospective study of 176 dogs with epistaxis, the condition was predominantly attributed to local causes (83% vs. 17% systemic) [8]. In the present case, we did not detect any mass, inflammation, infection, or foreign body in the nasal cavity and nasopharynx of the dog. However, the present dog's indirect systolic blood pressure was above the reference range, and therefore epistaxis might be attributable to hypertension. In an earlier veterinary medicine case, excessive and tortuous vessels were observed in the caudal rhinoscopy of a hypertensive cat with epistaxis [12]. In the present case, a nasopharyngoscopic examination revealed marked vascular engorgement in the nasal mucosa. Accordingly, the resection of the splenic MFH appeared sufficient to normalize the blood pressure and resolve epistaxis in the present canine patient.

In dogs, hypertension generally develops at an older age and more commonly affects males than females [13]. The most common diseases associated with canine hypertension are renal disease, cardiac left ventricular hypertrophy, hyperadrenocorticism, pheochromocytoma, and diabetes mellitus, whereas less commonly associated diseases include primary hyperaldosteronism, hyperthyroidism, obesity, and idiopathic hypertension [14]. In the present case, unfortunately, we were unable to perform evaluations of cardiac or hormonal factors (e.g., cortisol, dopamine, aldosterone, thyroxine); however, the hypertension resolved after splenectomy. Common clinical signs of hypertension in dogs include blindness or visual disturbances, although seizures and epistaxis may also present [14]. In hypertensive veterinary patients, risk of ocular injury increases when the systolic BP exceeds 180 mmHg [14, 15]. In the present case, no ocular lesions (e.g., retinal detachment, retinal hemorrhage, retinal perivascular edema, papilledema, vitreal hemorrhage, hyphema, secondary glaucoma, retinal degeneration) were observed, possibly because the episodes of hypertension exceeding 180 mmHg were transient and returned to normal values within a week.

The surgical resection of a MFH to control concurrent systemic hypertension in a dog has not previously been reported. In the present case, the hypertension was suspected to be caused by the MFH; therefore, its removal would theoretically reduce the blood pressure to within reference limits. Indeed, after splenectomy, the systolic blood pressure in the dog returned to normal and the epistaxis subsequently disappeared. The significance of the relationship between MFH and hypertensive epistaxis in the present case is unclear because epistaxis occurs even in healthy dogs. However, given the effectiveness of MFH resection in this dog, further investigations are needed to clarify the relationship between MFH and hypertensive epistaxis.

In older dogs, splenic masses are commonly occurred and may be malignant, benign, or non-neoplastic [16]. Several studies have reported that about 2/3 of canine splenic masses are malignant, and the most prevalent malignant splenic tumor is hemangiosarcoma [16, 17]. Additionally, various sarcomas, lymphoma, and MFH have been reported as malignant splenic masses [18, 19]. A diagnosis of MFH based on histological morphology is almost insufficient [20]. Therefore, for more accurate diagnosis, additional diagnostic methods are needed, including immunology and molecular approaches. The present study report diagnosis of MFH uses not only histological morphology, but also immunohistochemistry to investigate the origin of the tumor. In both humans and dogs, vimentin expression has been widely used to confirm the mesenchymal origins of tumors [21]. In this case, hematoxylin and eosin staining and immunoreactivity for vimentin led us to conclude that the tumor was a sarcoma and to make a final diagnosis of MFH. Furthermore, three types of MFH have been reported in dogs: giant cell, inflammatory, and storiform-pleomorphic [21]. Special staining techniques assisted classification of MFH, and several studies reported both histochemical staining and immunostaining including anti-actin, anti-desmin, anti-momonocytes/macrophages antibody were able to help in the classification of MFH into the three different subgroups in dogs [21, 22]. Additional diagnostic marker such as anti-S100 has been also reported to differentiate MFH from other malignant sarcoma [23]. However, definitive immunohistochemical staining patterns have not been clearly identified for MFH in veterinary medicine [21]. As multiple morphologic types may be detected in a single tumor, MFHs are usually classified by their predominant features. Accordingly, the tumor in the dog described here is most consistent with storiform-pleomorphic type MFH based on the histopathologic examination results. In human medicine, the variants of MFH have different clinical significances, and a MFH with marked inflammation is associated with a better prognosis, compared with the storiform–pleomorphic variant [24]. By contrast, the relationship between the histopathological variant and prognosis has not been reported in the context of veterinary medicine. Generally, veterinary cases of MFH have been reported as single and often locally invasive tumors, whereas metastasis is rare [1, 6]. In the present case, evidence of metastasis to the lung was evident from a CT examination at the time of the initial diagnosis. Additionally, the dog's condition began to deteriorate at 5 months after the initial presentation, at which time new, variously sized nodules were detected during an ultrasonographic examination of the liver.

In the present study, the nasal examinations which included CT and rhinoscopy, yielded no remarkable findings, and the cause of epistaxis remains unknown. We suggest two possibilities regarding hypertension and epistaxis in this dog with MFH. First, the dog might have previously exhibited hypertension and subsequent vascular abnormalities which is commonly referred to as a target-organ damage in the veterinary medicine [14], and would therefore have been prone to epistaxis, particularly in response to pain-induced abnormal blood pressure elevations caused by the massive splenic MFH. Second, idiopathic epistaxis might cause an arousal reaction because the nasal cavity is a region of rich

autonomous innervation [25], and this anxiety might manifest as transient hypertension. Accordingly epistaxis may have also been a potent trigger for hyperresponsiveness (e.g., hypertension) in the present canine case.

Conclusions

We report herein the clinical course of hypertensive epistaxis with the putative complication of splenic MFH in a dog. This is the first report of such a case in the literature. Although MFH is an extremely rare cause of the clinical signs observed in this dog, it should be considered in the differential diagnosis for uncontrolled epistaxis without clotting profile abnormalities. Furthermore, our findings warrant an investigation of biological behaviors in a larger number of cases and follow-up blood pressure evaluations in dogs with malignant tumors.

Endnotes

[1]Butophan Inj, Myungmoon Pharm, Seoul, Korea.

Abbreviations
CT: Computed tomography; MFH: Malignant fibrous histiocytoma

Authors' contributions
JHK: This author wrote the article and contributed to the clinical assessment, diagnosis, treatment and follow-up of the case. HJK: This author contributed to the initial clinical assessment and diagnostic work-up of the case, provided images, and helped to write the manuscript. SJL: This author contributed to the surgery and post-operative management of the case, and helped to write the manuscript. HYY: This author supervised the clinical assessment, diagnosis, and treatment of the case and helped to write the manuscript. All authors read and approved the final manuscript.

Authors' information
JHK is a clinical professor in veterinary internal medicine at Konkuk University Veterinary Teaching Hospital (KU-VTH). HJK is a DVM working in clinical veterinary internal medicine at KU-VHT under the supervision of JHK. SJL is a DVM working in clinical veterinary surgery at KU-VHT. HYY is an associated professor in veterinary surgery at Konkuk University.

Consent for publication
Not applicable.

Competing interests
The authors declare that they have no competing interests.

Author details
[1]Department of Veterinary Internal Medicine, Konkuk University Veterinary Medical Teaching Hospital, #120 Neungdong-ro, Gwangjin-gu, Seoul 143-701, Korea. [2]Department of Veterinary Surgery, College of Veterinary Medicine, Konkuk University, #120 Neungdong-ro, Gwangjin-gu, Seoul 143-701, Korea.

References

1. Gleiser CA, Raulston GL, Jardine JH, Gray KN. Malignant fibrous histiocytoma in dogs and cats. Vet Pathol. 1979;16:199–208.
2. Kerlin R, Hendrick M. Malignant fibrous histiocytoma and malignant histiocytosis in the dog—convergent or divergent phenotypic differentiation? Vet Pathol. 1996;33:713–6.
3. Schmidt ML, Rutteman GR, van Niel MH, Wolvekamp PT. Clinical and radiographic manifestations of canine malignant histiocytosis. Vet Q. 1993;15:117–20.
4. Liptak JM, Forrest LJ. Soft tissue sarcomas. In: Withrow SJ, Vail DM, Page RL, editors. Small animal clinical oncology. 5th ed. Philadelphia: WB Saunders; 2013. p. 356–80.
5. Kiran MM, Karaman M, Hatipoglu F, Koc Y. Malignant fibrous histiocytoma in a dog: a case report. Vet Med Czech. 2005;50:553–7.
6. Waters CB, Morrison WB, DeNicola DB, Widmer WR, White MR. Giant cell variant of malignant fibrous histiocytoma in dogs: 10 cases (1986-1993). J Am Vet Med Assoc. 1994;205:1420–4.
7. Pires M. Malignant fibrous histiocytoma in a puppy. Vet Rec. 1997;140:234–5.
8. Bissett SA, Drobatz KJ, McKnight A, Degernes LA. Prevalence, clinical features, and causes of epistaxis in dogs: 176 cases (1996–2001). J Am Vet Med Assoc. 2007;231:1843–50.
9. Strasser JL, Hawkins EC. Clinical features of epistaxis in dogs: a retrospective study of 35 cases (1999–2002). J Am Anim Hosp Assoc. 2005;41:179–84.
10. Schloendorff G. Severe arterial epistaxis in pheochromocytoma. Z Laryngol Rhinol Otol. 1962;41:700–3.
11. Talei A. Splenic hamartoma: a case report. Med J Islam Repub Iran. 1997;11:57–9.
12. Aoki T, Madarame H, Sugimoto K, Sunahara H, Fujii Y, Kanai E, Ito T. Diode laser coagulation for the treatment of epistaxis in a Scottish fold cat. Can Vet J. 2015;56:745–8.
13. Henik RA. Systemic hypertension and its management. Vet Clin North Am Small Anim Pract. 1997;27:1355–72.
14. Brown S, Atkins C, Bagley R, Carr A, Cowgill L, Davidson M, Egner B, Elliott J, Henik R, Labato M, Littman M, Polzin D, Ross L, Snyder P, Stepien R. Guidelines for the identification, evaluation, and management of systemic hypertension in dogs and cats. J Vet Intern Med. 2007;21:542–58.
15. Sansom J, Barnett KC, Dunn KA, Smith KC, Dennis R. Ocular disease associated with hypertension in 16 cats. J Small Anim Pract. 1994;35:604–11.
16. Grimes JA, Prasad N, Levy S, Cattley R, Lindley S, Boothe HW, Henderson RA, Smith BF. A comparison of microRNA expression profiles from splenic hemangiosarcoma, splenic nodular hyperplasia, and normal spleens of dogs. BMC Vet Res. 2016;12:272.
17. Spangler WL, Culbertson MR. Prevalence, type, and importance of splenic diseases in dogs: 1,480 cases (1985–1989). J Am Vet Med Assoc. 1992;200:829–34.
18. Hammond TN, Pesillo-Crosby SA. Prevalence of hemangiosarcoma in anemic dogs with a splenic mass and hemoperitoneum requiring a transfusion: 71 cases (2003–2005). J Am Vet Med Assoc. 2008;232:553–8.
19. Eberle N, von Babo V, Nolte I, Baumgartner W, Betz D. Splenic masses in dogs. Part 1: Epidemiologic, clinical characteristics as well as histopathologic diagnosis in 249 cases (2000–2011). Tierarztl Prax Ausg K Kleintiere Heimtiere. 2012;40:250–60.
20. Ko JS, Kim HJ, Choi YM, Kim JW, Park C, Do SH. Diagnostic approach to malignant fibrous histiocytomas of soft tissue in dogs: a case report. Vet Med Czech. 2013;58:621–7.
21. Morris JS, McInnes EF, Bostock DE, Hoather TM, Dobson JM. Immunohistochemical and histopathologic features of 14 malignant fibrous histiocytomas from flat-coated retrievers. Vet Pathol Online. 2002;39:473–9.
22. Do SH, Hong IH, Park JK, Ji AR, Kim TH, Kwak DM, Jeong KS. Two different types of malignant fibrous histiocytomas from pet dogs. J Vet Sci. 2009;10:169–71.
23. Makovicky P, Makovicky P, Nagy M, Nemeth P, Rajmon R. Differentiation of malignant fibrous histiocytoma and pleomorphic liposarcoma in dogs, using anti-S-100 protein antibody Immunohistochemical case report. Magyar Allatorvosok Lapja. 2012;134:101–5.
24. Enzinger FM, Weiss SW. Malignant tumors of uncertain histogenesis. In: Enzinger FM, Weiss SW, editors. Soft tissue tumors. 2nd ed. St. Louis: Mosby; 1988. p. 929–65.
25. Schmiedt CW, Creevy KE. Nasal planum, nasal caivity, and sinuses. In: Tobias KM, Johnston SA, editors. Veterinary surgery: small animal. 1st ed. St. Louis: Saunders; 2012. p. 1691–706.

18

A rare case of intracardiac fibrosarcoma with myxoid features inducing venous occlusion in a dog

Radu Andrei Baisan[1]* iD, Vasile Vulpe[1], Mircea Lazăr[2] and Sorin Aurelian Paşca[2]

Abstract

Background: In both humans and animals, cardiac fibrosarcoma is rare among primary cardiac malignant neoplasia. The overall prevalence of cardiac neoplasia in dogs is low, reported to be between 0.17% and 0.19% of hospital admissions. The aim of this report is to describe the clinical and pathological findings of a dog presenting signs of right sided congestive heart failure due to an intracardiac and venous obstructing mass, diagnosed by histopathology as cardiac fibrosarcoma with myxoid features.

Case presentation: A 7 years old male mix breed Husky weighing 23 kg was presented to our Veterinary Teaching Hospital the owner reporting weight loss, inappetence and exercise intolerance and on presentation exhibited breathlessness and an enlarged abdomen. A 5 minutes six leads electrocardiogram and cardiac ultrasonography were performed using standard, established techniques. Complete blood count, serum liver enzyme activities and renal parameters were assessed. Shortly after the cardiologic examination, the dog died and necropsy examination of the cardiovascular system revealed an elongated and branched mass attached dorsally to the endocardial insertion of the septal tricuspid valve leaflet. This mass extended retrogradely into the lumen of the cervical veins, obstructing the venous flow. Histological diagnosis of the mass was cardiac fibrosarcoma with myxoid features. Multiple metastases were found inside the lungs only.

Conclusion: This is the first report describing a right cardiac fibrosarcoma with myxoid features and venous obstruction in a dog. Cardiac fibrosarcoma is a rare finding, however should be considered when an intracardiac mass is diagnosed.

Keywords: Sarcoma, Dog, Metastasis, Right sided heart failure

Background

Fibrosarcoma is a rare, highly malignant tumour of mesenchymal cell origin. It derives from pathologically transformed spindle shaped fibroblasts with an excessively high division rate [1]. In both humans and animals, cardiac fibrosarcoma is rare among primary cardiac malignant neoplasia [2]. In dogs, approximately 1% of primary cardiac tumours are fibrosarcoma [3]. Fibrosarcoma with myxoid features had been described in human medicine as mxofibrosarcoma, however, veterinary literature describes this type of tumour as either fibrosarcoma or myxosarcoma. According to Milovancev et al. 2015, fibrosarcoma in dog resembles high grade myxofibrosarcoma, while myxosarcoma resembles low grade myxofibrosarcoma [4].

In dogs, the overall prevalence of cardiac neoplasia is low [5], reported to be 0.17% of hospital admissions [6]. Another retrospective large population study reported a prevalence of 0.19%, amounting to 1383 dogs with cardiac tumours out of a total population of 729,265 dogs [3]. Primary cardiac tumours in dogs include chemodectoma, chondrosarcoma, fibrosarcoma, hemangiosarcoma, leiomyosarcoma, lipofibroma, mesothelioma, myxofibroma, myxoma, rhabdomyosarcoma and ectopic thyroid sarcomas [7].

The aim of this report is to describe the clinical and pathological findings of a dog presenting signs of right sided congestive heart failure due to an intracardiac and

* Correspondence: andrei.baisan.mv@gmail.com;
baisan.andrei_mv@yahoo.com
[1]Department of Clinics, University of Agricultural Sciences and Veterinary Medicine "Ion Ionescu de la Brad", Aleea M. Sadoveanu no. 8, 700489 Iaşi, Romania
Full list of author information is available at the end of the article

venous obstructing mass, diagnosed by histopathology as cardiac fibrosarcoma with myxoid features. To author's knowledge, right sided cardiac fibrosarcoma with myxoid features extending into the venous system had not been reported in veterinary medicine to date. This case-report was structured according to proposed guidelines in the literature [8].

Case presentation

A 7 years old male mix breed Husky weighing 23 kg was presented to our Veterinary Teaching Hospital the owner reporting weight loss, inappetence and exercise intolerance and on presentation exhibited breathlessness and an enlarged abdomen. Physical examination revealed cyanotic mucosal membranes, severe subcutaneous edema in the head area, thorax and limbs and respiratory effort with a rate of 42 breaths per minute. Palpation of the abdomen revealed a positive ballottement reaction suggesting the presence of ascites. Cardiac sounds were muffled during auscultation and the femoral pulse was fast and weak. A 5 minutes six leads electrocardiogram (PolySpectrum ECG) and echocardiography (Esaote AU5), were performed using previously described methods [9, 10]. Complete blood count, serum liver enzyme activities and renal parameters were assessed.

Electrocardiography revealed a fast sinus rhythm of 140 bpm, absence of respiratory arrhythmia and low voltage QRS complexes (R wave in lead II = 0.09 mV), with a positive polarity in leads I, II, aVL, aVF and negative in leads III and aVR, with a left axis deviation.

A brief cardiac echocardiography revealed right atrial and ventricle enlargement with a hyperechoic heterogenous mobile mass of 4.26 × 2.64 cm inside the right ventricle extending into the right atrial cavity through the tricuspid annulus (Fig. 1). A subjective assessment of the left ventricle revealed thickened left ventricular septum and free wall and reduced lumen size, suggesting concentric hypertrophy. The left atrial cavity appeared normal. Also, free pleural fluid was observed. A complete echocardiographic examination was not possible because of the dog's clinical status. Red and white cell numbers were within the reference range and the haematocrit was mildly decreased Ht%: 38.4 (reference range 40–60%). Serum biochemistry revealed increased activity of serum alanin aminotransferase: 111 U/L (reference ranges 18–86 U/L), alkaline phosphatase: 203 U/L (reference range 12–121 U/L), normal total protein: 5.5 g/dL (reference range 5.4–7.5 g/dL) and increased BUN: 96 mg/dL (reference range 8–29 mg/dL).

Shortly after the cardiologic examination, the dog died and necropsy was performed. The necropsy revealed typical changes of right sided congestive heart failure. Severe cyanosis of oral mucosae, of the tongue and skin were observed. Also, generalized edema of the subcutaneous

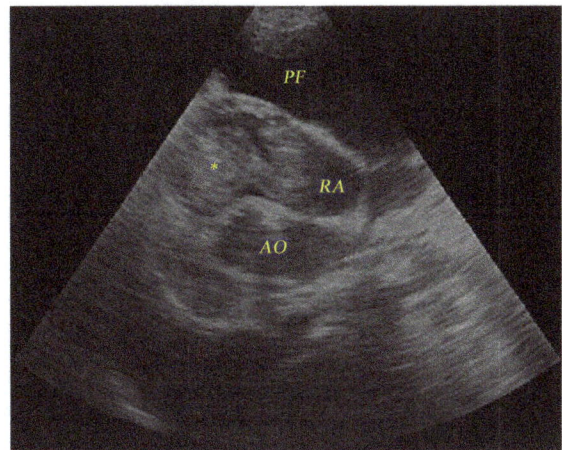

Fig. 1 Echocardiography of a dog with intracardiac mass: right parasternal long axis 5 chamber view – a hyperechoic mass (asterisk) is visible inside the right atrial cavity (RA). An anechoic area is visible around the heart represented by pleural fluid (PF); AO – aorta

tissue, more evident in the head area, ventral part of the body and limbs was observed. In both peritoneal and pleural cavities, a large amount (2.5 respectively 0.5 l) of free serous fluid was present. The lung had a pale appearance and higher density than normal at palpation, while the floating thest was negative, likely as a result of compression by pleural fluid.

Inside the right heart (atrium and ventricle), an elongated and branched mass with a smooth surface was observed. It extended from the right ventricle, retrograde to the right atrium, and then into the cranial vena cava, continued into the right brachiocephalic vein and split into the subclavian and external jugular vein. The subclavian branch was short. From the jugular vein, the tumour extended to the linguofacial and maxillary veins (Fig. 2a). The caudal vena cava and left brachiocephalic veins were enlarged, but no mass was found inside the lumen.

The mass was attached dorsally to the endocardial insertion of the septal tricuspid valve leaflet, suggesting a diagnosis of a primary endocardial tumour. The consistency was firm to elastic, with a smooth surface and an overall whitish colour with small red areas evident dispersed throughout the mass. The sectioned surface of this mass was nonhomogeneous, slightly fatty, with red and yellow striae inside.

The gross examination of the left heart revealed an apparently hypertrophied left ventricle with a reduced ventricular lumen (Fig. 2b). The mitral and aortic valves were normal, as well as the left ventricle outflow tract.

The liver, spleen and pancreas were increased in volume based on gross pathology inspection and a very dark red colour, presumably as a consequence of chronic venous congestion.

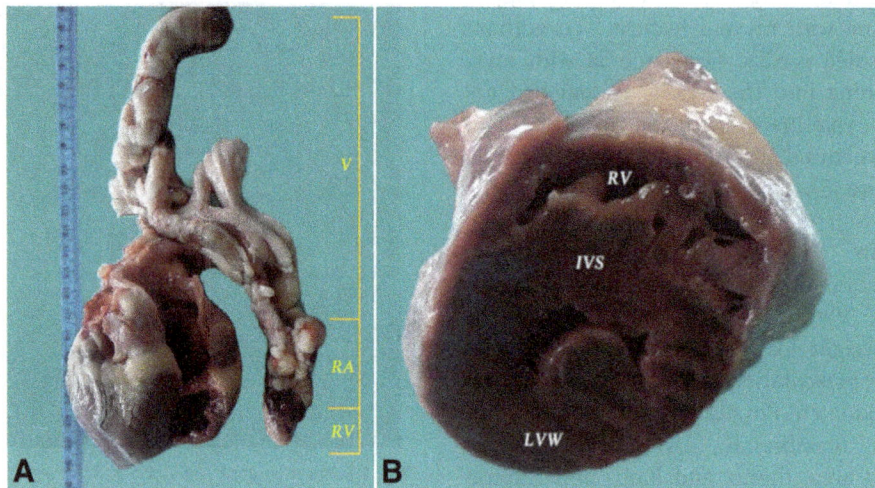

Fig. 2 a Gross pathology of the heart of a 7 years old male mix-breed Husky. The right heart is dissected and the intracardiac and intravascular mass is presented after the extraction from the heart and vein system showing the localization of the mass: RV – right ventricular mass, RA – right atrial mass, V – intravenous mass; **b** Gross pathology of the heart - section through the papillary muscles, demonstrating a severe concentric hypertrophy with decreased left ventricular cavity; LVW – left ventricular wall, IVS – interventricular septum, RV – right ventricle

During necropsy, multiple fragments were harvested from the intracardiac and intravascular locations of the mass as well as the connection of the mass and the endocardial insertion. Samples were also taken from liver, lung, pancreas, left and right kidney, spleen, brain, both of adrenal glands and myocardium.

Microscopic examination was performed on formalin-fixed and paraffin embedded tissues. The slides were routinely processed and stained with Masson's trichrome and alcian blue. Selected sections of the tumour were immunostained using the labelled CD34 (QBEnd-10; Dako), vimentin (Novocastra – Liquid mouse monoclonal antibody), desmin (Novocastra – Liquid mouse monoclonal antibody), CD31 (Novocastra – Lyophilized mouse monoclonal antibody), alpha – smooth muscle actin (Novocastra - Lyophilized mouse monoclonal antibody), epithelial membrane antigen (Novocastra - Liquid mouse monoclonal antibody), S-100 protein (Novocastra – Liquid mouse polyclonal antibody) and MUC1 (Novocastra – Lyophilized mouse monoclonal antibody).

Histological examination of the mass revealed a mixed tumour with two microscopical aspects: fibrosarcoma and myxoma. The two different types of the tumor were intercalated, resulting into a tumoral tissue organized in two structures with different architectures (Fig. 3a).

One type was organized in compact structure with spindle shaped cells. These cells had big, irregular and vesicular nuclei (anisokaryosis) with chromatin of a dusty appearance and a marked nucleolus, morphology corresponding to fibrosarcoma tumour. This type showed 8–12 mitotic figures per 400× field consistent with high grade of malignancy (Fig. 3b). The other type had an organisation typical of a myxomatous tumour,

formed by pleomorphic cells arranged in cords, trabeculae and small groups. The cells presented spindle, triangular and stellate shapes, anisokaryosis, low mitotic figures (1–3 per 400× field) and syncitia (Fig. 3c). Within the tumor, neoformation blood vessels and a very poor stroma were present. The myxoid matrix was strongly positive for alcian blue stain.

The examination of the contact area between the tumor and the atrial wall revealed tumoral cells among the myocardiocytes (Fig. 4a). Within the tumoral mass, extended areas of necrosis were observed, with the persistance of the tumoral arhitecture.

The microscopical lung metastasis had the same mixed structure as the primary tumor. A capsule-like structure represented by condensed lung tissue around the tumoral metastasis, lung atelectasis and compensatory emphysema near the metastasis were observed (Fig. 4b).

The fibrosarcomatous type of the cardiac tumor was positive for vimentin (Fig. 5a), S-100 protein and alpha-smooth muscle actin and negative for desmin, CD31, CD34, MUC1 and epithelial membrane antigen. The myxomatous type of the mass was positive for vimentin also (Fig. 5b), alpha-smooth muscle actin, weak positive for S-100 protein and negative for desmin, CD31, CD34, epithelial membrane antigen and MUC1. Desmin was positive only for myocardial tissue where the tumoral mass inserted.

No metastases were found in other organs except the lungs. However, lesions secondary to right sided congestion heart failure were observed in different organs. These lesions consisted of congestion and hypoxia-induced degeneration in the liver, spleen,

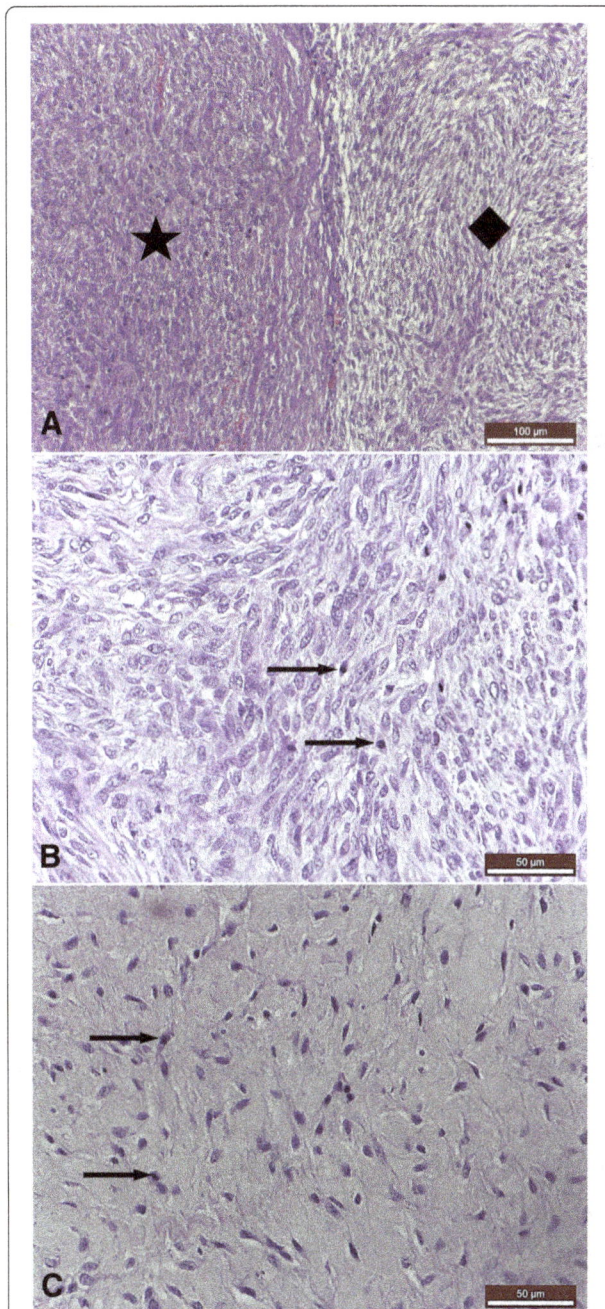

Fig. 3 a Histolgic aspects of the mixed intracardiac tumor. Two microscopical aspects are visible: compact structure with spindle shape cells (star) consistent with fibrosarcoma and a myxomatous aspect, formed by pleiomorphic cells with cords, trabeculae and small groups distribution (diamond). Fibrosarcoma with myxomatous features - primary tumour; **b** Histological aspect of the fibrosarcomatous area of the mass: multiple mitotic figures are visible on 400× field (arrow); **c** Histological aspect of the myxomatous area of the mass: few mitotic figures are visible on 400× field (arrow). Trichromic Masson stain

lobules, due to hypoxia, large groups of degenerated hepatocytes with pyknotic nuclei were observed. The kidney examination revealed distension of the interstitial capillaries, filled with red blood cells and proximal tubules epitelium degeneration secondary to hypoxia. Histopathological examination of the left ventricle wall revealed an increase in myocardiocytes size and a moderate congestion of the interstitial blood vessels.

Discussions and conclusions

This paper presents a very rare finding of a right sided congestive heart failure due to a massive cardiac fibrosarcoma with myxoid features associated with pulmonary metastasis in an adult dog. This is the first report of an intracardiac and intravenous obstructive fibrosarcoma with myxoid features in dog.

Several studies in veterinary medicine have reported intracardiac fibrosarcoma in dogs. One study reported a spherical mass of 0.5 cm in diameter in the right atrial surface of the atrial septum [11] while in another case, the tumour was well demarcated involving the subepicardial myocardium of the left ventricle [12]. One report described a large mass at the heart base in a Labrador filling approximately 80% of the left atrial lumen [13]. One paper described a primary malignant mixed mesenchymal tumour of the heart including fibrosarcoma, rhabdomyosarcoma, liposarcoma and chondrosarcoma [14]. Cardiac myxosarcoma in dogs are also very rare. One paper reported an extracardiac intrapericardial myxosarcoma of approximately 3 × 4.5 cm obstructing the right ventricular outflow tract [15].

The dog in this report was presented with severe signs of right sided cardiac heart failure, including peripheral edema and pleural and peritoneal free fluid due to the obstruction of the venous return flow. Electrocardiography revealed moderate sinus tachycardia with marked low voltage of the R-wave and left axis deviation. Tachycardia and low voltage of the R-wave are consistent with pleural and peritoneal effusion [16]. The left axis deviation may have been induced by the left ventricular hypertrophy. This condition have been commonly reported in cats with hypertrophic cardiomyopathy [16]. The increase in circulating liver enzyme activities was probably a consequence of the hepatic congestion secondary to the occlusion of the right ventricular inflow tract, in the absence of other histopathological changes [17]. Echocardiography revealed a hyperechoic mobile mass inside the right ventricle, continued inside the right atrium, consistent with an intracardiac tumour and obliterating the returning venous flow. Necropsy revealed that the mass inside the right ventricle extended into the right atrium and the venous system of the right side of the cranial mediastinum and neck, measuring a total length of 25 cm. The mass probably extended into the

pancreas and kidneys. Liver congestion was characterised by enlarged sinusoid capillaries, filled with agglutinated red blood cells and within the hepatic

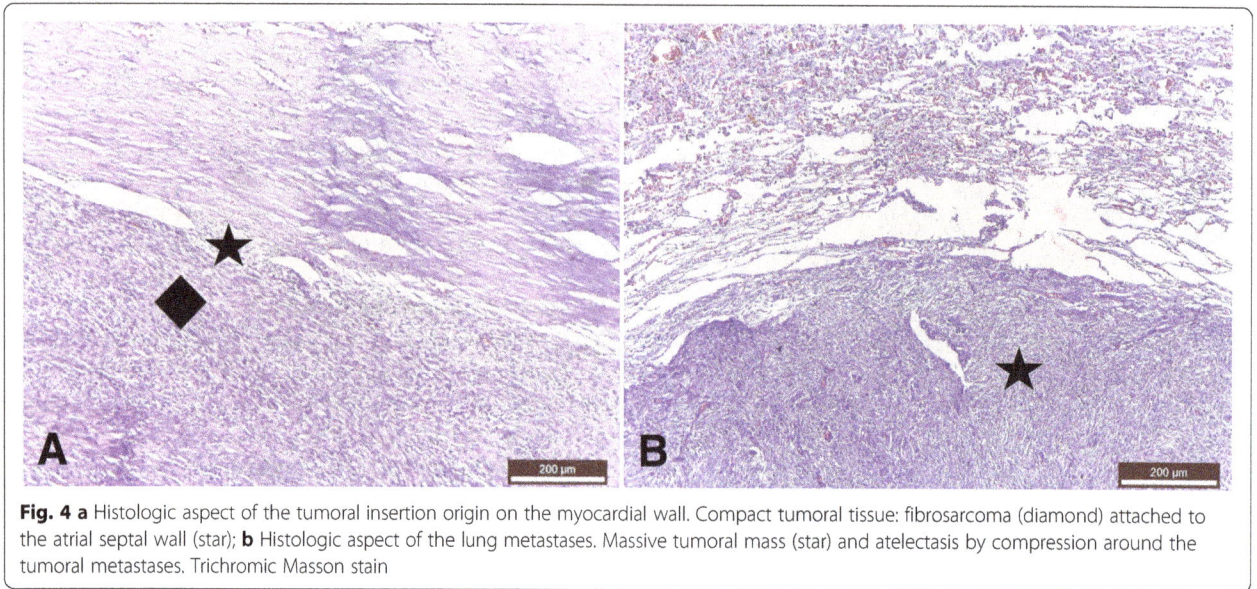

Fig. 4 a Histologic aspect of the tumoral insertion origin on the myocardial wall. Compact tumoral tissue: fibrosarcoma (diamond) attached to the atrial septal wall (star); **b** Histologic aspect of the lung metastases. Massive tumoral mass (star) and atelectasis by compression around the tumoral metastases. Trichromic Masson stain

right-sided venous system because of the alignment of the right brachiocephalic vein with cranial vena cava compared to the left one which detaches in an angle as it crosses the median plane towards the left side [18].

Histological examination revealed tumour tissue connections with the right atrial septal wall, dorsal to the insertion of the sepal tricuspid leaflet, proving that this mass developed from the heart in the first place and grew retrogradely into the right atrium and venous lumen. The morphological analysis of different type of cells from the mixed tissue mass, the immunohistochemical analysis and the different grades on malignancy based on the mitotic index, as well as the lung metastasis led to the diagnosis of a rare tumor: fibosarcoma with myxoid features

originating from the right atrial endocardial wall. Metastases of the same tissue were found only inside the lungs. This finding might be explained by the anatomical path of the blood stream from the right ventricle, on which tumour cells were carried into the lungs.

Echocardiography and gross examination of the heart at post mortem revealed apparent left ventricular hypertrophy in the absence of subaortic stenosis or any changes in the left ventricular outflow tract. These changes may be explained by the low preload of the left ventricle due to the presence of a small amount of blood in the pulmonary circulation. This mechanism has been also associated with cardiac tamponade and acute hypovolemia [19, 20]. In literature, this phenomenon is called

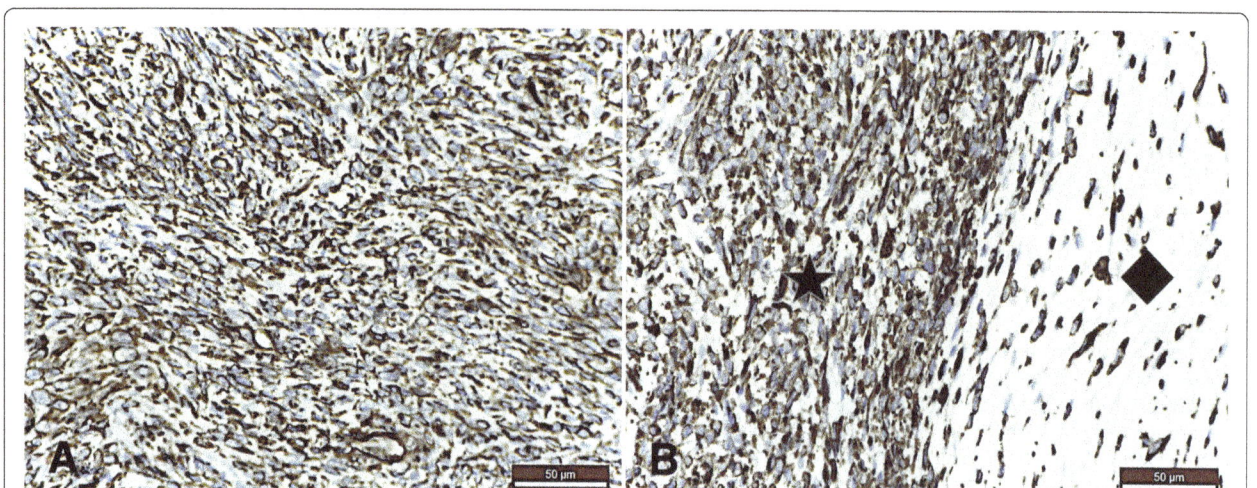

Fig. 5 a Immunohistochemical stain by vimentin of the tumour. Strong positive stain for vimentin of the fibrosarcomatous part of the mass; **b** two types of architecture are visible within the mass: on the left side of the field, condensed cellularity is visible (star) and on the right side of the field the cells are sparse (diamond) – the cytoplasm of the neoplastic cells stains for vimentin in both structures. Vimentin stain

pseudohypertrophy due to its transitory nature once blood reperfusion is achieved [21].

Fibrosarcoma with myxoid features, although a very rare finding, should be included in the differential diagnosis of intracardiac masses that may obliterate the blood flow and develop metastases in other organs.

Abbreviations
BUN: Blood urea nitrogen; Ht%: Haematocrit

Acknowledgments
Not applicable.

Funding
No funding was used for this study.

Authors' contributions
BRA performed the cardiologic examination, SAP and ML performed the necropsy and the histopathologic examination and interpretation, BRA, SAP and VV drafted and wrote the manuscript. All authors read and approved the final manuscript.

Consent for publication
The owner gave his written informed consent for publication by means of signing our official client acceptance form.

Competing interests
The authors declare that they have no competing interests.

Author details
¹Department of Clinics, University of Agricultural Sciences and Veterinary Medicine "Ion Ionescu de la Brad", Aleea M. Sadoveanu no. 8, 700489 Iaşi, Romania. ²Department of Pathology, University of Agricultural Sciences and Veterinary Medicine "Ion Ionescu de la Brad", Iaşi, Romania.

References

1. Augsburger D, Nelson PJ, Kalinski T, Udelnow A, Knosel T, Hofstetter M, Qin JW, Wang Y, Gupta AS, Bonifatius S, et al. Current diagnostics and treatment of fibrosarcoma -perspectives for future therapeutic targets and strategies. Oncotarget. 2017;8(61):104638–53.
2. Jyothirmayi R, Jacob R, Nair K, Rajan B. Primary fibrosarcoma of the right ventricle--a case report. Acta Oncol. 1995;34(7):972–4.
3. Ware WA, Hopper DL. Cardiac tumors in dogs: 1982-1995. J Vet Intern Med. 1999;13(2):95–103.
4. Milovancev M, Hauck M, Keller C, Stranahan LW, Mansoor A, Malarkey DE. Comparative pathology of canine soft tissue sarcomas: possible models of human non-rhabdomyosarcoma soft tissue sarcomas. J Comp Pathol. 2015; 152(1):22–7.
5. Treggiari E, Pedro B, Dukes-McEwan J, Gelzer AR, Blackwood L. A descriptive review of cardiac tumours in dogs and cats. Vet Comp Oncol. 2017;15(2): 273–88.
6. Ware WA. Cardiac neoplasia. In: Bonagura J, editor. Kirk's current veterinary therapy. Volume XII, edn. Philadelphia: WB Saunders; 1995. p. 873.
7. Sisson D, Thomas WP. Pericardial disease and cardiac tumors. In: Fox PR, Sisson D, Moise NS, editors. Textbook of canine and feline cardiology. edn. Philadelphia: Saunders; 1999. p. 679–701.
8. Gagnier JJ, Kienle G, Altman DG, Moher D, Sox H, Riley D. The CARE guidelines: consensus-based clinical case reporting guideline development. Glob Adv Health Med. 2013;2(5):38–43.
9. Tilley LP, Smith WWK Jr. Electrocardiography. In: Smith Jr WWK, Tilley L, Oyama M, Sleeper M, editors. Manual of Canine and Feline Cardiology. 5 edn. St Louis, Missouri: Elsevier; 2016. p. 49–76.
10. Thomas WP, Gaber CE, Jacobs GJ, Kaplan PM, Lombard CW, Moise NS, Moses BL. Recommendations for standards in transthoracic two-dimensional echocardiography in the dog and cat. Echocardiography Committee of the Specialty of cardiology, American College of Veterinary Internal Medicine. J Vet Intern Med. 1993;7(4):247–52.
11. Madarame H, Sato K, Ogihara K, Ishibashi T, Fujii Y, Wakao Y. Primary cardiac fibrosarcoma in a dog. J Vet Intern Med. 2004;66(8):979–82.
12. Speltz MC, Manivel JC, Tobias AH, Hayden DW. Primary cardiac fibrosarcoma with pulmonary metastasis in a Labrador retriever. Vet Pathol. 2007;44(3): 403–7.
13. Asakawa MG, Ames MK, Kim Y. Primary cardiac spindle cell tumor in a dog. Can Vet J. 2013;54(7):672–4.
14. Machida N, Kobayashi M, Tanaka R, Katsuda S, Mitsumori K. Primary malignant mixed mesenchymal tumour of the heart in a dog. J Comp Pathol. 2003;128(1):71–4.
15. Karlin ET, Yang VK, Prabhakar M, Gregorich SL, Hahn S, Rush JE. Extracardiac intrapericardial myxosarcoma causing right ventricular outflow tract obstruction in a dog. J Vet Cardiol. 2018;20(2):129–35.
16. Santilli RA, Perego M. Electrocardiography of the dog and cat. Milano: EDRA LSWR; 2014.
17. Atkins CE, Keene BW, McGuirk SM. Investigation of caval syndrome in dogs experimentally infected with Dirofilaria immitis. J Vet Intern Med. 1988;2(1): 36–40.
18. Spătaru C. Anatomia animalelor: sistemul circulator, sistemul nervos. Iaşi: Ed. Alfa; 2013.
19. Di Segni E, Preisman S, Ohad DG, Battier A, Boyko V, Kaplinsky E, Perel A, Vered Z. Echocardiographic left ventricular remodeling and pseudohypertrophy as markers of hypovolemia. An experimental study on bleeding and volume repletion. J Am Soc Echocardiogr. 1997;10(9):926–36.
20. Di Segni E, Beker B, Arbel Y, Bakst A, Dean H, Levi A, Kaplinsky E, Klein HO. Left ventricular pseudohypertrophy in pericardial effusion as a sign of cardiac tamponade. Am J Cardiol. 1990;66(4):508–11.
21. Di Segni E, Feinberg MS, Sheinowitz M, Motro M, Battler A, Kaplinsky E, Vered Z. Left ventricular pseudohypertrophy in cardiac tamponade: an echocardiographic study in a canine model. J Am Coll Cardiol. 1993;21(5): 1286–94.

19

A methodological approach for deep learning to distinguish between meningiomas and gliomas on canine MR-images

Tommaso Banzato[1], Marco Bernardini[1,2], Giunio B. Cherubini[3] and Alessandro Zotti[1]* (ID)

Abstract

Background: Distinguishing between meningeal-based and intra-axial lesions by means of magnetic resonance (MR) imaging findings may occasionally be challenging. Meningiomas and gliomas account for most of the total primary brain neoplasms in dogs, and differentiating between these two forms is mandatory in choosing the correct therapy. The aims of the present study are: 1) to determine the accuracy of a deep convolutional neural network (CNN, *GoogleNet)* in discriminating between meningiomas and gliomas in pre- and post-contrast T1 images and T2 images; 2) to develop an image classifier, based on the combination of CNN and MRI sequence displaying the highest accuracy, to predict whether a lesion is a meningioma or a glioma.

Results: Eighty cases with a final diagnosis of meningioma ($n = 56$) and glioma ($n = 24$) from two different institutions were included in the study. A pre-trained CNN was retrained on our data through a process called transfer learning. To evaluate CNN accuracy in the different imaging sequences, the dataset was divided into a training, a validation and a test set. The accuracy of the CNN was calculated on the test set. The combination between post-contrast T1 images and CNN was chosen in developing the image classifier (trCNN). Ten images from challenging cases were excluded from the database in order to test trCNN accuracy; the trCNN was trained on the remainder of the dataset of post-contrast T1 images, and correctly classified all the selected images. To compensate for the imbalance between meningiomas and gliomas in the dataset, the Matthews correlation coefficient (MCC) was also calculated. The trCNN showed an accuracy of 94% (MCC = 0.88) on post-contrast T1 images, 91% (MCC = 0.81) on pre-contrast T1-images and 90% (MCC = 0.8) on T2 images.

Conclusions: The developed trCNN could be a reliable tool in distinguishing between different meningiomas and gliomas from MR images.

Keywords: Convolutional neural network, Meningioma, Glioma, Magnetic resonance imaging, Histopathology

Background

Brain neoplasms are a primary concern in adult dogs, with an overall reported prevalence of 4.5% [1]. Treatment options for brain tumours in dogs include symptomatic management, chemotherapy, surgery, radiation therapy, surgery combined with chemotherapy and/or radiation therapy [2]. When symptomatic management or radiation therapy is chosen as the treatment option, histopathological analysis of the lesions is usually not performed and the diagnosis is based only on interpretation by the imaging expert [3]. Although some imaging features may be used to increase or decrease suspicion of a particular tumour type, the distinction between meningeal-based and intra-axial lesions may occasionally be challenging [4]. Meningiomas and gliomas account for most of the total primary brain neoplasms in dogs [1], and differentiating between these two forms is mandatory in choosing the correct therapy.

* Correspondence: alessandro.zotti@unipd.it
[1]Department of Animal Medicine, Production and Health, University of Padua, Viale dell'Università 16, AGRIPOLIS, Legnaro, 35020 Padua, Italy

The role of diagnostic imaging grows progressively more important as the demand for high quality veterinary care constantly increases. In such a scenario, a thorough standardisation in interpretation of diagnostic images becomes ever more desirable. The possible applications of a texture analysis-based approach on other diagnostic imaging techniques such as MRI [5] or computed tomography [6] have only seldom been investigated in veterinary medicine. On the other hand, several studies exploring the use of texture analysis to establish the relationship between ultrasonography and pathology have been published [7–13]. The main purpose of these studies was to overcome the inherent limitations of ultrasonography in identifying subtle changes in the appearance of parenchymal organs (mainly kidney and liver) caused by degenerative pathologies.

In the present work we have tried to take advantage of CNNs in the extraction and analysis of complex data patterns in order to distinguish between meningiomas and gliomas in pre- and post-contrast T1 images and T2 images. Furthermore, we have developed an image classifier, which could be prospectively used in a clinical scenario, to predict whether a lesion is a meningioma or a glioma; such a classifier is based on the combination of CNN and MRI sequence displaying the highest accuracy.

Materials and methods
Cases selection
The databases of two different institutions [Portoni Rossi Veterinary Hospital (Institution 1), Zola Predosa, Italy; Dick White Referrals, Six Mile Bottom, UK (Institution 2)] were retrospectively searched between January 2011 and January 2018 for dogs having an MRI scan showing an intracranial space-occupying lesion and a final histopathological diagnosis of either meningioma or glioma. No a-priori selection based on the histopathological classification of the lesions was made at this stage.

MR imaging
The MRI scans were performed with a 0.4 T open-type permanent magnet (Hitachi Aperto, Hitachi Medical Corporation, Japan) at Institution 2, and with a 0.22 T open-type permanent magnet (MrV, Paramed Medical Systems, Genova, Italy) at Institution 1. Different imaging protocols were used at the two institutions. Only MRI scans including a T2W fast spin-echo series (repetition time, 13 to 120 ms; echo time, 290 to 7790 ms; matrix, 512×512 pixels) and pre- and post-contrast (gadolinium-based medium) T1W spin-echo series (repetition time, 13 to 26 m; echo time, 462 to 880 ms; matrix, 512×512 pixels) were included in the study. All images were acquired with 3- to 5-mm slice thickness

with a 10% gap, while the signal-to-noise ratio was improved using 2 to 4 averages for each acquisition.

Dataset preparation
All the MRI studies were exported in a .jpg format from the original digital imaging communication in medicine (DICOM) format. Pre- and post-contrast T1 and T2 sequences were included in the study. Images belonging to different imaging sequences were analysed separately. Dorsal, sagittal and transverse scans were selected to increase the number of available images. All lesion-containing images were divided into two different folders based on the final histopathological diagnosis (meningioma or glioma). Thereafter, the images were cropped so that only the lesion and a small portion of the surrounding tissues were included. Lastly, the images were resized, using a photo editing program (PhotoshopCC, Adobe Sytems Incorporated, USA), to a 224×224-pixel format to match the CNN requirements.

Deep learning model
Due to the limited size of our database, we retrained a pre-trained CNN called GoogleNet [14] on our images, a process called "transfer learning". The built-in MATLAB (MATLAB and Statistics Toolbox Release 2017b, The MathWorks, Inc., Natick) toolbox for neural networks was used for the experiment. GoogleNet was trained on a large-scale image database [ImageNet database (www.image-net.org)] comprising approximately 1.2 million everyday images belonging to 1000 different categories. GoogleNet is an extremely deep neural network (it comprises 144 different layers) and is composed of several layer types with specific functions. An in-depth description of the structure of GoogleNet is beyond the purposes of this paper but a general description of how CNNs work is useful to its clarity. The basic components of a CNN are: convolutional layers, pooling layers and dense layers. Convolutional layers extract a large number of features from the images and create maps of the distribution of these features throughout the image. Deeper convolutional layers are able to detect more complex features (Fig. 2). Pooling layers are used to reduce data volume, decreasing the size of the feature maps while retaining the most important information. The dense layers are the classification layers and are the equivalent of a classical artificial neural network; a set of interconnected neurons that analyse an input and generate an output to make predictions on new data.

The features (along with their weights and biases) derived from the ImageNet database were then adjusted on the new dataset to predict the labels of the new images (transfer learning).

Evaluation of the classification performance of GoogleNet in the different MRI sequences

To prevent overfitting (i.e. poor generalisation performance), the images in the dataset were randomly divided into a training set, a validation set and a test set, respectively comprising 70%, 15% and 15% of the images. The validation set was used to fine-tune the network parameters and the test set was used to test network accuracy. If only a training set and a test set are used, there is a high risk of over-adapting the network to the test data, with consequent poor generalisation performance (overfitting). The network parameters were set as follows: LearnRateSchedule = piecewise, MaxEpochs = 120. An early stopping function was used to further prevent overfitting; if accuracy in the validation set stopped increasing for five consecutive epochs (an epoch is a complete iteration of the network throughout the training set), the learning phase was terminated [15]. Accuracy of a CNN is measured by the loss (or cost) function: the loss function measures the difference between the CNN output and the real label of the data. The lower the cost function value, the higher the network performance. When the loss stops decreasing, the CNN has reached the optimal solution (meant as the best possible accuracy given the network, dataset and settings) for the classification problem. The learn rate defines how large the network steps to reach the optimal solution are; if the steps are too big the optimal solution may be skipped, if the steps are too small the network could take an unreasonable amount of time to train. We programmed the network to adapt the learn rate to the learning process so that the learn rate decreased the closer the network got to the optimal solution. Classification accuracy was then displayed as the percentage of correctly labelled images in the test set and as a confusion matrix for the real and predicted image category. In order to account for the random distribution of the images in the training, validation and test sets, the analyses were repeated five times.

A cross-classification table method was used to calculate the accuracy of the trained classifier. Accuracy was calculated as the percentage of correctly classified cases. To compensate for the different distribution of the cases between the two classes (the total number of meningiomas was more than twice that of gliomas), additional metrics of accuracy, such as sensitivity, specificity, Cohen's Kappa (CK), and the Matthews correlation coefficient (MCC) [16], were calculated. The data are reported as median with the limits of the overall range.

Development of the trained classifier (trCNN)

To develop and test our trained classifier we asked one of the authors (MB, board- certified neurologist) to select five cases in which, based on the imaging reports, lesion location (intra- or extra- axial) made it difficult to assess. Ten images (five belonging to meningioma cases and five to glioma cases) were selected and excluded from the database used to retrain the network. GoogleNet was then retrained on the entire set of images (minus the ten selected images) (trCNN) and later used to predict the labels for the 10 previously excluded images.

Results

Eighty cases were included in the study. Twenty-four cases had a final diagnosis of glioma (Institution 1 $n = 14$; Institution 2 $n = 10$) and 56 of meningioma (Institution 1 $n = 23$; Institution 2 $n = 33$). Forty-five meningioma cases included in the present study (Institution 1 $n = 18$; Institution 2 $n = 27$) were also part of a previous study (Banzato et al., 2017) on texture image analysis. Complete results of the histopathological analysis are reported in Table 1. Six of the 56 meningioma cases were discarded because the lesions were completely cystic and only an insufficient amount of tissue was available for analysis.

The complete CNN workflow is reported in Fig. 1. A schematic representation of the analytical procedure, along with the analysis output, is reported in Fig. 2.

GoogleNet displayed the best performance on post-contrast T1 images, with a 94% accuracy (range: 89–98%). Sensitivity was 0.94 (range: 0.87–0.97),

Table 1 Complete histopathological results of the cases included in the study

Histopathological type	Number of cases
Gliomas (n = 24)	
Oligodendroglioma	12
Astrocytoma	8
Glioblastoma	3
Oligoastrocytoma	1
Meningiomas (n = 56)	
Papillar	11
Transitional	9
Atypical	6
Meningothelial	4
Fibroblastic	4
Psammomatous	3
Syncytial	3
Lipomatous	3
Meningoendothelial	3
Chordoid	2
Anaplastic	2
Other (biphasic, cystic, malignant, microcystic, osteoid, vacuolar, vascular)	6

Exported the DICOM images in .jpg and created the database for the analysis (each imaging sequence was analyzed separately)

Crop the images to fit GoogleNet requirements (224 x 224 pixel RGB images)

Divide the images in two folders based on the results of histopatological analysis

Load Googlenet

Divide the dataset into a training set (70%), a validation set (15%), and a test set (15%)

Retrain GoogleNet on the training set

Validate the accuracy on the validation set

Measure network diagnostic accuracy on the test set

Fig. 1 Workflow used for the experiment

specificity was 0.94 (range 0.82–1), CK was 0.87 (range: 0.78–0.97), and MCC was 0.88 (range: 0.78–0.97).

The classification performance of GoogleNet on pre-contrast T1 images was lower, with a 91% accuracy (range: 88–92%). Sensitivity of 91% (range: 88–100%), specificity of 91% (range: 88–96%), CK of 0.81 (range: 0.75–0.86) and MCC of 0.81 (range: 0.75–0,86) were recorded.

GoogleNet had the poorest performance on T2W images, with a 90% (range: 89–93%) accuracy. Sensitivity was 89% (range: 83–96%), specificity was 91% (range: 83–97%), CK was 0.8 (range: 0.77–0.85) and MCC was 0.8 (range: 0.77–0,85).

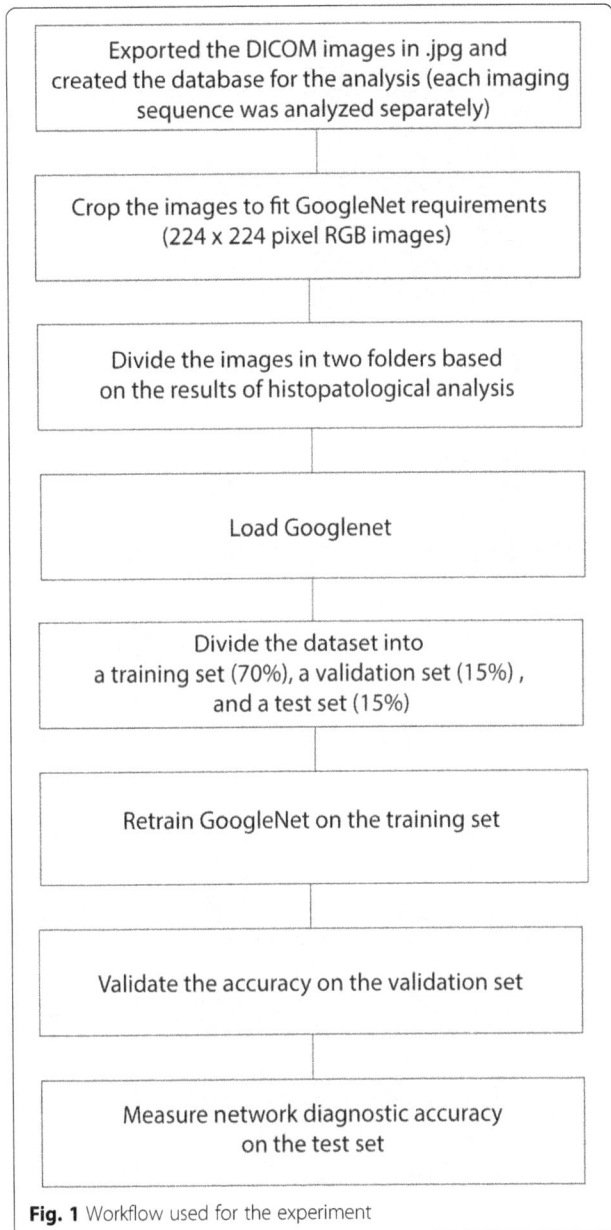

Lastly, the trCNN correctly classified all the 10 images (from 3 glioma and 2 meningioma cases) that had previously been excluded from the database.

Discussion

Several image analysis techniques have been proposed both in human [17] and veterinary medicine [10] in recent years. One of the main advantage of deep learning among other image-analysis techniques (such as texture analysis) is that deep learning algorithms can be trained directly on the images and, once developed, can be applied to new images to make predictions [18]. A specialised class of deep-learning architectures, the so-called convolutional neural networks (CNNs), are considered the state-of-the-art algorithms for image analysis and classification [19]; a substantial number of different applications are being developed in medical imaging for structure detection, image segmentation, and computer-aided diagnosis [20]. Deep learning is also gaining popularity in medical imaging for other tasks such as: the automated creation of study protocols, improving image quality while decreasing radiation dose in CT; improving image quality and reducing scan time in MRI; plus many others [21]. The increasing availability of computers with great computational powers, as well as the scope to easily create and share large datasets, are acting as boosters for the development of deep-learning-based applications in the medical-imaging field, and the routine use of some applications assisting the radiologist's decision-making process is likely to be seen in the near future [22]. Recently, the possibility of using deep learning to detect degenerative liver disease in canine patients from ultrasonographic images has been explored [23].

GoogleNet displayed a very high accuracy on all the imaging sequences (more than 90% of the images were correctly labelled) in discriminating between meningiomas and gliomas, suggesting that the use of transfer learning was an appropriate solution to our classification problem. In testing our trCNN, the test-cases were selected based on the opinion of MB (co-author, board-certified neurologist), since one of the aims of this study was to evaluate trCNN performance in those cases that resulted as challenging for expert radiologists. In particular, in our experience, it is far more common for a glioma to resemble an extra-axial neoplasm rather than for a meningioma to resemble an intra-axial lesion. Prospectively, use of the CNN developed in this study might help the clinician in the distinction between intra-and extra axial lesions.

The most important limitations of this work are its relatively low number of cases and the imbalance between glioma (24) and meningioma cases (56). However, it is the authors' opinion that such an imbalance did not act as a major limitation, due to the high

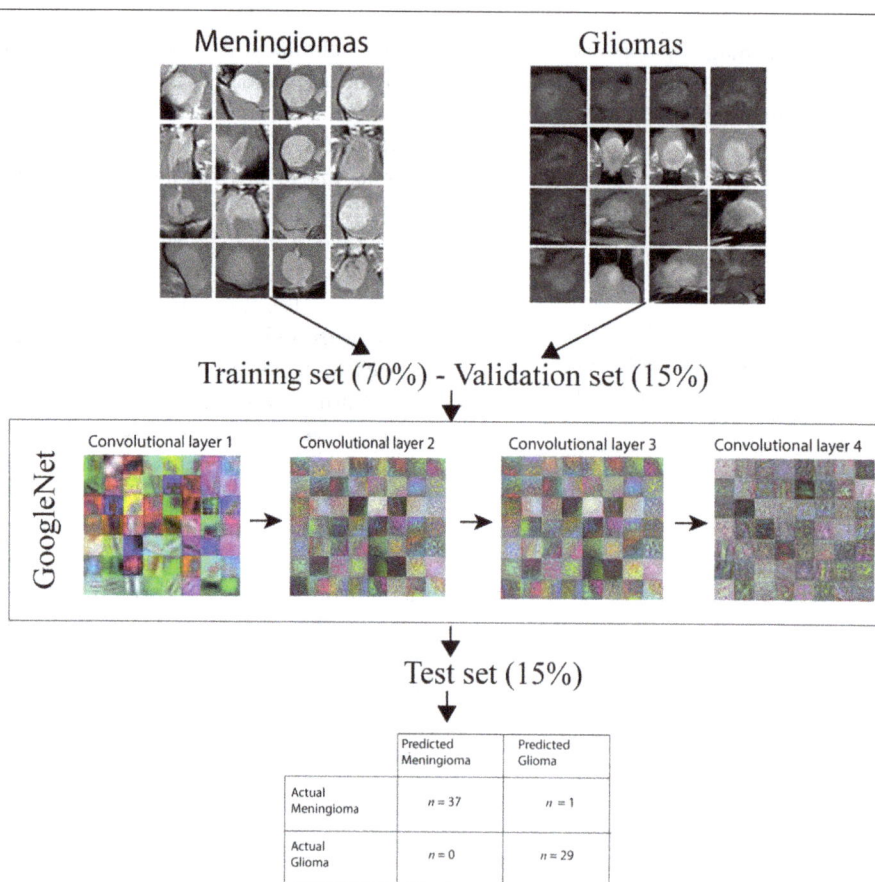

Fig. 2 Simplified representation of the analytical method used in the experiment and analytical output. The images are divided into two folders based on the results of the histopathological analysis. Thereafter, the dataset is divided into a training, a validation and a test set. The training and the validation sets are used for the transfer-learning procedure with GoogleNet. A schematic and simplified representation of the output of the first convolutional layers is reported. Please note that the features represented become more complex during convolutions. Lastly, the retrained GoogleNet convolutional deep neural network is used to predict the labels for the test set. A confusion matrix is generated as a final output. n = number of images

classification accuracy displayed by the trCNN. GoogleNet classification performance was carefully evaluated using metrics of accuracy, such as MCC, which were specifically developed to assess the performance of a classifier on heavily imbalanced databases. In particular, MCC takes values in the interval $[-1, 1]$, with 1 showing a complete agreement, -1 a complete disagreement, and 0 showing that the prediction was uncorrelated with the ground truth [24]. The MCC of GoogleNet applied on post-contrast T1 images was 0.88 (range: 0.78–0.97), indicating a very high agreement between the real and the predicted histopathological classes of the images.

Based on the data reported in Table 1, it is remarkable that the model proposed here showed excellent classification results despite the intrinsic variability of histological subtypes in both gliomas and meningiomas. Further studies, preferably including a larger number of patients from various institutions, are needed to determine the real generalisation performance of our trCNN.

Another important limitation is that, with the model we proposed, only two histopathological classes of brain tumours were included in the study and the trCNN had to classify each lesion as meningioma or glioma regardless of the actual nature of the lesion. However, the aim of this methodological study is not to propose a ready-to-use clinical test but to explore, retrospectively, the capacity of CNNs to distinguish between the two most common primary brain tumours in the dog. The excellent classification results achieved by our trCNN suggest that CNNs could become useful tools for both neuro-radiologists and clinicians in planning the correct therapeutic protocol. The next step towards development of a routine clinical application should include more categories of brain disease (both neoplastic and non-neoplastic) to further test the accuracy of deep learning in an actual clinical scenario.

Conclusions

The results reported in the present study suggest that CNNs could be a reliable tool in distinguishing between different meningiomas and gliomas from MR images. Further studies, possibly including a larger number of cases and histopathological categories, are required to determine the performance of CNNs in a clinical scenario.

Abbreviations

CK: Cohen's Kappa; CNN: Convolutional neural network; MCC: Mathews correlation coefficient; MR: Magnetic resonance; trCNN: Trained convolutional neural network

Funding

The present paper is part of a project funded by two research grants from the University of Padova, Italy:

1) Junior Research Grant from the UniPD (2015), funded for a total amount of € 48.000
2) Supporting Talents in Research@University of Padua, funded for a total amount of € 180.000, with a project entitled: "Prediction of the histological grading of human meningiomas using MR images texture and deep learning: a translational application of a model developed on spontaneously occurring meningiomas in dogs".

In addition, the authors would like to thank the NVIDIA Corporation (CA, USA) for donation of the GPU card used in this study.

Authors' contributions

TB and AZ conceived and designed the study, developed the deep-learning model, and drafted the manuscript. MB and GBC provided the MRI cases, drafted and revised the manuscript. All authors prepared and approved the final manuscript.

Consent for publication

Not applicable.

Competing interests

The authors declare that they have no competing interests.

Author details

[1]Department of Animal Medicine, Production and Health, University of Padua, Viale dell'Università 16, AGRIPOLIS, Legnaro, 35020 Padua, Italy. [2]Portoni Rossi Veterinary Hospital, Via Roma 57, Zola Predosa, 40069 Bologna, Italy. [3]Dick White Referrals, Six Mile Bottom, Cambridgeshire CB8 0UH, UK.

References

1. Song RB, Vite CH, Bradley CW, et al. Postmortem evaluation of 435 cases of intracranial neoplasia in dogs and relationship of neoplasm with breed, age, and body weight. J Vet Intern Med. 2013;27:1143–52.
2. Hu H, Barker A, Harcourt-Brown T, et al. Systematic review of brain tumor treatment in dogs. J Vet Intern Med. 2015;29:1456–63.
3. Keyerleber MA, Mcentee MC, Farrelly J, et al. Three-dimensional conformal radiation therapy alone or in combination with surgery for treatment of canine intracranial meningiomas. Vet Comp Oncol. 2015;13:385–97.
4. Bentley RT. Magnetic resonance imaging diagnosis of brain tumors in dogs. Vet J. 2015;205:204–16.
5. Banzato T, Bernardini M, Cherubini GB, et al. Texture analysis of magnetic resonance images to predict histologic grade of meningiomas in dogs. Am J Vet Res. 2017;78:1156–62.
6. Marschner CB, Kokla M, Amigo JM, et al. Texture analysis of pulmonary parenchymateous changes related to pulmonary thromboembolism in dogs – a novel approach using quantitative methods. BMC Vet Res. 2017;13:219.
7. Zotti A, Banzato T, Gelain ME, et al. Correlation of renal histopathology with renal echogenicity in dogs and cats: an ex-vivo quantitative study. BMC Vet Res. 2015;11:99.
8. Banzato T, Bonsembiante F, Aresu L, et al. Relationship of diagnostic accuracy of renal cortical echogenicity with renal histopathology in dogs and cats, a quantitative study. BMC Vet Res. 2017;13:24.
9. Banzato T, Fiore E, Morgante M, et al. Texture analysis of B-mode ultrasound images to stage hepatic lipidosis in the dairy cow : a methodological study. Res Vet Sci. 2016;108:71–5.
10. Starke A, Haudum A, Weijers G, et al. Noninvasive detection of hepatic lipidosis in dairy cows with calibrated ultrasonographic image analysis. J Dairy Sci. 2010;93:2952–65.
11. Weijers G, Starke A, Thijssen JM, et al. Transcutaneous vs. intraoperative quantitative ultrasound for staging bovine hepatic steatosis. Ultrasound Med Biol. 2012;38:1404–13.
12. Banzato T, Zovi G, Milani C. Estimation of fetal lung development using quantitative analysis of ultrasonographic images in normal canine pregnancy. Theriogenology. 2017;96:158–63.
13. Banzato T, Gelain ME, Aresu L, et al. Quantitative analysis of ultrasonographic images and cytology in relation to histopathology of canine and feline liver: an ex-vivo study. Res Vet Sci. 2015;103:164–9.
14. Szegedy C, Liu W, Jia Y, et al. Going deeper with Convolutions. arXiv: 14094842. 2014. https://arxiv.org/abs/1409.4842.
15. Akata Z, Perronnin F, Harchaoui Z, et al. Good practice in large-scale learning for image classification. Pami. 2014;36:507–20.
16. Boughorbel S, Jarray F, El-Anbari M. Optimal classifier for imbalanced data using Matthews correlation coefficient metric. PLoS One. 2017;12:1–17.
17. Nogueira MA, Abreu PH, Martins P, et al. Image descriptors in radiology images: a systematic review. Artif Intell Rev. 2016;47:1–29.
18. LeCun Y, Bengio Y, Hinton G. Deep learning. Nature. 2015;521:436–44.
19. Litjens G, Kooi T, Bejnordi BE, et al. A survey on deep learning in medical image analysis. Med Image Anal. 2017;42:60–88.
20. Shen D, Wu G, Suk H. Deep learning in medical image analysis. Annu Rev Biomed Eng. 2017;19:221–48.
21. Lakhani P, Prater AB, Hutson RK, et al. Machine learning in radiology: applications beyond image interpretation. J Am Coll Radiol. 2017;15:1–10.
22. Dreyer KJ, Geis JR. When machines think: Radiology's next frontier. Radiology. 2017;285:713–8.
23. Banzato T, Bonsembiante F, Aresu L, et al. Use of transfer learning to detect diffuse degenerative hepatic diseases from ultrasound images in dogs: a methodological study. Vet J. 2018;233:35–40.
24. Watson PF, Petrie A. Method agreement analysis: a review of correct methodology. Theriogenology. 2010;73:1167–79.

20

Evaluation of Ki-67 expression in feline non-ocular melanocytic tumours

Silvia Sabattini[1]* (iD), Andrea Renzi[1], Francesco Albanese[2], Marco Fantinati[1], Antonella Rigillo[1], Francesca Abramo[3], Raimondo Tornago[4], Giovanni Tortorella[2], Maria Massaro[2], Teresa Bruna Pagano[2], Julia Buchholz[5] and Giuliano Bettini[1]

Abstract

Background: Melanomas are rare in cats. The eye is the most commonly involved site, whereas few data are available about feline non-ocular melanomas (NOMs). Ki-67 thresholds with prognostic relevance have been established for canine melanomas, but not in cats. This study was undertaken to investigate the relationship between Ki-67 index, tumour characteristics, and clinical outcome in feline NOMs.

Histologic samples were retrospectively reviewed. Amelanotic tumours were admitted upon immunohistochemical positivity for Melan A or S100. Evaluated parameters included morphological diagnosis, histotype, junctional activity, degree of pigmentation, vascular invasion, lymphocytic infiltrate, necrosis, mitotic count (MC) and Ki-67 index. Pigmented tumours were bleached before evaluation. Clinical and follow-up information were retrieved via telephone interviews with the referring veterinarians.

Results: Fifty tumours located in skin ($n = 33$) and mucosae ($n = 17$) were included. Forty-eight percent and 95% of amelanotic tumours ($n = 21$) stained positive for Melan A and S100, respectively. Most achromic tumours were mucosal ($P < 0.001$, Fisher's exact test) and presented a spindle cell morphology ($P = 0.002$; Fisher's exact test). MC and Ki-67 index were significantly correlated ($P < 0.001$; $R = 0.67$; Spearman's rank correlation); median values were 15 (range, 0–153) and 28% (range, 1–78%), respectively. Both were significantly higher in spindle cell melanomas, in tumours lacking junctional activity and in poorly-pigmented tumours. Follow-up information was available for 33 cats (66%). Variables related with a poor clinical outcome included mucosal location, tumour size, spindle, balloon and signet ring cell histotypes, low pigmentation, MC > 5, Ki-67 > 20% and lack of treatment administration. On multivariable analysis, only tumour histotype and treatment retained prognostic significance.

Conclusions: Although the majority of feline NOMs behave aggressively, Ki-67 index, together with other parameters, may contribute to prognostic assessment. Prospective studies on homogeneous populations are warranted to identify reliable threshold values for this marker.

Keywords: Feline, Melanoma, Ki-67 index, Proliferative activity, Mitotic count, Prognosis

Background

Non-ocular melanocytic neoplasms (NOMs) are extremely rare in cats, accounting for 2.7% of all skin tumours and less than 1% of oral tumours [1, 2].

The few studies reporting the clinical evolution of NOMs and investigating factors of potential prognostic interest have so far generated conflicting results [1, 3–6].

The most cited parameters associated with a worse outcome include eyelid or mucosal location, achromic phenotype and epithelioid morphology [1, 3, 4, 6] whereas tumours arising on the ear pinna may exhibit a more favourable prognosis [4].

The relative number of tumour cells positive for the nuclear protein Ki-67 (Ki-67 index, tumour growth fraction) is an acknowledged prognostic factor for canine melanoma [7–9]. In this species, the Ki-67 index has been demonstrated to be significantly different between benign and malignant melanocytic neoplasms, and

---

* Correspondence: silvia.sabattini@unibo.it
[1]Department of Veterinary Medical Sciences, Alma Mater Studiorum University of Bologna, Via Tolara di Sopra, 50, 40064 Ozzano Emilia, (BO), Italy
Full list of author information is available at the end of the article

negatively correlated with survival. Consequently, thresholds holding a prognostic value have been established for both cutaneous and oral canine melanocytic neoplasms, and the assessment of the growth fraction has become part of the routine histology practice for these tumours [7–9].

This is the first study investigating the relevance of the growth fraction in feline melanocytic tumours. The primary goal was to evaluate the relationship between Ki-67 index and tumour characteristics, including anatomic location, size, histologic malignancy, predominant histotype and mitotic count. Secondly, we aimed to evaluate whether the Ki-67 index was related to clinical outcome and survival times in a subset of cats with available follow-up information.

Results

Demographic information and tumour characteristics

Fifty feline melanocytic tumours fulfilled the inclusion criteria. Breeds included 42 Domestic Shorthairs, 3 Persians, 2 Siamese, 1 Maine Coon, 1 Devon Rex and 1 Chartreux. There were 26 castrated males (52%) and 24 spayed females (48%), with a mean age of 11 ± 4 years (range, 2–19). Information regarding hair colour and living environment were available for 33 cats (66%). Most represented coat colours included grey tabby ($n = 10$), red tabby ($n = 8$), black solid or bicolor black-white ($n = 5$), brown tabby ($n = 4$) and calico ($n = 4$). Cats had outdoor access in 18 out of 33 cases (54%).

Thirty-three tumours (66%) were located in the skin; including ear pinna ($n = 7$), eyelids ($n = 4$), face ($n = 4$), trunk ($n = 11$), limbs ($n = 3$) and digits ($n = 4$). Eleven out of 20 (55%) of these cats had no outdoor access. Seventeen tumours (34%) were in a mucosal location or in a mucocutaneous junction (oral mucosa, $n = 10$; lip, $n = 6$; nasal mucosa, $n = 1$). Median tumour diameter before fixation was 1.3 cm (range, 0.3–4). Regional lymph node metastases had been cytologically or histologically identified at diagnosis in 5 cutaneous melanomas (2 digital and one each on eyelid, ear pinna and trunk).

Histology and immunohistochemistry

Forty-three cases (86%; 27 cutaneous and 16 mucosal) were diagnosed as malignant melanomas and 7 (14%; 6 cutaneous and 1 oral) as melanocytomas. According to the prevalent histotype, there were 12 epithelioid, 8 spindle cell, 5 balloon cell, 1 signet ring cell and 17 mixed melanomas (Figs. 1, 2 and 3). Melanocytomas belonged to the composite epithelioid ($n = 3$) or mixed ($n = 4$) subtypes. Twenty-one tumours (42%) were completely amelanotic; all but one of them (95%) were positive to S100, whereas 10 cases (48%) expressed

Melan A, including the S100-negative tumour. The remaining tumours, including all the melanocytomas, had either a degree of pigmentation below ($n = 18$; 36%) or above ($n = 11$; 22%) 50%. Seventy-six percent of the mucosal tumours were achromic versus 24% of the cutaneous tumours ($P < 0.001$; Fisher's exact test). Eighty-seven percent of spindle cell melanomas were amelanotic versus 25% of epithelioid or mixed types ($P = 0.002$; Fisher's exact test).

Junctional activity, lymphocytic infiltrate and necrosis were observed in 34%, 38% and 16% of cases, respectively. Vascular invasion was identified in 7 tumours (14%) with epithelioid or balloon cell differentiation (Table 1).

Median MC and Ki-67 index were 15 (range, 0–153) and 28% (range, 1–78%), respectively. These parameters were correlated ($P < 0.001$; $R = 0.67$; Spearman's rank correlation). MC was significantly higher in tumours diagnosed as malignant, in spindle cell tumours, in those lacking junctional activity and in those with a percentage of pigmented cells below 50%. Ki-67 index was significantly higher in all of the above and in tumours larger than 1.3 cm (Table 1).

Clinical course

Follow-up information was available for 33 cats (66%; with 21 cutaneous and 12 oral tumours). Eighteen (54%) underwent surgery; one received radiation therapy and 2 cats underwent a multimodal approach consisting of radiotherapy plus dose-intense chemotherapy (carboplatin, doxorubicin) and surgery plus metronomic chemotherapy (cyclophosphamide, thalidomide). In the cats receiving surgery, margins were histologically clean in 14 cases (74%) and infiltrated in 5 (26%). The remaining 12 cats (36%) only received palliative care.

At the end of the study, 10 cats (30%) were alive, after a median follow-up time of 140 days (95% CI, 64–401). Four cats (12%) had died for tumour-unrelated causes (chronic renal failure, $n = 2$; diabetes, $n = 1$; intestinal mast cell tumour, $n = 1$) after a median of 656 days (95% CI, 446–1175) and 19 cats (58%) had died of melanoma, with a median OS of 150 days (95% CI, 94–206).

For both MC and Ki-67 index, it was not possible to identify cut-off values to satisfactorily separate tumours with benign and aggressive biologic behaviour. When applying threshold values similar to those reported for canine melanoma (5 for MC and 20% for Ki-67 index), both were significantly associated with survival (Table 2).

Other variables significantly associated with shorter survival times included mucosal location, large tumour size, spindle, balloon or signet ring cell histotypes; less than 50% of pigmented neoplastic cells and lack of treatment (Table 2). Cats with clean surgical margin had a significant better outcome than cats with infiltrated

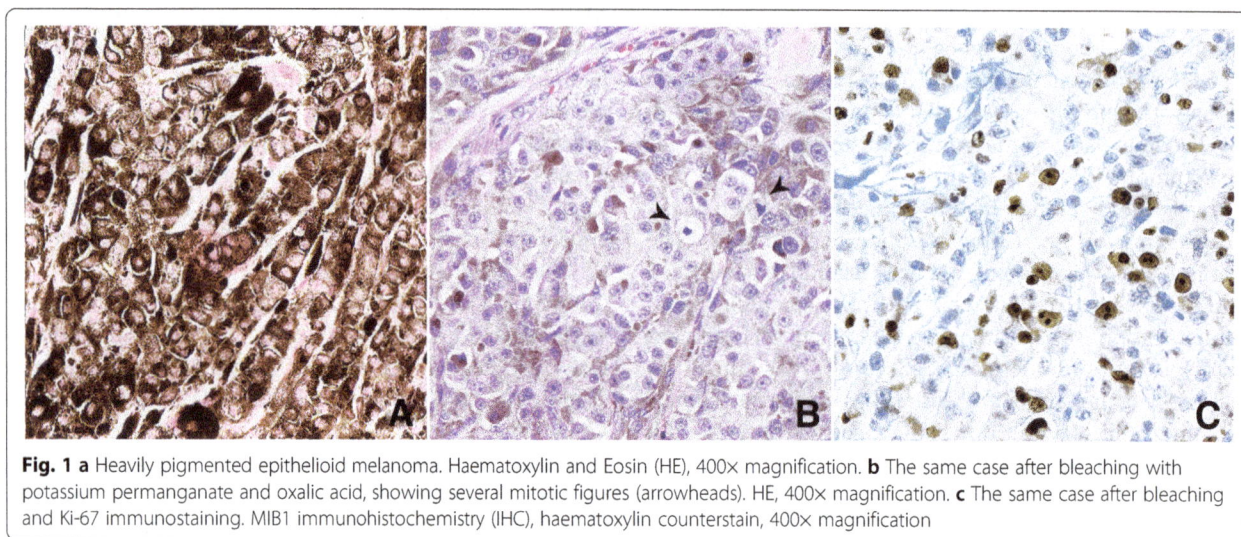

Fig. 1 a Heavily pigmented epithelioid melanoma. Haematoxylin and Eosin (HE), 400× magnification. **b** The same case after bleaching with potassium permanganate and oxalic acid, showing several mitotic figures (arrowheads). HE, 400× magnification. **c** The same case after bleaching and Ki-67 immunostaining. MIB1 immunohistochemistry (IHC), haematoxylin counterstain, 400× magnification

margins ($P < 0.001$; log-rank test) On multivariable survival analysis, only tumour histotype and treatment administration retained prognostic significance (Table 3).

Discussion

The majority of feline NOMs are reported to be malignant, but definitive information about clinical and histologic prognostic factors are lacking, mostly due to the low frequency of these neoplasms.

This is the second largest study on feline NOMs and the first investigating the prognostic relevance of Ki-67 in this species.

Although the observed age range was extremely wide, the majority of subjects were aged, confirming previous reports [1, 5, 10]. According to several authors, melanomas with primary auricular localization would affect younger subjects and be associated with a better outcome [1, 4–6]. This finding was not supported by our

results, since only one of 7 cats with pinnal melanoma was under 10 years of age, and 3 cats out of 4 experienced rapid disease progression.

Apparently, a greater proportion of feline malignant melanomas arises in the skin, as compared with dogs, and the involved region has not a prominent role in the assessment of prognosis [1, 5]. Conversely, mucosal location seems to be associated with a worse prognosis, possibly due to a greater difficulty to obtain adequate local tumour control.

While being an acknowledged promoting factor for human and equine melanoma, ultraviolet (UV) light exposure was only hypothesized to play a role in feline cutaneous melanoma, mainly due to the common occurrence of these tumours on the head and ears [5, 6]. In the present study, the 50% of cats with cutaneous melanoma had no outdoor access, making the causative role of solar exposure less likely. Cats with orange, red, calico

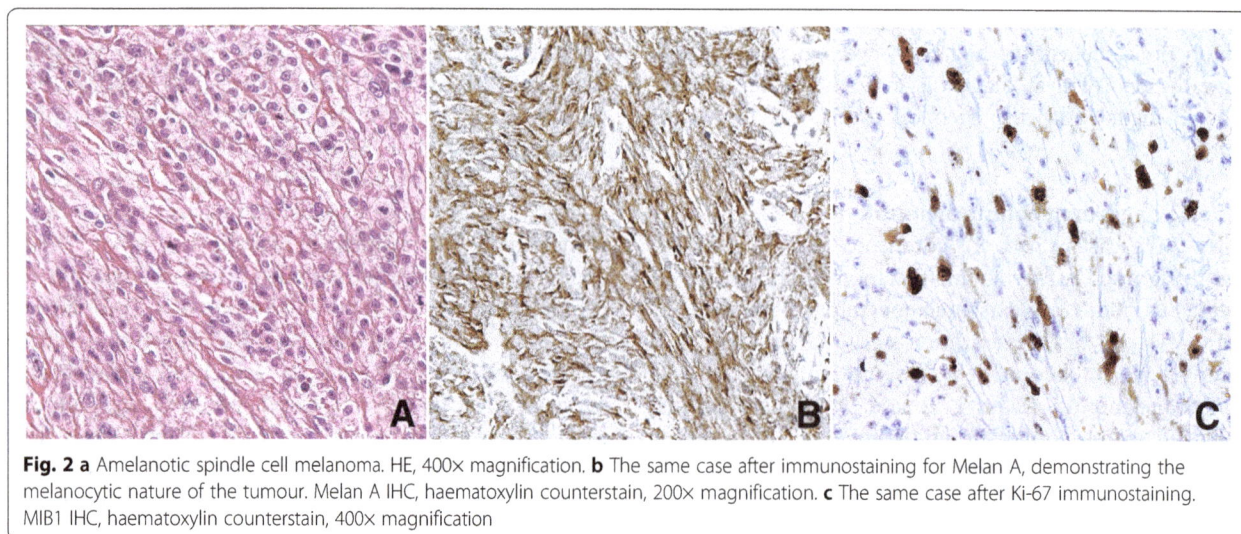

Fig. 2 a Amelanotic spindle cell melanoma. HE, 400× magnification. **b** The same case after immunostaining for Melan A, demonstrating the melanocytic nature of the tumour. Melan A IHC, haematoxylin counterstain, 200× magnification. **c** The same case after Ki-67 immunostaining. MIB1 IHC, haematoxylin counterstain, 400× magnification

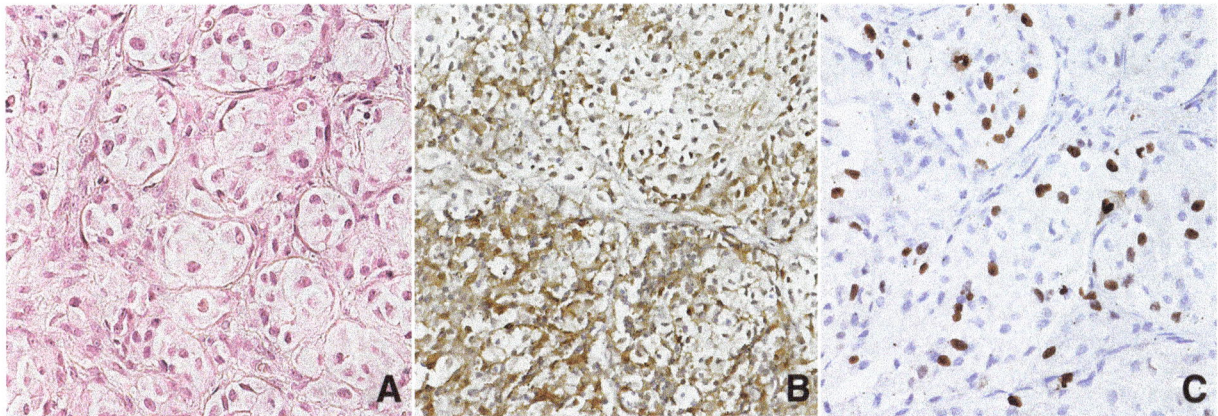

Fig. 3 a Amelanotic balloon cell melanoma. HE, 400× magnification. **b** The same case after immunostaining for S100, demonstrating the melanocytic nature of the tumour. S100 IHC, haematoxylin counterstain, 200× magnification. **c** The same case after Ki-67 immunostaining. MIB1 IHC, haematoxylin counterstain, 400× magnification

or silver coat are associated with a higher incidence of developing intraepidermal melanocytic hyperplasia (lentigo) on their lips, gums, eyelids and/or nose [11]. This is a benign condition that has not been reported to evolve to malignant melanoma, however, notably, 67% of the cats in this study were the above colours. Case-control studies could be helpful to clarify the role of UV radiation and hair color in feline NOMs.

The elective therapy for feline melanoma remains complete surgical excision. In the study by Chamel et al., (2016), cats undergoing surgery survived significantly longer than those receiving no treatment or medical treatment only. In the same study, complete surgical margins were not associated with a survival advantage [6]. In the present study, the median survival time of subjects receiving treatment was 3 times higher than those receiving a palliative treatment, but the presence of clean surgical margins was significantly correlated with a better prognosis.

Another previously reported negative prognostic factor which was confirmed by our results is the lack of melanin. The degree of pigmentation is a well acknowledged prognostic factor also in canine melanoma [9]. Indeed, the absence of melanin pigment could be associated with loss of differentiation and acquisition of a molecular phenotype with increased invasiveness and metastatic potential [2, 6].

Completely amelanotic melanomas are likely under-diagnosed in cats, due to difficulties in their identification. Depending on their morphological features, they can be misdiagnosed as undifferentiated carcinomas, sarcomas or round cell tumours (e.g. lymphoma, progressive histiocytosis, or atypical mast cell tumours). In this study, immunohistochemical positivity to at least one of Melan A and S100 was required for all amelanotic tumours, even in the presence of convincing morphological features. These are the only validated markers to confirm the melanocytic nature of a tumour in cats, however their limited diagnostic utility is acknowledged [6, 12]. As expected, less than 50% of amelanotic melanomas in this study were positive for Melan A, confirming the poor sensitivity of this marker. In contrast, almost all the amelanotic melanomas stained positively for S100, a highly sensitive but poorly specific marker.

In the literature, epithelioid, spindle cell, mixed, signet ring and balloon cell type of melanomas have been described in cats [10]. The relevance of tumour histotype in predicting the clinical behaviour of feline NOMs has been disputed, with some authors reporting a worse prognosis associated with epithelioid melanomas [4]. In the present study, spindle, signet ring and balloon cell histotypes were significantly associated with a poorer prognosis in comparison with epithelioid and mixed melanomas. Moreover, epithelioid tumours were characterized by lower proliferative activity and a higher degree of pigmentation.

Although Ki-67 index has been previously evaluated in 4 cats with ocular and extra-ocular melanomas [13], the prognostic relevance of proliferative activity has never been reliably assessed in this species. In the present study, Ki-67 index was significantly correlated with other prognostic variables, including tumour size, spindle cell histotype, lack of pigmentation and MC, and values greater than 20% were ultimately correlated with a worse outcome. However, the same statistical correlations were also observed for MC, suggesting that the immunohistochemical assessment of Ki-67 index in feline NOMs may not add much more to the plain assessment of MC on HE-stained sections.

Table 1 Relationship between proliferation indices (mitotic count and Ki-67 index) and clinicopathologic variables in 50 cases of feline non-ocular melanocytic tumors

Variables	Number of cases	Median mitotic count (range)	P	Median Ki-67 index (range)	P
Tumor location			0.396		0.984
skin	33	15 (0–153)		29% (1–78%)	
mucosae	17	15 (2–48)		22% (10–68%)	
Largest diameter[a]			0.052		0.014*
≤ 1.3 cm	28	10 (0–40)		18% (1–78%)	
> 1.3 cm	22	17 (3–153)		31% (14–77%)	
Morphological diagnosis			< 0.001*		< 0.001*
melanocytoma	7	2 (0–4)		6% (1–18%)	
melanoma	43	17 (1–153)		30% (6–78%)	
Prevalent histotype			0.002*		0.005*
spindle cell	8	28 (16–153)		38% (20–54%)	
others	42	12 (0–40)		25% (1–78%)	
Junctional activity			0.005*		0.026*
present	17	11 (0–27)		22% (1–61%)	
absent	33	21 (0–153)		32% (2–78%)	
Pigmentation			< 0.001*		< 0.001*
≥ 50%	11	3 (0–27)		8% (1–29%)	
< 50% or absent	39	17 (1–153)		31% (9–78%)	
Vascular invasion			0.353		0.565
present	7	19 (4–36)		32% (10–47%)	
absent	43	13 (0–153)		27% (1–78%)	
Lymphocytic infiltrate			0.299		0.14
present	19	17 (2–40)		31% (11–78%)	
absent	31	12 (0–153)		25% (1–68%)	
Necrosis			0.166		0.29
present	8	22 (4–153)		33% (10–71%)	
absent	42	13 (0–48)		27% (1–78%)	

*Significant
[a]Median value as cut-off

Nevertheless, with both markers, we failed to identify a threshold value to satisfactorily identify tumours with a worse clinical outcome and, after adjustment with other clinicopathological variables in a multivariable model, prognostic significance was not retained. It must be reminded that the retrospective setting of this study resulted in not standardized staging procedures, treatment plans and follow-up schedules, making comparisons difficult. Almost all cats were treated in first opinion practices by a wide range of practitioners with different levels of experience, reflecting the clinical management of the majority of cats with this disease. Prospective studies are encouraged to assess the prognostic utility of the Ki-67 index on more cases with complete clinical staging, receiving gold standard treatments and with long term follow-up information.

Conclusions

This study confirms a poor prognosis of the majority feline NOMs, although a certain degree of variability can be observed, with a better outcome observed for small, pigmented skin tumours removed with complete surgical margins. Contrarily to previous studies, the epithelioid morphology appears to be associated with a less malignant biologic behaviour. MC and Ki-67 index may contribute, with the aforementioned variables, to the prognostic assessment of feline NOMs. Reliable threshold values for both markers need to be identified in prospective, standardized studies.

Methods
Inclusion criteria

Lesions histologically diagnosed as feline non-ocular melanoma/melanocytoma or with melanoma among

Table 2 Relationship between overall survival (OS) and clinicopathological variables in 33 cases of feline non-ocular melanocytic tumors with available follow-up information

Variables	Number of cases	Median OS (95% CI)[c]	P
Tumor location			0.036*
Skin	21	197 (133–261)	
Mucosae	12	72 (48–96)	
Largest diameter[a]			0.006*
≤ 1.3 cm	14	689 (79–1299)	
> 1.3 cm	19	75 (11–139)	
Morphological diagnosis			0.109
Melanocytoma	3	Not reached	
Melanoma	30	156 (91–221)	
Prevalent histotype			0.014*
Spindle, balloon and signet ring cell	10	48 (0–115)	
Epithelioid	9	689 (0–1444)	
Mixed	14	156 (125–187)	
Junctional activity			0.412
Present	10	136 (101–171)	
Absent	23	197 (120–273)	
Pigmentation			0.015*
≥ 50%	8	Not reached	
< 50% or absent	25	119 (29–208)	
Vascular invasion			0.809
Present	6	176 (0–405)	
Absent	27	156 (77–235)	
Lymphocytic infiltrate			0.838
present	12	176 (39–313)	
absent	21	156 (92–219)	
Necrosis			0.681
present	7	197 (48–346)	
absent	26	156 (116–196)	
Mitotic count[b]			0.013*
≤ 5	9	689 (0–1451)	
> 5	24	119 (32–206)	
Ki-67 index[b]			0.036*
≤ 20%	10	689 (0–1460)	
> 20%	23	119 (34–204)	
Treatment			< 0.001*
Yes	21	689 (12–1366)	
No	12	59 (20–98)	

CI confidence interval
*Significant
[a]Median value
[b]Cutoff value based on data analysis and canine melanoma literature
[c]Days

Table 3 Multivariable analysis of variables potentially related to overall survival (OS) in 33 cases of feline non-ocular melanocytic tumors with available follow-up information

Variables	Hazard ratio	95% CI	P
Mucosal location	2.26	0.71–7.19	0.165
Largest diameter > 1.3 cm[a]	3.46	0.7–17.06	0.128
Spindle-, balloon cell and signet ring histotypes	3.48	1.04–11.57	0.042*
Pigmentation < 50%	1.69	0.09–32.56	0.730
Mitotic count >5[b]	6.77	0.36–128.02	0.202
Ki-67 index > 20%[b]	0.14	0.01–2.05	0.152
Lack of treatment	4.22	1.18–15.05	0.027*

CI confidence interval
*Significant
[a]Median value
[b]cutoff value based on data analysis and canine melanoma literature

differential diagnoses were retrospectively retrieved from the archives of the pathology service of the Departments of Veterinary Medical Sciences (University of Bologna, Italy) and of Veterinary Sciences (University of Pisa, Italy), and from a private veterinary diagnostic laboratory (La Vallonea, Rho, Italy). Only primary tumours were considered for inclusion: local recurrences and nodal/distant metastases were removed from the selection.

Histologic sections from each case were reviewed for diagnosis confirmation. Amelanotic tumours were included only upon immunohistochemical positivity to at least one melanocytic marker with validated diagnostic utility in cats, including melan-A (1:400; A103 clone, Dako, Glostrup, Denmark) and S100 (Catalogue number: Z0311;1:2400; rabbit polyclonal, Dako) [12]. The immunohistochemical analysis was performed as part of the study at the Department of Veterinary Medical Sciences, University of Bologna.

Histology

All samples for histologic examination were fixed in 10% neutered-buffered formalin, processed by routine methods, embedded in paraffin wax, sectioned at 4 µm and stained with haematoxylin and eosin (HE). The evaluated histologic features included morphological diagnosis (melanocytoma or malignant melanoma, according to the WHO guidelines) [14], prevalent histotype (epithelioid, spindle cell, balloon cell, signet ring cell or mixed), junctional activity, degree of pigmentation (more than 50% of pigmented cells, less than 50% or absent), vascular invasion, lymphocytic infiltrate, necrosis and mitotic count (MC). MC was assessed as the number of mitotic figures in a 2.37 mm^2 area (10 fields with a 40× objective and a 10× ocular with a field number of 22 mm), according to the standards proposed by Meuten et al., 2016 [15]. The count was performed in

10 consecutive non-overlapping high-power fields (HPFs), starting from an area of high mitotic activity. Fields with necrosis or inflammation were skipped. All histologic evaluations were performed by consensus by two of the authors (SS and AR).

Bleaching of melanin

The bleaching of melanin was performed on all the tumours with approximately more than 25% of pigmented cells before assessing MC and performing Ki-67 immunohistochemistry (IHC).

Briefly, 4 μm tissue sections were exposed to treatment with 2.5 g/L potassium permanganate (Merck, Darmstadt, Germany) for 5 min, followed by 50 g/L oxalic acid (Merck) for 5 min at room temperature.

To evaluate the effects of bleaching on tissue immunoreactivity, Ki-67 labelling was carried out on serial sections of an amelanotic melanoma, with and without bleaching. No differences in labelling intensity or distribution were observed, and it was therefore concluded that the bleaching method did not interfere with the assessment of tumour growth fraction.

Ki-67 immunohistochemistry

Tumour sections were immunolabelled for Ki-67 by using a commercial anti-human primary antibody (MIB-1 clone, Dako) with validated reactivity in feline tissues [16].

Endogenous peroxidase activity was blocked by incubation for 30 mins with 0.3% hydrogen peroxide in methanol. For antigen retrieval, slides were microwaved in citrate buffer (pH 6.0) for 4 cycles of 5 mins, at 750 W. Sections were incubated overnight at 4 °C in a humid chamber with the primary antibody diluted 1:600 in a blocking solution (10% goat serum in phosphate-buffered saline). Binding sites of primary antibody were identified using a biotinylated goat anti-mouse secondary antibody (1:200 in blocking solution, Dako) with an incubation step of 30 min at room temperature. Sections were then incubated with a commercial streptavidin-biotin-peroxidase kit (Vectastain Elite ABC Kit, Vector Laboratories, Burlingame, CA, USA) and 3,3'-diaminobenzidine (DAB tablets, Diagnostic BioSystems, Pleasanton, CA, USA) was used as chromogen. Counterstain was performed with Papanicolaou's haematoxylin.

Feline intestinal mucosa was used as positive control for MIB-1. Negative controls were obtained by omitting the primary antibody.

The evaluation of Ki-67 immunolabelling was performed by two authors (SS, MF), without knowledge of the case outcome. Five high-power (400×) fields selected within the areas of highest Ki-67 positivity were photographed. Areas with severe inflammation or necrosis were avoided. In every image, the number of neoplastic cell nuclei with positive labelling and the total number of neoplastic cells were assessed manually with a digital cell counter (ImageJ, National Institutes of Health, Bethesda, MD, USA). Ki-67 index was calculated as the mean percentage of labelled neoplastic cells in the 5 photographed fields.

Clinical information

Patient records were reviewed to collect signalment, tumour location and tumour size (largest diameter).

Referring veterinarians and/or owners were contacted for additional information, including hair colour, living environment (indoor/outdoor), clinical presentation, presence of metastases, treatment, survival and patient status.

The availability of these data was not among inclusion criteria.

Statistical analysis

Data were analysed by use of a commercial software program (SPSS Statistics v19, IBM, Armonk, NY, USA); P values ≤ 0.05 were considered significant.

When appropriate, data sets were tested for normality by use of the D'Agostino and Pearson omnibus normality test. Values were expressed as mean ± standard deviation in case of normal distribution, or as median with a range in case of non-normal distribution.

The relationships between the following variables were investigated: tumour location, tumour size, morphological diagnosis, prevalent histotype, junctional activity, degree of pigmentation, vascular invasion, lymphocytic infiltrate, necrosis, MC and Ki-67 index. The distributions of qualitative and quantitative variables were assessed by Fisher's exact test and Student's T/Mann-Whitney U test, respectively. The correlation between MC and Ki-67 index was evaluated by means of the Spearman's rank correlation coefficient.

Overall survival (OS) was defined as the time (days) from the date of diagnosis to the last reported date on which the patient was seen alive. The patient status was recorded as alive, dead because of melanoma-unrelated causes or dead because of melanoma-related causes. Survival estimates are presented as medians with the corresponding 95% confidence intervals (95% CI).

The log-rank test was applied to compare survival distributions. Single variables analysed for prognostic relevance included tumour location, tumour size, morphological diagnosis, prevalent histotype, junctional activity, degree of pigmentation, vascular invasion, lymphocytic infiltrate, necrosis, MC, Ki-67 index and received treatment. Significant variables were further tested in a multivariable Cox proportional hazard model.

Abbreviations
CI: Confidence interval; HE: Haematoxylin and eosin; HPF: High-power field; IHC: Immunohistochemistry; MC: Mitotic count; NOM: Non-ocular melanomas; OS: Overall survival; UV: Ultraviolet

Acknowledgements
The authors wish to thank Drs Patrizia Pircher, Roberta Gamba, Roberta Schiavone, Patrizia Giancristofaro and the other veterinary practitioners who provided clinical histories and follow-up information for the cases in this study.

Funding
The authors received no specific financial support for this research.

Authors' contributions
SS carried out histological evaluations, data analysis and drafted the manuscript; AR1, MF, AR2, FA1, GT, TBP and FA2 contributed to the histological/immunohistochemical evaluations and helped writing the manuscript; GB conceived and supervised the study; RT and JB gave a significant contribution to the collection of cases, medical data and follow-up information and revised the manuscript providing critical feedback. MM performed laboratory analyses and assisted SS in final data analysis. All authors read and approved the final manuscript.

Consent for publication
Not applicable.

Competing interests
The authors declare that they have no competing interests.

Author details
[1]Department of Veterinary Medical Sciences, Alma Mater Studiorum University of Bologna, Via Tolara di Sopra, 50, 40064 Ozzano Emilia, (BO), Italy. [2]"La Vallonea" laboratory, Via Giuseppe Sirtori, 9, 20017 Rho, MI), Italy. [3]Department of Veterinary Sciences, University of Pisa, Viale delle Piagge, 1, 56124 Pisa, Italy. [4]"Città di Bolzano" veterinary clinic, Via Resia, 20, 39100 Bolzano, Italy. [5]Radiation Oncology Consultant, Unterrenggstrasse 36, CH-8135 Langnau am Albis, Switzerland.

References
1. Miller WH, Scott DW, Anderson WI. Feline cutaneous melanocytic neoplasms: a retrospective analysis of 43 cases (1979–1991). Vet Dermatol. 1993;4:19–26.
2. Stebbins KE, Morse CG, Goldschmidt MH. Feline oral neoplasia: a ten-year survey. Vet Pathol. 1989;26:121–8.
3. Patnaik AK, Mooney S. Feline melanoma: a comparative study of ocular, oral and dermal neoplasms. Vet Pathol. 1988;25:105–12.
4. Goldschmidt MH, Liu SMS, Shofer FS. Feline dermal melanoma: a retrospective study. In: Ihrke PJ, editor. Advances in veterinary dermatology. Oxford: Pergamon Press; 1993. p. 285–91.
5. Luna LD, Higginbotham ML, Henry CJ, Turnquist SE, Moore AS, Graham JC. Feline non-ocular melanoma: a retrospective study of 23 cases (1991-1999). J Feline Med Surg. 2000;1:173–81.
6. Chamel G, Abadie J, Albaric O, Labrut S, Ponce F, Ibisch C. Non-ocular melanomas in cats: a retrospective study of 30 cases. J Feline Med Surg. 2016;19:351–7.
7. Laprie C, Abadie J, Amardeilh MF, Net JL, Lagadic M, Delverdier M. MIB-1 immunoreactivity correlates with biologic behaviour in canine cutaneous melanoma. Vet Dermatol. 2001;12:139–47.
8. Bergin IL, Smedley RC, Esplin DG, Spangler WL, Kiupel M. Prognostic evaluation of Ki67 threshold value in canine oral melanoma. Vet Pathol. 2011;48:41–53.
9. Smedley RC, Spangler WL, Esplin DG, Kitchell BE, Bergman PJ, Ho H-Y, Bergin IL, Kiupel M. Prognostic markers for canine melanocytic neoplasms: a comparative review of the literature and goals for future investigations. Vet Pathol. 2011;48:54–72.
10. van der Linde-Sipman JS, de Wit MML, van Garderen E, Molenbeek RF, van der Velde-Zimmermann D, de Weger RA. Cutaneous malignant melanomas in 57 cats: identification of (amelanotic) signet-ring and balloon cell types and verification of their origin by immunohistochemistry, electron microscopy, and in situ hybridization. Vet Pathol. 1997;34:31–8.
11. Scott DW. Lentigo simplex in orange cats. Compan Anim Pract. 1987;1:23–5.
12. Ramos-Vara JA, Miller MA, Johnson GC. Melan-a and S100 protein immunohistochemistry in feline melanomas: 48 cases. Vet Pathol. 2002;39:127–32.
13. Roels S, Tilmant K, Ducatelle R. PCNA and Ki67 proliferation markers as criteria for prediction of clinical behavior of melanocytic tumours in cats and dogs. J Comp Pathol. 1999;121:13–24.
14. Goldschmidt MH, Dunstan RW, Stannard AA, von Tscharner C, Walder EJ, Yager JA. Melanoma. In: Schulman YF, editor. Histological classification of epithelial and melanocytic tumors of the skin of domestic animals. Washington: World Health Organization Collaborating Center, Armed Force Institute of Pathology; 1998. p. 38–40.
15. Meuten DJ, Moore FM, George JW. Mitotic count and the field of view area: time to standardize. Vet Pathol. 2016;53:7–9.
16. Sabattini S, Giantin M, Barbanera A, Zorro Shahidian L, Decasto M, Zancanella V, Prata D, Trivigno E, Bettini G. Feline intestinal mast cell tumours: clinicopathological characterisation and KIT mutation analysis. J Feline Med Surg. 2016;18:280–9.

21

An evaluation of TAZ and YAP crosstalk with TGFβ signalling in canine osteosarcoma suggests involvement of hippo signalling in disease progression

Anita K. Luu[1], Courtney R. Schott[2], Robert Jones[1], Andrew C. Poon[1], Brandon Golding[1], Roa'a Hamed[1], Benjamin Deheshi[3], Anthony Mutsaers[1], Geoffrey A. Wood[2*] and Alicia M. Viloria-Petit[1*]

Abstract

Background: Osteosarcoma (OSA) is the most common bone cancer in canines. Both transforming growth factor beta (TGFβ) and Hippo pathway mediators have important roles in bone development, stemness, and cancer progression. The role of Hippo signalling effectors TAZ and YAP has never been addressed in canine OSA. Further, the cooperative role of TGFβ and Hippo signalling has yet to be explored in osteosarcoma. To address these gaps, this study investigated the prognostic value of TAZ and YAP alone and in combination with pSmad2 (a marker of active TGFβ signalling), as well as the involvement of a TGFβ-Hippo signalling crosstalk in tumourigenic properties of OSA cells in vitro. An in-house trial tissue microarray (TMA) which contained 16 canine appendicular OSA cases undergoing standard care and accompanying follow-up was used to explore the prognostic role of TAZ, YAP and pSmad2. Published datasets were used to test associations between *TAZ* and *YAP* mRNA levels, metastasis, and disease recurrence. Small interfering RNAs specific to TAZ and YAP were utilized in vitro alone or in combination with TGFβ treatment to determine their role in OSA viability, proliferation and migration.

Results: Patients with low levels of both YAP and pSmad2 when evaluated in combination had a significantly longer time to metastasis (log-rank test, $p = 0.0058$) and a longer overall survival (log rank test, $p = 0.0002$). No similar associations were found for TAZ and YAP mRNA levels. In vitro, TAZ knockdown significantly decreased cell viability, proliferation, and migration in metastatic cell lines, while YAP knockdown significantly decreased viability in three cell lines, and migration in two cell lines, derived from either primary tumours or their metastases. The impact of TGFβ signaling activation on these effects was cell line-dependent.

Conclusions: YAP and pSmad2 have potential prognostic value in canine appendicular osteosarcoma. Inhibiting YAP and TAZ function could lead to a decrease in viability, proliferation, and migratory capacity of canine OSA cells. Assessment of YAP and pSmad2 in larger patient cohorts in future studies are needed to further elucidate the role of TGFβ-Hippo signalling crosstalk in canine OSA progression.

Keywords: Canine osteosarcoma, Hippo signalling, TGFβ, YAP1, TAZ, WWTR1, Prognostic marker, Metastasis

* Correspondence: gewood@uoguelph.ca; aviloria@uoguelph.ca
[2]Department of Pathobiology, Ontario Veterinary College, University of Guelph, 50 Stone Road East, Guelph, ON N1G 2W1, Canada
[1]Department of Biomedical Sciences, Ontario Veterinary College, University of Guelph, 50 Stone Road East, Guelph, ON N1G 2W1, Canada
Full list of author information is available at the end of the article

Background

Osteosarcoma (OSA) is the most commonly diagnosed primary cancer of the bone in both humans and dogs, but it is about fourteen times more common in dogs, with an estimated incidence of 13.9/100,000 [1]. Most canine OSAs develop in large and giant dog breeds, are appendicular in location, and tend to develop pulmonary metastasis [1]. The standard of care (SOC) for canine osteosarcoma (OSA) currently consists of limb amputation or limb-sparing surgery and chemotherapy. With this treatment, the median survival time is 8–12 months and metastasis to the lungs is primarily responsible for patient's mortality [2, 3]. As such, there has been an increased focus on discovering novel prognostic markers and molecular targets to improve patient outcome.

Transforming growth factor beta (TGFβ) exists in three different isoforms (TGFβ 1, 2 and 3). All of these, in addition to other members of the TGFβ superfamily of secreted proteins (in particular bone morphogenetic proteins/BMPs), have been implicated in bone formation, remodeling and bone metastasis [4, 5]. The three TGFβ isoforms classically signal via the Smad pathway, involving Smad2/3 and Smad4. This is initiated by TGFβ binding to a TGFβ receptor type II (TβRII) homodimer, which facilitates the formation of a complex with a TGFβ receptor type I (TβRI) homodimer. In this tetrameric complex, TβRII (a constitutively active kinase) phosphorylates and activates TβRI, leading to the recruitment of the receptor-activated Smads (R-Smads), Smad2 and Smad3. Smad 2/3 recruitment to the TβR complex leads to their c-terminal phosphorylation and subsequent activation by TβRI, which enables them to form a complex with the co-Smad, Smad4. The R-Smads and co-Smad complex then translocates to the nucleus to modulate gene expression through cooperation with other transcription factors, co-activators, and co-repressors (reviewed in [6]).

In respect to OSA, several studies support an important role of TGFβ in the invasive/aggressive behavior of both human and canine OSA. Human OSA patients with high levels of TGFβ3 in tumour tissue have a shorter disease-free survival, whereas human patients with high grade OSA had significantly greater tumour expression of TGFβ1 when compared to low-grade OSA patients [7, 8]. In addition, TGFβ signalling promotes growth, migration, and invasiveness in both human and canine OSA cell lines [9–11], and TGFβ1 induces de-differentiation of OSA cells into self-renewing cancer stem cells [12]. Given the demonstrated roles of cancer stem cells in resistance to various therapy modalities, such as conventional chemotherapy, radiotherapy, and molecular targeted therapy, these latter findings suggest that high TGFβ signalling in OSA, apart from promoting metastasis, could additionally contribute to patient mortality by driving therapy resistance [13].

The transcriptional modulator, referred to as WW domain-containing transcription regulator 1 (WWTR1), also known as transcriptional co-activator with a PDZ binding motif (TAZ, the acronym we will use from now on), has been shown to be important for regulating Smad (the downstream mediator of TGFβ signalling) transcriptional activity [14]. Both TAZ and its paralogue YAP1 (Yes-associated protein 1) act as co-activators for a number of transcription factors, and were first known for their role in the Hippo pathway [15]. However, later studies indicated that they also facilitate nuclear sequestration of Smads and subsequent transcriptional activity [14, 15]. This crosstalk between TGFβ and Hippo signalling might be particularly important in osteosarcoma biology. TAZ mediates mesenchymal stem cell differentiation into osteoblasts via its association with Runx2 [16, 17], as well as osteogenic differentiation of bone marrow stromal cells downstream of TGFβ [18]. Further, TAZ is required to maintain self-renewal of embryonic stem cells [14, 19], and was shown to confer invasive properties, self-renewal capacity and chemoresistance to cancer cells [20, 21]. Recent findings indicate that TAZ mediates TGFβ-induced carcinoma progression, through the promotion of metastasis and the cancer stem cell phenotype [22].

The role of Hippo signalling in sarcomas is also well documented. TAZ and YAP were both found to be commonly activated in human sarcomas, with 2/3 of sarcomas harboring nuclear TAZ and 1/2 harboring nuclear YAP [23]. In this study, high levels of TAZ mRNA were found to be associated with reduced overall survival in dedifferentiated liposarcoma [23]. With regard to OSA, high TAZ/YAP expression in tumour tissue samples was found to correlate with poor overall survival in human OSA [24], and an in vitro study showed that YAP promotes chemoresistance in human OSA cell lines [25]. Treatment of human OSA cells with chemotherapeutics doxorubicin and methotrexate was shown to cause degradation of MST1/2 and decreases in LATS1/2 protein levels, the upstream regulators of TAZ/YAP. This subsequently caused an increase in nuclear YAP levels, promoting cell proliferation and chemoresistance [25]. The nuclear localization of Hippo mediators is important for their ability to interact with TEAD (TEA domain DNA-binding family of transcription factors) and activate downstream gene targets to promote proliferation, survival and invasiveness [25].

In veterinary oncology and to the best of our knowledge, TAZ has only been explored in canine mammary tumours, where it was observed that high grade (grade III) tumours had high nuclear expression of TAZ [26]. In vitro, canine mammary tumours strongly express TAZ and disruption of TAZ/YAP-TEAD with verteporfin treatment induces cell apoptosis and reduces migratory and invasive properties [27].

Thus, based on the aforementioned evidence, we hypothesized that levels of nuclear phosphorylated Smad2 (pSmad2, indicative of activated TGFβ signalling), TAZ, YAP or combinations of these markers, will associate with established markers of poor prognosis, metastatic disease and overall patient survival in canine OSA. Furthermore, TAZ and YAP depletion will decrease cell migration and proliferation in canine OSA cell lines. To address these hypotheses, this study employed a pilot tissue microarray (TMA) containing 41 OSA tumour samples, 16 of which were derived from patients with appendicular OSA that were treated with the SOC and had accompanying follow-up. We also investigated the TGFβ-TAZ/YAP relationship in vitro, using siRNA specific to TAZ and YAP in combination with TGFβ treatment to determine its role in promoting tumourigenic properties. Results show that low levels of YAP and pSmad2 combined associate with longer time to metastasis and longer overall survival, while both TAZ and YAP depletion, and TGFβ signalling activation, impacted cell viability, proliferation and migration of OSA cell lines in a cell line-dependent manner.

Results
Clinical data
A total of sixteen appendicular canine OSA patients that underwent SOC were considered in patient analyses. Specifically, the SOC consisted of limb amputation or limb-sparing surgery and 1 to 6 cycles of carboplatin (depending on the patients), which was administered every 3 weeks at a dose of 300 mg/m^2 IV, starting 10–14 days post surgery. The patient data set had a larger representation of male (75%) as compared to female (25%) patients. The average age and weight of patients plus standard deviation, were 8.01 ± 1.73 years and 37.1 ± 10.3 kg, respectively at the time of diagnosis. Alkaline phosphatase (ALP) status and classification of "high", "low" or "normal" was determined by serum biochemistry test at the time of diagnosis; 25% of patients had high ALP. Of all 16 patients with follow-up, 62.5% were classified as high for pSmad2 levels, while 37.5% were classified as low for pSmad2 levels. This distribution was similarly observed for patients when considering YAP levels: 64% and 36% of patients were classified as having high and low YAP levels, respectively. In terms of TAZ levels, 56.3% of patients were classified as having high TAZ levels and 44.7% were classified as having low TAZ levels. All patient data and their corresponding classification for ALP, pSmad2, TAZ, and YAP expression are indicated in Table 1. Histologic grade classification by the two existing systems for canine OSA is also included.

pSmad2, TAZ and YAP Immunolabelling
To determine antibody specificity, immunoblotting was performed on canine OSA cell lines. The immunoblot for YAP demonstrates a prominent band at the expected position of

Table 1 Clinical and histopathological characteristics of appendicular OSA cases included in metastasis and survival analyses

Case	BREED	SEX	Age Dx (Y)	Weight Dx (kg)	Location	ALP Status	Survival Days	Metastasis	pSmad2 Levels	TAZ Levels	YAP Levels	Grade Kirp	Grade Louko
1	Standard Poodle	CM	10.55	23.6	right proximal tibia	N	91	84	High	High	N/A	3	3
2	Doberman	SF	5.99	32.4	right distal femur	H	116	93	High	High	Low	2	3
3	Rottweiler	M	6.30	53.0	left proximal humerus	H	130	N/A	High	Low	Low	2	1
4	Australian Shepherd	CM	8.32	24.6	right proximal humerus	N	148	78	High	High	High	2	2
5	Rottweiler	CM	8.26	50.0	right distal radius	H	165	131	High	Low	High	2	2
6	Greyhound	SF	8.87	26.0	right distal femur	N	215	N/A	High	Low	High	3	2
7	Mixed breed	CM	8.30	37.4	left distal radius	N	218	167	Low	High	High	2	1
8	Rottweiler	CM	4.66	53.4	left proximal humerus	N	282	182	Low	High	High	2	3
9	Golden Retriever	CM	10.99	32.2	left proximal tibia	N	294[a]	247	Low	Low	High	2	1
10	Mixed breed	CM	10.02	42.0	left distal tibia	N	301	N/A	High	High	High	2	1
11	Mixed breed	CM	7.25	51.0	left distal tibia	N	381	N/A	High	High	High	2	2
12	Doberman	SF	5.91	41.0	right distal radius	N	485[a]	485[a]	High	Low	High	3	3
13	Mixed breed	CM	8.03	28.4	left proximal femur	N	605	604	Low	Low	Low	2	1
14	Greyhound	CM	9.02	29.4	right distal femur	N	1005	1005[a]	High	High	N/A	2	1
15	Mixed breed	CM	8.25	37.2	left proximal femur	N	1386	1386[a]	Low	High	Low	2	1
16	Greyhound	SF	7.43	32.4	left distal tibia	H	1091[a]	1091[a]	Low	Low	Low	2	1

MC male castrated, *FS* female spayed, *ALP* alkaline phosphatase status, *H* high, *N* normal, *L* low; Kirp, Grade assigned using criteria as explained in Kirpensteijn et al. [28]; Louko, Grade assigned using criteria as explained in Loukopoulos et al. [29];
N/A Data not available
[a]Data was censored for Kaplan-Meier analysis

65 kDa, with possible reactivity with TAZ. Similarly for TAZ, the immunoblot shows a prominent band at the expected position (55 kDa), with some possible reactivity with YAP and other possible lower and higher molecular weight forms of TAZ (Additional file 1: Figure S1); pSmad2 showed only one band at the expected molecular weight (60 KDa), which was significantly enhanced by TGFβ1 treatment, as expected (data not shown). In tumour tissue, pSmad2 immunolabelling was predominantly nuclear, while TAZ and YAP were found to be both cytoplasmic and nuclear. As expected, the intensity and level of staining for the markers of interest were variable amongst tumour cores from different cases. Representative images for high and low for pSmad2, TAZ and YAP expression, and their respective negative control (no primary antibody) are shown in Fig. 1b.

No associations between pSmad2, TAZ, or YAP levels, and patient characteristics, histologic grade or alkaline phosphatase status

Using a chi square test, no significant associations were found between pSmad2, TAZ, and YAP levels and breed, or sex (Table 2). When considering histologic grade or ALP status at the time of diagnosis, no significant associations were found between pSmad2 levels, TAZ or YAP, and either the Kirpensteijn et al. [28] or the Loukopoulos et al [29] grading system, or the ALP status (Table 3).

Correlations of pSmad2, TAZ and YAP levels and metastasis and overall survival

No significant differences were found in the time to metastasis and overall survival for patients that expressed high levels of pSmad2, TAZ or YAP compared to those that expressed low levels of these markers when they were evaluated alone (Fig. 2a). Interestingly, when pSmad2 and YAP were evaluated in combination and reclassified into four groups (Fig. 2b), there was a significant difference observed amongst the groups in the time to metastasis (log-rank/Mantel-Cox test, $p = 0.0058$) and overall survival (log rank/Mantel-Cox test, $p = 0.0002$). These trends were not observed when pSmad2 and TAZ were evaluated in combination for time to metastasis nor overall survival. The results obtained suggest that

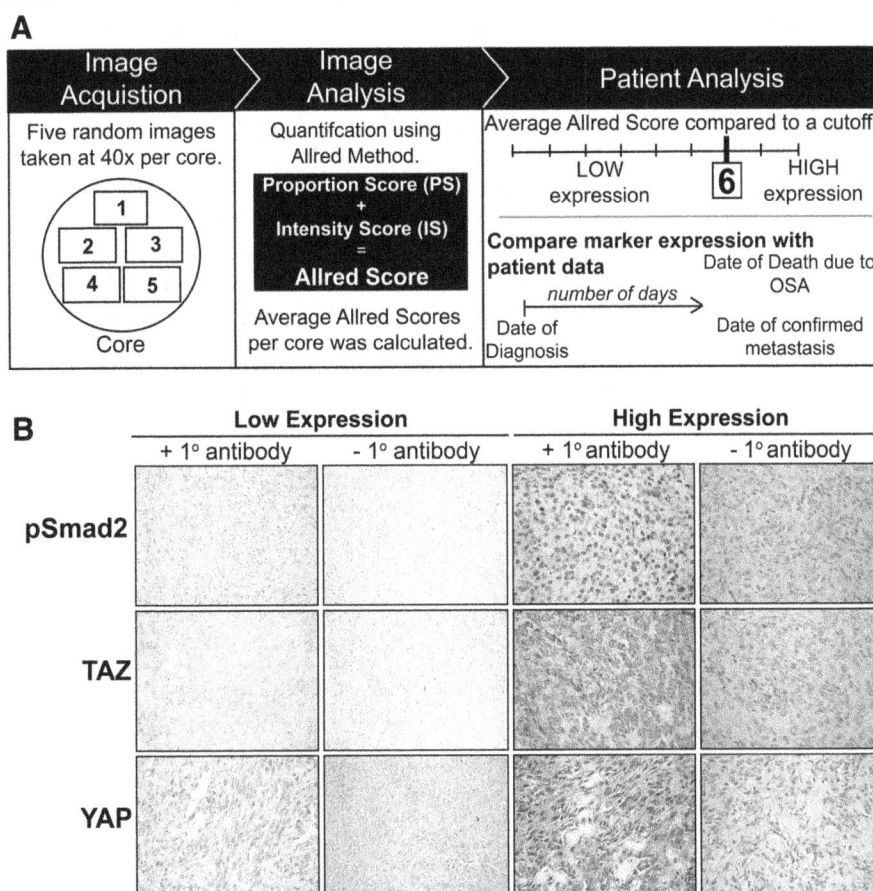

Fig. 1 Workflow of TMA quantification and pSmad2, TAZ and YAP in canine OSA immunolabelling. Workflow for TMA image acquisition, analysis and patient analysis described in (a). Representative images of low and high pSmad2, TAZ and YAP immunolabeling (+ 1° antibody) and respective negative controls (- 1° antibody) in canine OSA tumour tissue at 40X (b)

Table 2 Associations between pSmad2, TAZ and YAP levels and patient sex and breed

Patient Characteristic	pSmad2 High	Low	p value	TAZ High	Low	p value	YAP High	Low	p value
				Sex					
Castrated Male	6	5	0.5589	8	3	0.1296	7	2	0.2382
Male (Intact)	1	0		0	1		0	1	
Spayed Female	3	1		1	3		2	2	
Breed			0.2101			0.1967			0.8030
Non-Mixed	8	3		5	6		6	3	
Mixed	2	3		4	1		3	2	

canine patients with low levels of both pSmad2 and YAP have a later time to metastasis and a longer overall survival.

No association between *TAZ/WWTR1* or *YAP* mRNA levels and metastasis development, recurrence, and overall survival in human and canine OSA

To investigate whether the associations suggested by our analysis of TAZ and YAP proteins in canine OSA could also be observed in human OSA, we compared TAZ and YAP mRNA levels among different groups of patients using datasets from previously published studies that were deposited in the Gene Expression Omnibus (GEO) public database. We did not observe significant differences in TAZ or YAP mRNA levels in primary tumours derived from patients that develop versus patients that did not developed metastasis after tumour resection in two independent datasets, Kobayashi et al. 2010 (accession # GSE14827 [30]) and Namlos et al. 2012, (accession # GSE32981 [31]) (Figs. 3a and 4a, left and right plots, respectively). Similarly, we did not observe significant differences in TAZ or YAP mRNA levels in primary tumour tissue as compared to tissue from actual metastases in one data set Namlos et al. 2012, (accession # GSE32981 [31]) (Figs. 3a and 4a, respectively, right plot), or between tumours derived from patients that did not recur after treatment as compared to patients that recurred (Kelly et al. 2013, accession # GSE39058 [32]) (Figs. 3b and 4b, respectively). Analysis of one available dataset for canine OSA showed no association between TAZ or YAP mRNA levels and overall survival (Scott et al. 2011, accession # GSE27217 [33]) (Figs. 3c and 4c, respectively). Similarly, no associations with metastasis, recurrence, or OS were found when we used the same data sets to look for correlations between the aforementioned parameters and TAZ or YAP mRNA levels in combination with the mRNA level of genes in a TGFβ signature [34] comprised of *TGFB1* itself plus the following: *COL1A1, COL6A1, COL6A3, MMP11, MMP14* and *POSTN*

Table 3 Associations between pSmad2, TAZ and YAP levels and established prognostic factors

Histopathological Characteristics	pSmad2 High	Low	p value	TAZ High	Low	p value	YAP High	Low	p value
Tumour Grade									
Kirpensteijn et al. (2002) [28]									
1	0	0	0.1366	0	0	0.3747	0	0	0.2549
2	7	6		8	5		7	5	
3	3	0		1	2		2	0	
Loukopoulos et al. (2007) [29]			0.0907			0.6832			0.1629
1	3	5		4	4		3	4	
2	4	0		2	2		4	0	
3	3	1		3	1		2	1	
Serum ALP[a] Status			0.5510			0.1457			0.0524
High	3	1		1	3		8	2	
Normal	7	5		8	4		1	3	
Low	0	0		0	0		0	0	

[a]ALP: Alkaline phosphatase

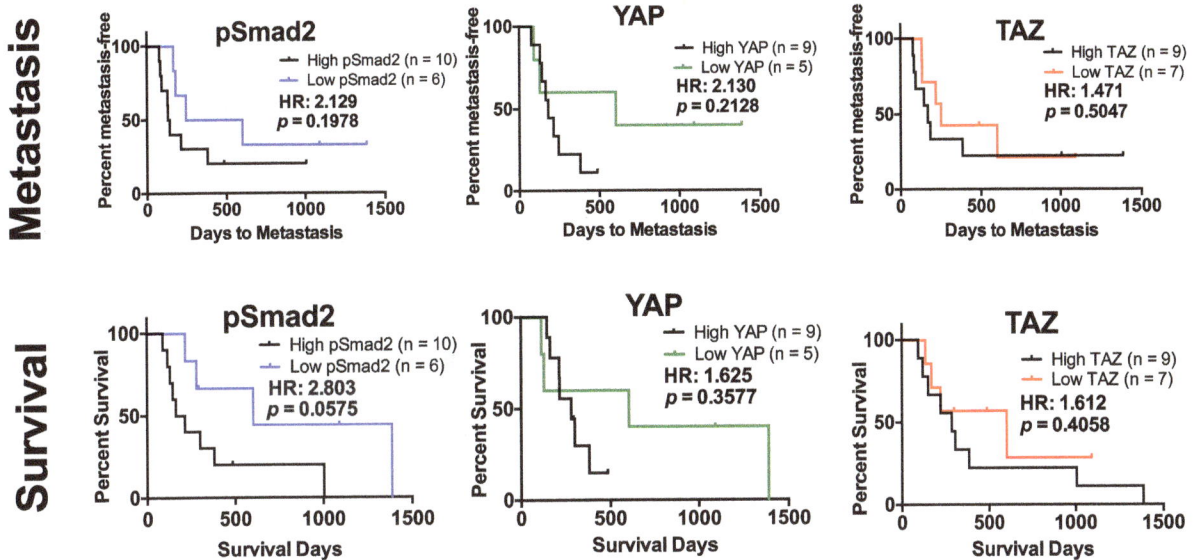

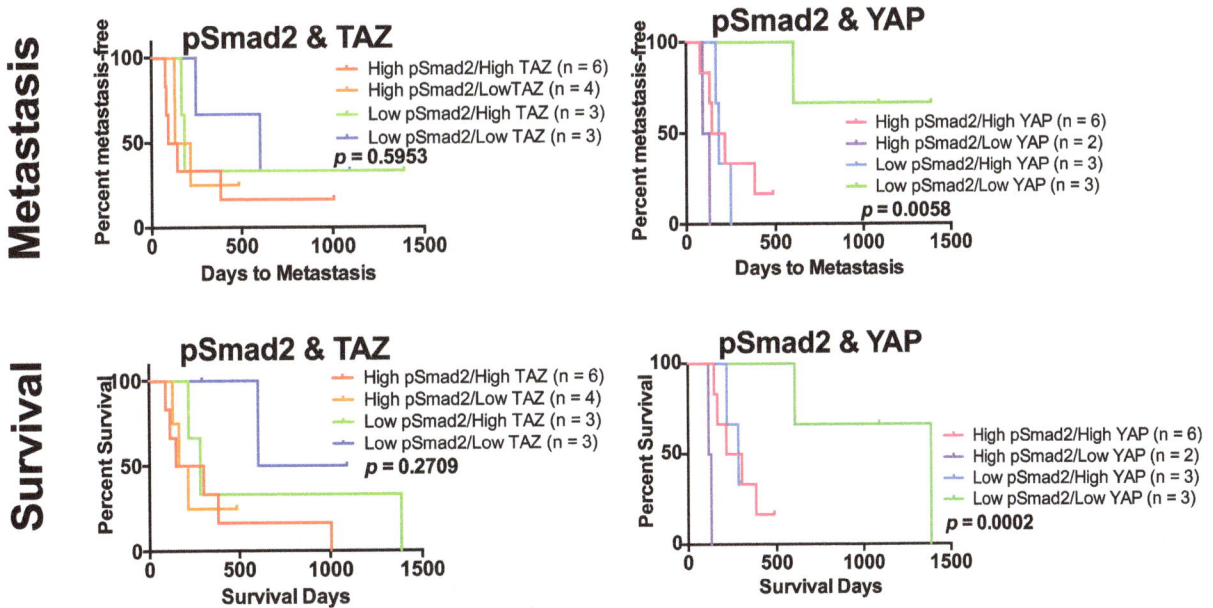

Fig. 2 Kaplan-Meier plots depicting the correlation pSmad2, TAZ and YAP levels and time to metastasis and overall survival. No significant difference was found between the number of days to metastasis and overall survival when considering pSmad2, TAZ and YAP alone (**a**) or pSmad2 and TAZ in combination (**b**, left). Significant difference in time to metastasis and overall survival was observed when considering pSmad2 and YAP in combination (**b**, right). All statistical analyses were performed using the log-rank (Mantel-Cox) test

(data not shown). To further explore whether the associations observed in the TMA analyses reflect a role for TAZ and/or YAP in canine OSA and whether or not their function is influenced by canonical TGFβ signaling activation, in vitro studies were completed.

Characterization of TGFβ signalling and hippo pathway mediators in canine osteosarcoma cell lines

To first determine the presence of both TGFβ receptors, as well as the degree of Smad activation in response to exogenous TGFβ and its effects on Hippo pathway mediators, TAZ and YAP, immunoblotting analyses was completed on

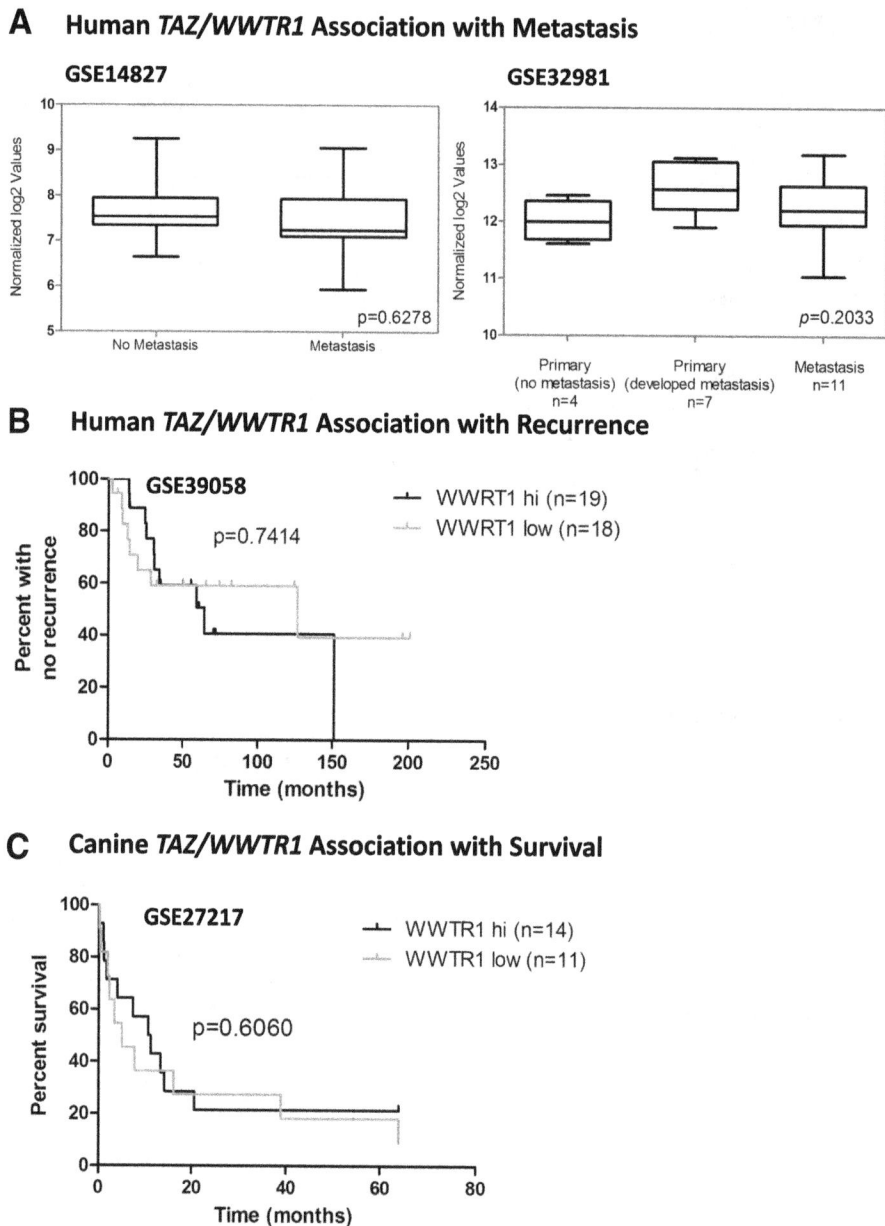

Fig. 3 Associations between TAZ mRNA levels and metastasis, recurrence or OS. No significant differences were observed in TAZ mRNA levels in human patients that did not develop metastases, compared to patients that did metastasize (**a**, left panel). Similarly, no statistical significance was achieved when comparing TAZ mRNA levels in non-metastatic primary tumours versus primary tumours that developed metastasis, or between primary tumours and metastases (**a**, right panel). No significant differences were observed in recurrence for human patients with high versus low TAZ mRNA (**b**), or for OS in canine patients with hi versus low TAZ mRNA (**c**)

four canine OSA cell lines, two derived from primary tumours (OVC-cOSA-75 and OVC-cOSA-78), and two derived from metastatic colonies (OVC-cOSA-31 and D17). As expected, all cell lines expressed both TβRI and TβRII. The primary cell lines appeared to have higher levels of TβRI when compared to the metastatic cell lines, while there were no obvious patterns when considering TβRII levels (Fig. 5a). To

determine the extent of canonical TGFβ signalling activation, the levels of phosphorylated (active) Smad2 and Smad3 were determined after 5 ng/mL of TGFβ treatment. All cell lines robustly responded to exogenous TGFβ1 as demonstrated by the large increase in phosphorylated Smad3 and Smad2 (pSmad3 and pSmad2, shown in Fig. 5b and c, respectively). TAZ levels increased in response to TGFβ1 treatment (significantly so for

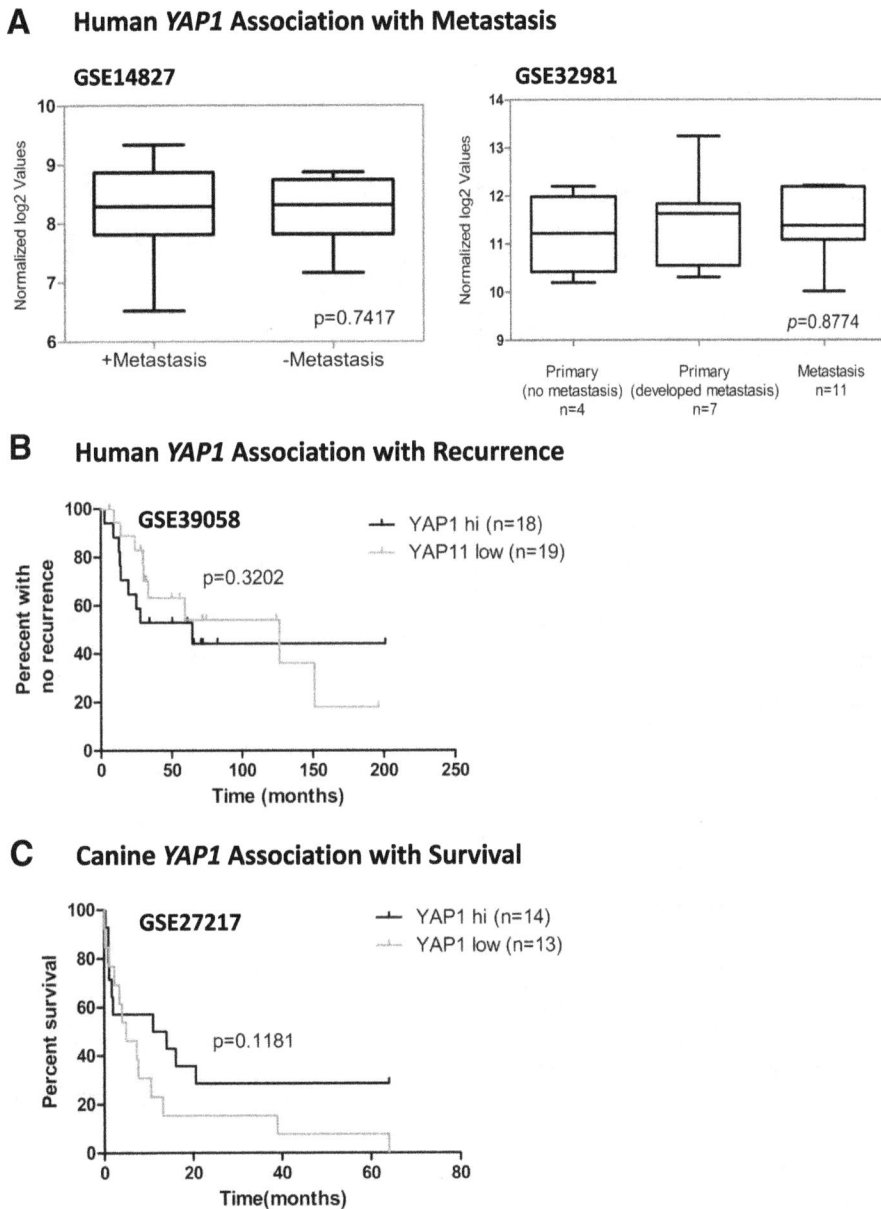

Fig. 4 Associations between YAP1 mRNA levels and metastasis, recurrence or OS. No significant differences were observed in YAP mRNA levels in human patients that did not develop metastases, compared to patients that did metastasize (**a**, left panel). Similarly, no statistical significance was achieved when comparing YAP mRNA levels in non-metastatic primary tumours versus primary tumours that developed metastasis, or between primary tumours and metastases (**a**, right panel). No significant differences were observed in recurrence for human patients with high versus low YAP mRNA (**b**), or for OS in canine patients with hi versus low YAP mRNA (**c**)

OVC-cOSA-75 and OVC-cOSA-78 cell lines only), while YAP levels remained fairly similar between treatment groups (Fig. 5d).

Cell-line dependent effects of TAZ and YAP depletion on cell viability

To determine the role of Hippo pathway mediators and TGFβ signaling on OSA cell viability, TAZ and YAP were depleted in three cell lines using siRNA (siTAZ and siYAP),

and the cells were subsequently treated or not with TGFβ, followed by exposure (or not) to Doxorubicin, a drug commonly used for SOC of canine osteosarcoma [2], and one that in our hands has been reliable for in vitro experimentation. TAZ knockdown significantly reduced viability of D17 cells relative to control (Ctrl) both in the absence and presence of Doxorubicin, and both in the presence or absence of TGFβ for cells that were not treated with Doxorubicin, but has no effect on the other two cell lines (Fig. 6a). In

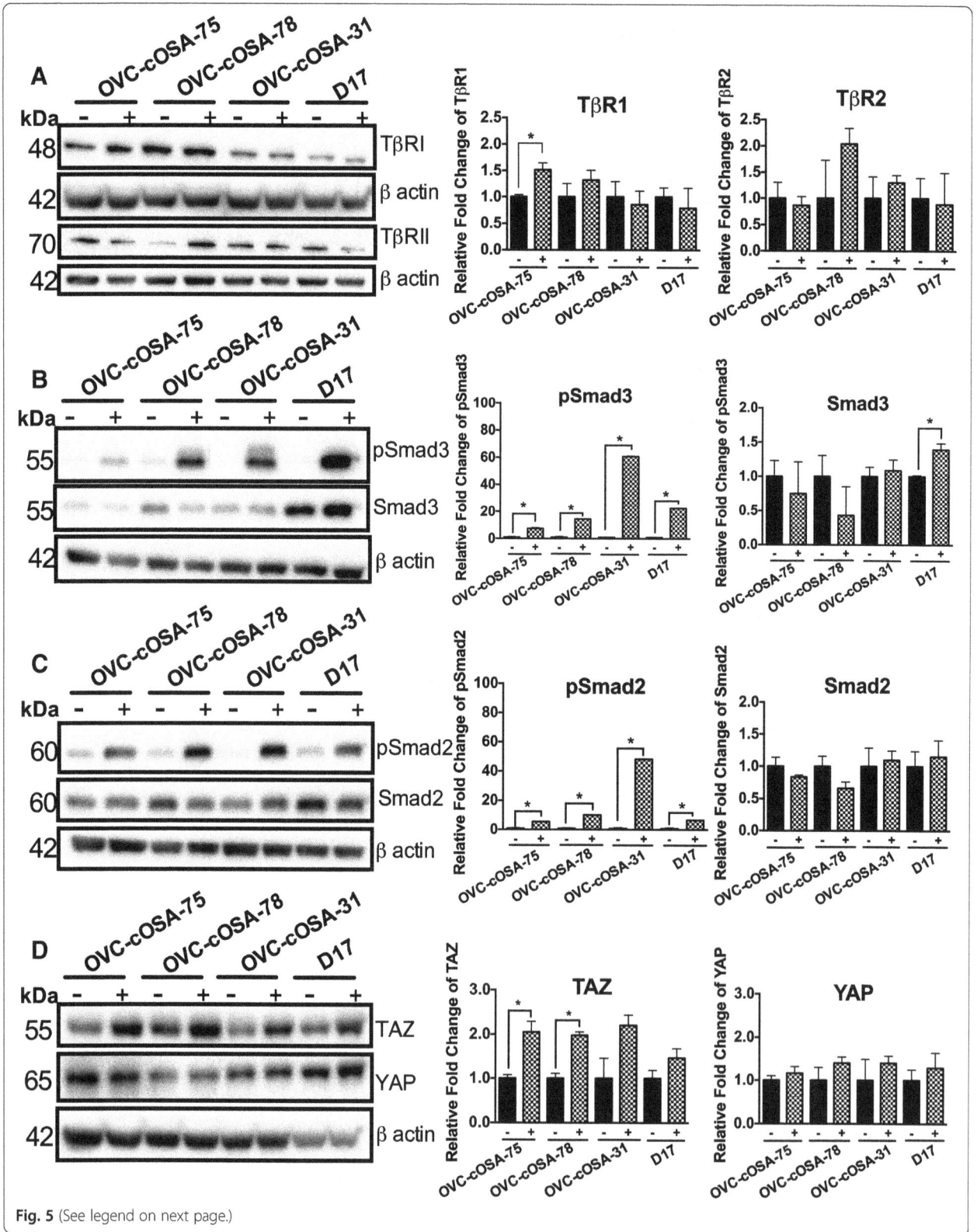

Fig. 5 (See legend on next page.)

(See figure on previous page.)
Fig. 5 All canine OSA cell lines express TGFβRI, TGFβRII, respond to TGFβ1 treatment and have basal levels of Hippo mediators TAZ and YAP. Cells were serum starved for 6 h and either stimulated with 5 ng/mL TGFβ1 (+) or not (−) for 24 h. Representative immunoblots and densitometry analysis showing the levels of TGFβRI and TGFβRII (**a**), pSmad3 and Smad 3 (**b**), pSmad2 and Smad2 (**c**) and TAZ and YAP (**d**), n = 3. Phospho-protein levels were normalized to native protein levels, and all native protein levels were normalized to β actin (loading control) and compared to the control (−) to determine relative differences. Independent t-test was used to determine significant differences between control and treated groups, * indicates p < 0.05, ** indicates p < 0.010, error bars depict average ± SEM

contrast, YAP knockdown significantly reduced cell viability in all three cell lines relative to control (Ctrl), and this occurred both in the presence or absence of doxorubicin, and in the presence or absence of TGFβ, for OVC-cOSA-75 and OVC-cOSA-31, but not for D17, where the effect was only significant in the absence of doxorubicin and in the absence of TGFβ (Fig. 6b). Taken together, these results suggest that YAP is a key mediator of canine OSA cell viability and can influence their response to chemotherapy, while TAZ role is more limited.

Cell-line dependent effects of TAZ and YAP depletion on cell proliferation

Since a reduction in cell viability caused by YAP or TAZ knockdown in various OSA cell lines could result from an effect on cell survival, cell proliferation, or both, we next focused on assessing the role of TAZ, YAP, and TGFβ signalling on cell proliferation exclusively. For this purpose, we depleted TAZ and YAP with siRNA (siTAZ and siYAP) and subsequently cultured the cells in the presence or absence of TGFβ1 under serum starvation conditions for

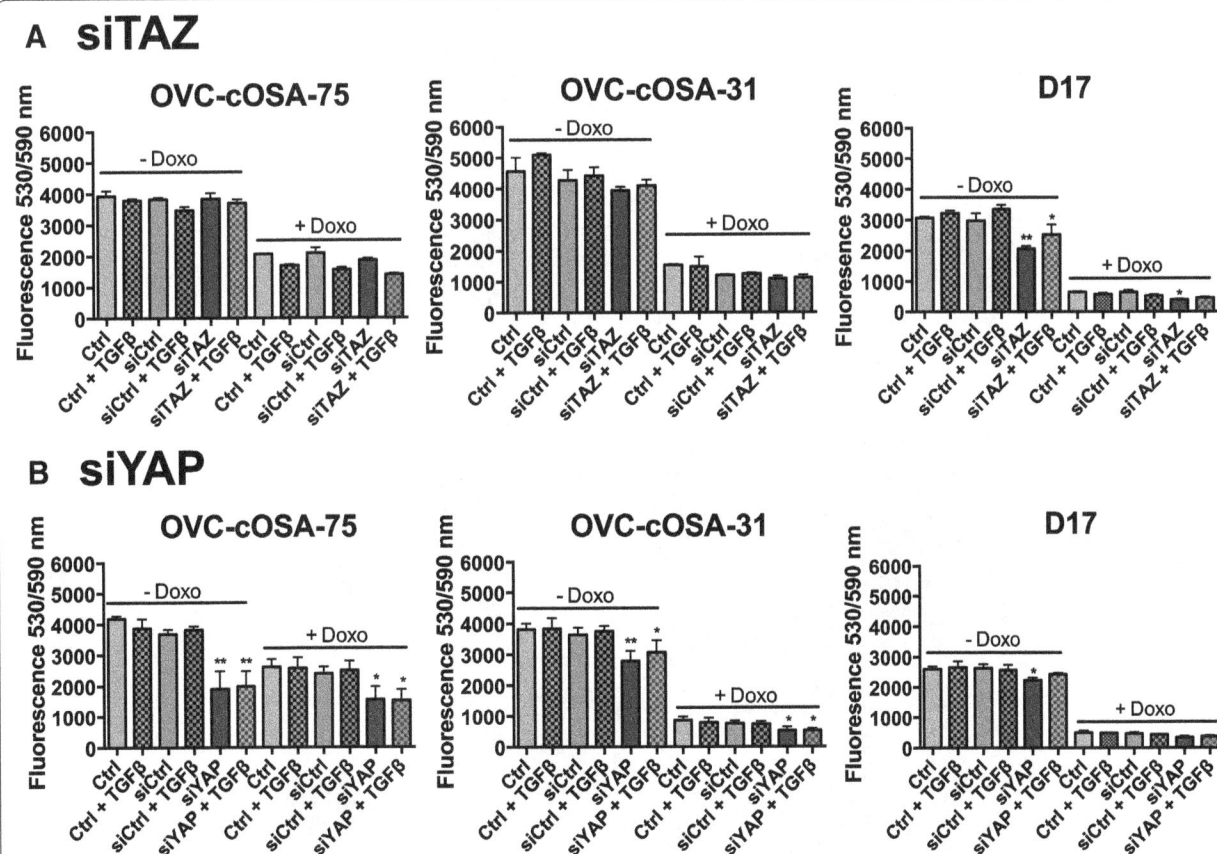

Fig. 6 Effect of TAZ or YAP knockdown plus and minus TGFβ on cell viability of canine OSA cell lines. Graphs depict the fluorescence readings at 530/590 nm when TAZ (**a**) or YAP (**b**) was depleted in OVC-cOSA-75, OVC-cOSA-31, and D17 cells, which were stimulated or not with 5 ng/mL TGFβ in the presence (+ Doxo) or absence (−Doxo) of Doxorubicin. Readings were first blank-corrected to fluorescence values obtained for the media only control. Bars depict the average ± SEM from two independent experiments plated in duplicate. Asterisks depict statistical differences as determined by a one-way ANOVA (Kruskal-Wallis test) with Dunn-Sidak correction to identify significant differences relative to control within each, the −Doxo and + Doxo treatment groups; * indicates p < 0.05, ** indicates p < 0.010. TAZ knockdown decreased cell viability in the D17 cell line both in the presence and absence of Doxorubicin. YAP knockdown decreased cell viability in the presence (OVC-cOSA-75, OVC-cOSA-31) and absence (all three cell lines) of Doxorubicin

optimal canonical signaling activation (the effectiveness of siRNAs at downregulating TAZ and YAP expression can be seen in Additional file 2: Figure S2 and Additional file 3: Figure S3). The mitotic marker phospho-histone H3 (pHH3) was used to fluorescently label proliferating cells (Fig. 7). All cell lines demonstrated a low basal proliferating rate ($\sim$ 1–2%) under serum starvation conditions as seen in the untreated control (Ctrl) and siRNA control (siCtrl) groups. TAZ depletion decreased the relative percentage of pHH3 positive cells in the D17 cell line, while having no significant effect on the OVC-cOSA-75, OVC-cOSA-78, and OVC-cOSA-31 cell lines. Also in the D17 cell line, TGFβ treatment significantly increased pHH3 positivity, better visualized when comparing the siCtrl and

siCtrl + TGFβ groups (p = 0.0479). However, when TAZ was depleted alone and in combination with TGFβ treatment, there was a reduction in pHH3 positivity, which became significant when comparing siCtrl + TGFβ to siTAZ (p = 0.0029), and to siTAZ + TGFβ groups (p = 0.011). This was not observed for OVC-cOSA-75, OVC-cOSA-78 and OVC-cOSA-31 (Fig. 7a). In terms of YAP, there was no statistically significant change observed in pHH3 positivity upon knockdown in any of the cell lines (Fig. 7b), although a slight decrease in pHH3 positivity was seen in OVC-cOSA-31 and D17 cells relative to Ctrl and siCtrl, and this was both in the absence or presence of TGFβ treatment (Fig. 7b). These results suggest that TAZ (and possibly YAP), mediate cell proliferation in OSA cell lines in a cell

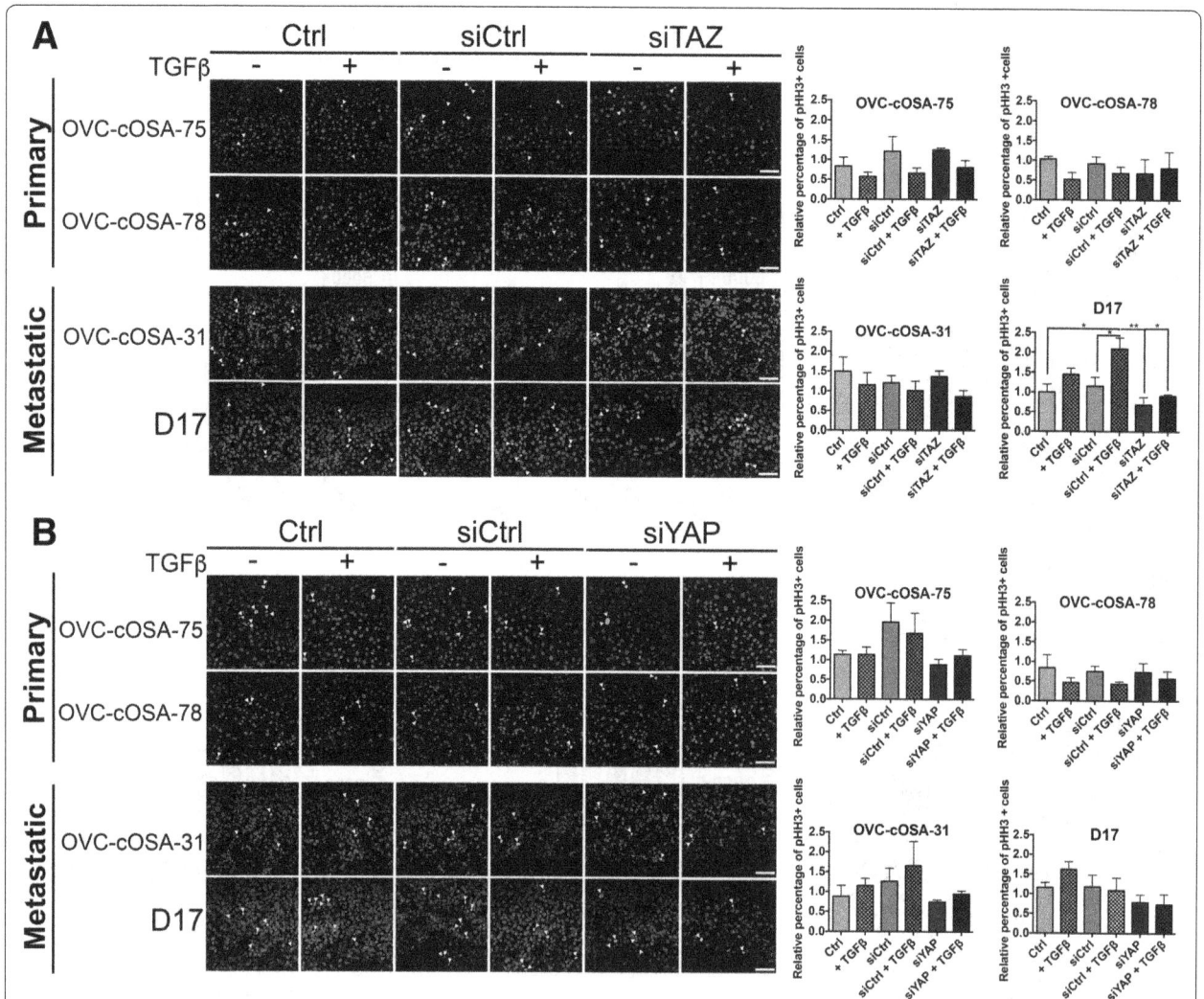

Fig. 7 Effect of TAZ or YAP knockdown plus and minus TGFβ on cell proliferation of canine OSA cell lines. Representative immunofluorescence images of the mitotic marker phosphor-histone H3 (pHH3) taken at 20X objective lens for primary tumour-derived cell lines (a), and metastatic cell lines (b). Graphs depict the relative percentage of pHH3 positivity cells, as determined by dividing the number of pHH3 cells by the number of cells in the field of view. Five images were taken per experimental group and averaged. Error bars depict average ± SEM from three independent experiments. Scale bar = 100 μm. Asterisks depict statistical differences as determined by a two-way ANOVA with post-hoc Tukey-Kramer, * indicates p < 0.05, ** indicates p < 0.010, *** indicates p < 0.0010

line-dependent manner and in both the presence and absence of activated TGFβ signalling.

TAZ and TGFβ signaling crosstalk in D17 cells

The above described effects of TAZ knockdown on D17 cells, where reducing TAZ levels not only inhibited proliferation in the absence of TGFβ, but also blocked the growth-stimulatory effects of this cytokine, were suggestive of a crosstalk between TGFβ signaling and TAZ, whereby low levels of TAZ can negatively modulate protumorigenic properties of TGFβ in this cell line. To explore this possibility, we conducted the same experiment in the presence and absence of a specific inhibitor of the TGFβ receptor type I (referred to here as LY), which blocks the activation of canonical (Smad) TGFβ signaling. LY treatment reduced the levels of TAZ in D17 cells (Fig. 8a), suggesting that basal TAZ expression in D17 cells is dependent on TGFβ signaling, possibly resulting from the capacity of D17 cells to secrete its own TGFβ (autocrine signalling), as these experiments were performed under serum starvation conditions. Although the results were not statistically significant due to high variability among the replicates, the average percentage of proliferating cells under TGFβ stimulation was equally reduced by TAZ knockdown independently of whether or not TGFβ signaling was blocked (compare siCtrl + TGFβ versus siTAZ + TGFβ and versus siTAZ + TGFβ + LY in Fig. 8b). These results support the existence of a crosstalk between TGFβ signalling and TAZ in D17 cells, whereby TAZ expression is modulated by TGFβ. However, TGFβ signaling inhibition does not significantly enhance the effect of TAZ knockdown in cell proliferation.

Cell line dependent effects of TAZ and YAP in cell migration

To determine the role of TAZ, YAP, and TGFβ signalling in cell migration, the Transwell assay was performed. TAZ depletion, alone or in combination with TGFβ treatment, did not have an effect on the migratory

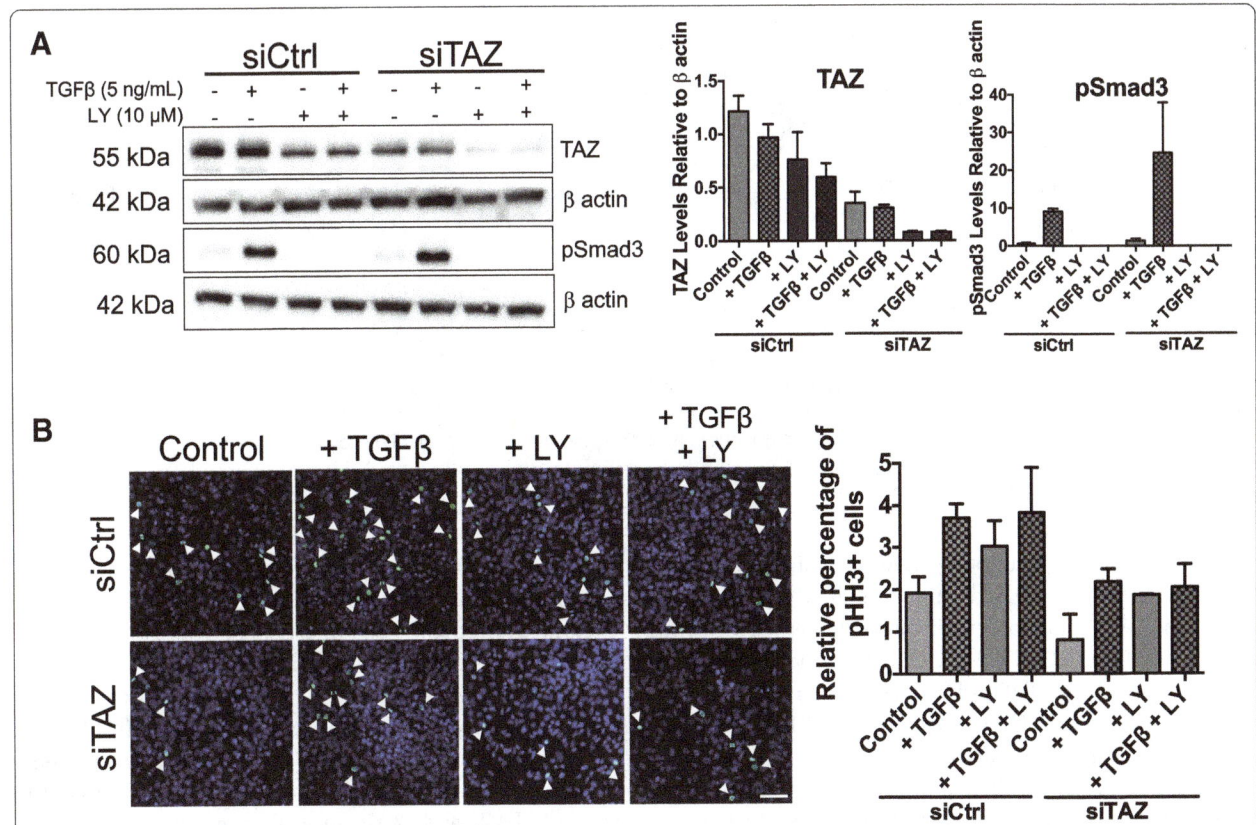

Fig. 8 Effect of TGFβ receptor I inhibition by LY2157299 on TAZ levels and cell proliferation in D17 cells. Representative immuoblots and densitometry analysis of TAZ and pSmad3 protein levels when TAZ levels were depleted (siTAZ) or not (siCtrl), and cells were treated with nothing (Control), 5 ng/mL TGFβ (+ TGFβ), 10 μM of LY2152799 (+ LY) or combination treatment (+ TGFβ + LY). Experimental groups were normalized to loading control β-actin. Graphs depict the average fold change in TAZ or pSmad3 expression relative to siCtrl non-treated group ± SEM from two independent experiments (**a**). LY inhibited Smad3 phosphorylation and decreased TAZ levels compared to non-LY treated cells, suggesting that suppressing active TGFβ signaling could decrease TAZ levels in D17 cells. **b** Representative immunofluorescence images of the mitotic marker phospho-histone H3 (pHH3) taken at 20X objective lens and graph depicting the relative percentage of pHH3 positive cells; bars depict average ± SEM from three independent experiments. Scale bar = 100 μm

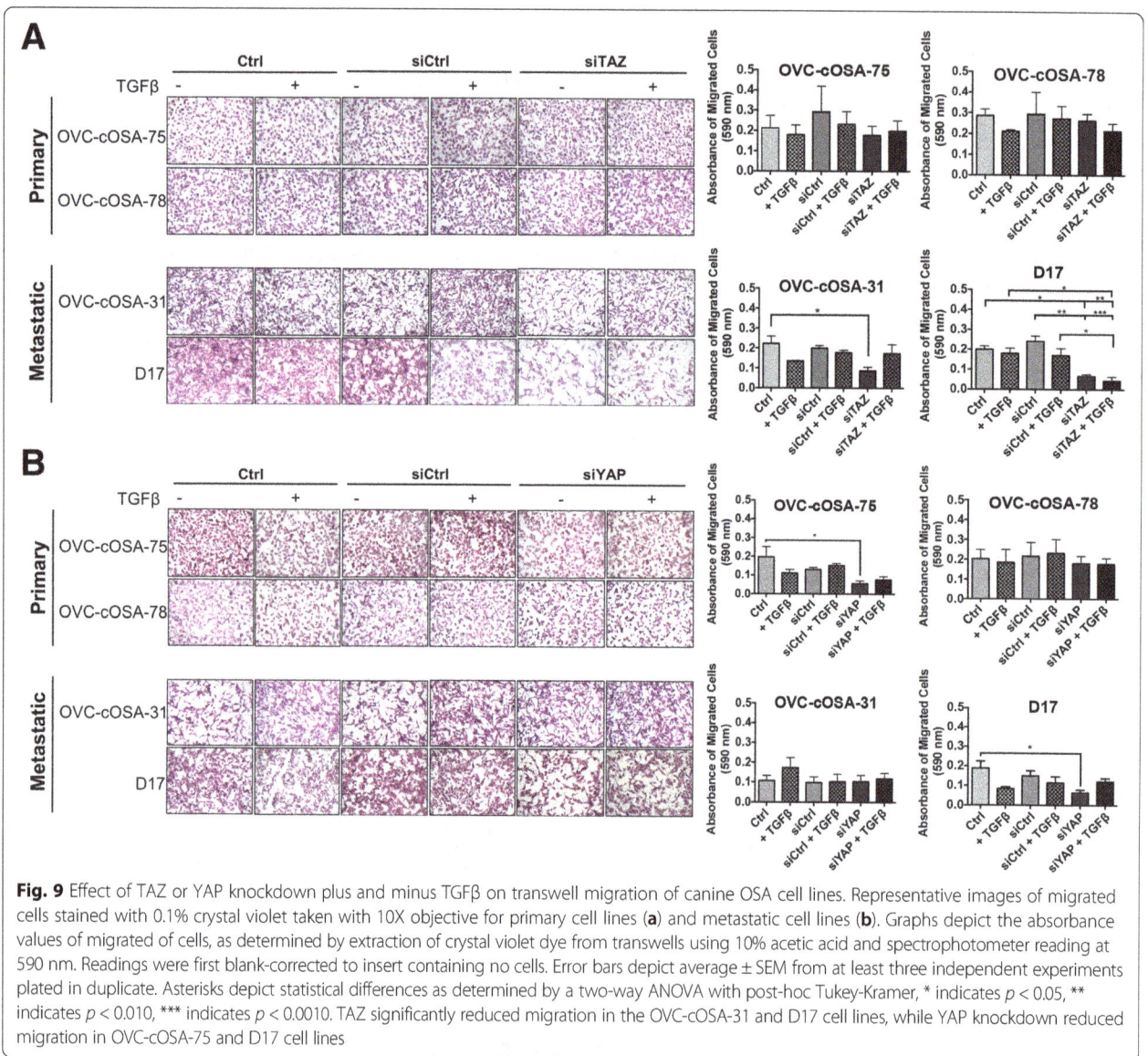

Fig. 9 Effect of TAZ or YAP knockdown plus and minus TGFβ on transwell migration of canine OSA cell lines. Representative images of migrated cells stained with 0.1% crystal violet taken with 10X objective for primary cell lines (**a**) and metastatic cell lines (**b**). Graphs depict the absorbance values of migrated of cells, as determined by extraction of crystal violet dye from transwells using 10% acetic acid and spectrophotometer reading at 590 nm. Readings were first blank-corrected to insert containing no cells. Error bars depict average ± SEM from at least three independent experiments plated in duplicate. Asterisks depict statistical differences as determined by a two-way ANOVA with post-hoc Tukey-Kramer, * indicates $p < 0.05$, ** indicates $p < 0.010$, *** indicates $p < 0.0010$. TAZ significantly reduced migration in the OVC-cOSA-31 and D17 cell lines, while YAP knockdown reduced migration in OVC-cOSA-75 and D17 cell lines

behavior of primary tumour-derived cell lines (Fig. 9a), but significantly decreased migration in the metastatic cell lines. TAZ depletion significantly decreased cell migration in the OVC-cOSA-31 cell line when compared to the control ($p = 0.03$). However, when knockdown was combined with TGFβ in OVC-cOSA-31, cell migration increased to levels similar to those of the controls. In the D17 cell line, TAZ depletion resulted in a significant reduction in cell migration as compared to Ctrl ($p = 0.0191$) and siCtrl ($p = 0.0024$). When TAZ depletion was combined with TGFβ treatment (siTAZ + TGFβ), there was a significant decrease when compared to Ctrl + TGFβ ($p = 0.0169$), and the siCtrl group alone or in combination with TGFβ ($p = 0.0009$ and $p = 0.0267$, respectively) (Fig. 9a). These results suggest that TAZ mediates migratory properties independent of TGFβ

signalling activation in D17 cells. YAP depletion did not have a noticeable effect on cell migration in the primary tumour-derived OSA cell line OVC-cOSA-78, and in the metastasis-derived OVC-cOSA-31 (Fig. 9b). However, YAP depletion significantly reduced migration in primary tumour-derived OVC-cOSA-75 ($p = 0.0210$), and metastasis-derived D17 cells ($p = 0.0296$), when compared to Ctrl (Fig. 9b). These results suggest that the role of TAZ and YAP in cell migration is cell line dependent, with predominant effects on TAZ in the metastatic cell lines that may or may not be modulated by TGFβ signalling activation.

Discussion

Canine osteosarcoma is an aggressive, highly metastatic disease that lacks reliable prognostic factors. Due to the reported independent roles of TGFβ signalling and TAZ/YAP in promoting OSA progression, as well as their ability to crosstalk, this study aimed to investigate their cooperative role in canine OSA. To explore this possibility, we first employed a trial tissue microarray that contained 16 appendicular canine OSA patients that underwent SOC treatment. It was found that a majority of patients (approximately 60%) had high levels of pSmad2, TAZ and YAP expression. The high levels of nuclear pSmad2 observed in a high proportion of the tumours indicate active canonical signalling in canine OSA, and this is in agreement with previous reports implicating TGFβ signalling in both human [35, 36] and canine [11] OSA pathogenesis. Our choice for assessing total TAZ and YAP levels, including both nuclear and cytoplasmic protein, was based on the prominent role that proteasome-dependent degradation plays in the regulation of TAZ activity (reviewed in Yu et al. 2015 [37]). The proportion of TAZ and YAP positive tumours we observed using Allred's scoring method, 56% and 64%, respectively, was similar to the 60% reported for total combined TAZ/YAP expression in conventional human OSA, and to the 67% reported for nuclear TAZ expression in high grade human OSA [23, 24].

There were no significant associations found between high pSmad2, TAZ or YAP levels and ALP status, nor between pSmad2, TAZ or YAP levels and histologic grade (Table 3). We recently reported that neither of the commonly used grading systems for canine OSA, nor serum ALP, are predictive for clinical outcome following SOC treatment [38]. Although we conducted the current study before the results of our grading study were complete, it is not surprising that we did not find correlations between expression levels of pSmad2, TAZ, or YAP, and grade or serum ALP. No previous studies looked for associations between TGFβ signalling status, TGFβ serum levels, TAZ or YAP and the aforementioned grading systems for canine OSA. A study in human OSA patients found a significant association between high levels of tumour TGFβ1 and high histologic grade [7]. Similarly, in human OSA, YAP1 expression has been correlated with high Enneking stages (II and III) [39].

The prognostic value of serum ALP, on the other hand, has been reiterated in recent canine osteosarcoma studies [40–42], although, as mentioned above, our recently published study found no predictive value of serum ALP in canine OSA patients receiving SOC [38]. However, the lack of associations observed between ALP status and pSmad2, TAZ, or YAP levels, is in agreement with previous reports that investigated OSA cells derived from dogs with known ALP status. Specifically, OSA cells derived from canine patients with differing serum ALP levels displayed no differences in migration,

invasion and chemosensitivity when evaluated in vitro [43]. Similarly, Rodrigues and colleagues reported that serum ALP is not associated with specific gene expression patterns or intrinsic differences between patient-derived OSA cells [44]. Yet, different gene expression profiles were shown to be useful in separating canine OSA patients into short and long-term survivors [45]. These findings suggest that serum ALP levels may not provide insight on osteosarcoma cell behavior as it relates to molecular and signalling profiles. Taken together with the above-discussed controversies, our data might prove useful to future studies aimed at establishing the prognostic utility or ALP or tumour grading.

There were no significant differences in time to metastasis or overall patient survival when the markers of interest were evaluated independently. Although not statically significant, when considering the Kaplan-Meier curves in Fig. 2a, the borderline significant p value for pSmad2 (in relation to overall survival) and the divergent curves, suggest that patients with high levels of YAP or pSmad2 have a shorter time to metastasis and overall survival. However, these trends were not observed when considering TAZ levels alone. Interestingly, when pSmad2 and YAP were evaluated in combination (Fig. 2b, right), there was a significant difference in time to metastasis ($p = 0.0058$) and overall survival ($p = 0.0002$), with a better outcome observed in patients with lower levels of both markers. When TAZ and pSmad2 levels were considered in combination, the trends improved compared to when TAZ levels were evaluated alone, but not compared to when pSmad2 was evaluated alone. This suggests that TAZ may not have the strength that pSmad2 or YAP have as potential prognostic factors.

Of note, the potential association between YAP, metastasis and survival appears to be limited to protein levels, as we did not observe any associations with metastasis, survival or recurrence when we looked at mRNA levels of *TAZ/WWTR1* or *YAP1* alone or in combination with a TGFβ signature, using published datasets (Figs. 3 and 4, and data not shown). This is in agreement with the lack of reports of similar associations in human OSA, and possibly reflects the fact that a major determinant of whether or not TAZ and YAP protein levels are sustained to ultimately lead to a cellular response depends on post-translational modifications, such as phosphorylation events, which direct the proteasome-dependent degradation of these transcriptional co-activators. This is in turn controlled by complex signaling networks that activate or inhibit the Hippo signaling cascade, and can also be different for YAP as compared to TAZ (reviewed in [46]).

Since we recognized the limitations in interpreting the TMA findings due to the small sample size, we explored further the relationship between TAZ, YAP and TGFβ signalling in vitro using four independently derived canine OSA cell lines: two originating from a primary tumour (OVC-cOSA-75 and OVC-cOSA-78) and two derived from metastatic, secondary tumours (OVC-cOSA-31 and D17). We utilized siRNAs specific to TAZ and YAP (siTAZ, siYAP) and treated or not treated these cells with TGFβ1, to investigate the biological function of this crosstalk.

We first sought to characterize the response of cell lines to TGFβ1 treatment, and to look at basal and activated levels of canonical mediators pSmad2, Smad2, pSmad3, Smad3, and the effect of TGFβ signalling activation on TAZ and YAP levels. As expected and in agreement with previous studies [11], all cell lines expressed both receptors (Fig. 5a) and responded to TGFβ1 treatment as indicated by the increase in Smad3 and Smad2 phosphorylation (Fig. 5b and c). Also in agreement with the literature is the observed increase in TAZ protein levels in response to TGFβ1 treatment [14], while this was not seen for YAP.

We first examined the effect of TAZ and YAP knockdown in cell viability in the presence or absence of chemotherapy and in the presence of absence of active TGFβ signaling. The results showed that both TAZ and YAP modulate cell viability, but the effect of TAZ was limited to the D17 cell line (Fig. 6). As the Hippo pathway and TGFβ signalling have been documented to be important cell cycle regulators [47, 48], and to understand better whether the effects of knockdown on cell viability reflected changes in cell proliferation, we investigated the role of TGFβ-Hippo signalling on mitotic activity by examining pHH3 fluorescent labeling. Interestingly, TGFβ treatment did not have a significant effect on the percentage of mitotically active cells in the majority of cell lines, with the exception of D17. In agreement with the results when examining cell viability, TAZ knockdown significantly decreased the percentage of mitotically active cells only in the D17 cell line, where it also inhibited the growth promoting effect of TGFβ (Fig. 7a). This effect could possibly reflect the fact that exogenous TGFβ does not significantly enhance TAZ levels in D17 cells, where TAZ expression might be induced by TGFβ produced by the cells themselves (Fig. 8). The intrinsic levels of TAZ in this cell line thus appear to contribute to both, its basal proliferation and that induced by exogenous TGFβ, either by influencing canonical signal outcome (via facilitating Smad nuclear retention or transcriptional activity), or by interfering with non-canonical signaling.

YAP knockdown did not significantly reduce the percentage of mitotically active cells in any of the cell lines tested, although a slight decrease was observed in the metastatic cell lines in relation to both controls (Fig. 7b). Previous cell cycle analyses demonstrated that YAP1

knockdown decreases cell proliferation by arresting cells in the G0/G1 phase while decreasing the number of cells in the S phase [49]; however, the proportion of cells in the G2/M phase was similar when comparing the YAP knockdown and control group. These results suggest that YAP may have a more dominant role in mediating cell cycle progression (which is in line with its ability to induce expression of cyclin D1) [49], and could explain why the effects of YAP knockdown on proliferation did not reach significance in our study, as pHH3 positivity reflects the number of mitotically active cells. Taken together with the consistent reduction of viability across cell lines upon YAP knockdown (Fig. 6b), and the significance of such effects in the presence of Doxorubicin, our results suggest a key role for YAP in canine osteosarcoma survival and possibly in proliferation, and are in agreement with the associations of YAP with time to metastasis and overall survival suggested by the TMA analysis.

The results of the Transwell assay showed that TAZ knockdown significantly decreased cell migration in both of the metastasis-derived cell lines, D17 and OVC-cOSA-31 (Fig. 9a), and in D17 this was also significant in the presence of TGFβ. YAP knockdown, on the other hand, inhibited migration of two cell lines independently of their primary or secondary site of origin (Fig. 9b), and similar to what was observed for TAZ, this effect on migration was only significant for one cell line in the presence of TGFβ. Taken together with the effect of TAZ knockdown only in the viability and proliferation of D17 cells, these results suggest that TAZ effects of OSA cells were specific to metastasis-derived cell lines, and whether or not active TGFβ signaling modulates the effect that TAZ or YAP has in OSA cell migration is cell line dependent.

A role for TAZ in migration of canine OSA cells is in agreement with a previous report in human osteosarcoma, in which TAZ was found to mediate migratory and colony forming ability of OSA cells [50]. TAZ role in migration was found to be mediated, at least in part, via a positive feedback loop involving miR-135b [50]. TAZ induced the expression of miR-135b, and miR-135b overexpression was able to rescue the pro-tumourigenic functions in cells with depleted TAZ. A similar interaction was reported between miR-224 and TAZ [51]. The significant effect of YAP depletion on the migratory behavior of canine OSA cells is also in agreement with a previous report by Zhang and colleagues, who demonstrated that YAP1 depletion decreased invasiveness in human OSA [39].

Interestingly, when comparing the patient data with the results observed in vitro, the results obtained were not completely congruent. YAP and pSmad2 showed a potential prognostic value, but not TAZ. However, in vitro, TAZ appeared to have a functional role in modulating migration and cell proliferation in metastasis-derived cell lines. A possibility for the observed discrepancy could be due to the small patient sample size in the TMA. Although the median survival time for all patients considered was 292 days, similar to previous reports for canine appendicular OSA undergoing SOC (~ 300 days) [52], increasing the sample size could lead to greater power to recognize significant trends. In addition, although the TMA was an advantageous technique to determine the expression of these markers and its potential prognostic value, it only allows for the evaluation of a small portion of tumour tissue. A small tumour sample may not be able to fully recapitulate the marker expression of the tumour, and OSA is notoriously heterogeneous. Another possibility could be that the total levels (nuclear and cytoplasmic) of TAZ and YAP, and not their nuclear levels, were investigated in the tumour tissue. Given that TAZ and YAP are transcription factors, its nuclear retention is important for mediating oncogenic properties [53], and have indeed been associated with poor progression free survival in OSA [24]. Thus, determining correlations between nuclear TAZ and YAP alone or in combination with pSmad2 could yield different results.

Another possibility for the observed discrepancies could be the complexity in regulatory inputs for TAZ and YAP. All in vitro experiments were completed under serum deprivation conditions, and mechanical and environmental inputs were not considered, whereas patient tissue samples provided a realistic representation of microenvironmental effects. Furthermore, only viability, proliferation, and migration were evaluated. The function of TAZ and YAP in mediating other metastasis and drug-response associated traits, such as cellular survival and stemness, should be evaluated in future studies. Nonetheless, this pilot study demonstrated that Hippo mediators, in particular YAP, mediates canine OSA cell viability and migration independent of active TGFβ signalling, and YAP and pSmad2, alone and in combination, could potentially be used as a prognostic factor. Future studies should evaluate these molecules in larger canine patient cohorts, as well as determine the effects of TAZ and YAP knockdown and/or pharmacologic targeting of these transcription factors as well as TGFβ, on additional traits of OSA progression.

Conclusions

To the best of our knowledge, this was the first study to investigate TGFβ-Hippo signalling crosstalk in canine OSA. Assessment of pSmad2, TAZ and YAP proteins alone or in combination in a trial TMA suggests a potential benefit of using pSmad2 and YAP combined as prognostic markers for canine OSA, with low levels of both possibly indicating better prognosis. This requires further testing in a more robust patient cohort. The in vitro results indicate that both YAP and TAZ modulate metastasis-associated properties of canine osteosarcoma, with the effects of TAZ on proliferation and migration being more specific to cell lines derived from metastases. The impact of microenvironment-derived TGFβ on TAZ/YAP-dependent cellular outcomes, such as viability, migration and proliferation is context-dependent. Additional mechanistic studies with a larger number of cell lines and combined TGFβ signalling blocking strategies are required to better understand the role of TGFβ-Hippo signalling crosstalk in canine OSA.

Methods

Antibodies and TGFβ

Antibodies used in this study included: YAP (#14074), β actin (#4967S), pSmad2 (#3108), and Smad2 (#5339) or Smad2/3 (#5678) for pSmad2 normalization (all from Cell Signaling Technology, New England Biolabs, Ltd., Whitby, ON, Canada). TβR1 (v-22) (#sc-398) was purchased from Santa Cruz Biotechnology Inc. (Dallas, TX, USA). TβRII (ab612143), anti-Histone H3 (phospho S10, ab5176), pSmad3 (ab52903), and Smad3 (ab28379) were purchased from Abcam. TAZ/WWTR1 antibody (HPA007415) and secondary antibody, goat anti-rabbit IgG-peroxidase (A0545), were purchased from Sigma-Aldrich (Oakville, ON, Canada). rhTGFβ1 (PHG9204) was purchased from Invitrogen, Life Technologies (Burlington, ON, Canada). LY2157299 (Cayman Chemicals) was purchased from Cedarlane (Burlington, ON, Canada). Doxorubicin (Accord Healthcare, Kirkland, QC, Canada) was obtained from the Ontario Veterinary College Pharmacy.

TMA construction

Cases were selected from the Ontario Veterinary College Health Sciences Centre (OVC-HSC) database. Formalin fixed paraffin embedded (FFPE) tissues for the selected cases were retrieved from the Animal Health Laboratory archive. Specific areas of the FFPE tissue for each individual case were selected for coring using the guidance of haematoxylin and eosin stained histologic sections. A single 1.0 mm core was taken from each donor paraffin block and transferred into the recipient block using a Pathology Devices TMArrayer™ (Pathology Devices, Westminster, MD, USA). The recipient block contained 101 available positions that included canine tissue cores from: 31 primary appendicular OSAs with 7 matched metastatic sites, 10 axial OSAs with 2 matched metastatic sites, a selection of other tumours, and normal tissue. After the TMA was constructed, a glass slide was placed on top of the block and was placed in an oven at 55 °C for 15 min to bind the cores into the surrounding paraffin. The TMA block was left to cool before removing the slide and covering the surface of the block with a paraffin wax seal. The TMA block was cut at 4 µm, then each section was mounted on a positively charged slide and baked in an oven overnight at 37 °C.

Antibody specificity

To determine antibody specificity, TAZ and YAP immunoblotting was completed on lysates obtained from 5 cell lines grown under standard conditions (see culture conditions in corresponding section below). These included three in-house derived cell lines (OVC-cOSA-31, OVC-cOSA-75, and OVC-cOSA-78), as well as D17 and Abrams (Additional file 1: Figure S1). The latter cell lines were a generous gift from Dr. Anthony Mutsaers (Department of Biomedical Sciences, University of Guelph), although D17 is also commercially available. For the pSmad2 immunoblotting, the same cell lines were serum starved for 6 h and either treated or not treated with 5 ng/mL TGFβ1 for 24 h prior to lysate collection.

Immunohistochemistry of TMAs

Verification of antibody specificity, as well as optimization of antigen retrieval time and antibody concentration was first performed, according to manufacturer's instructions, resulting in the protocol described next. First, slides were deparaffinized in 3 xylene washes (2 min each), and subsequently hydrated in 3 washes in 100% isopropanol (2 min each), and one wash in 70% isopropanol (2 min) and deionized water (2 min). Slides were then blocked in 3% hydrogen peroxide for 20 min to prevent endogenous peroxidase activity and rinsed with deionized water for 5 min. Antigen retrieval was performed with Sodium Citrate buffer pH 6.0 (Invitrogen, Burlington, ON, Canada) at 95 °C for 15 and 10 min for the pSmad2 and TAZ TMA, respectively. Following a cool-down step at room temperature for 30 min, slides were subsequently washed 3 times with Tris Buffer Saline containing 0.1% Tween (TBST), pH = 7.4 (Fisher Scientific, Ottawa, Canada) for 2 min each. To prevent antibody nonspecific binding, slides were incubated with 5% normal goat serum (Vector Laboratories, Burlington, ON, Canada) diluted in phosphate buffered saline (PBS) (Lonza, Walkersvilla, MD, USA) for one hour at room temperature in a humidified chamber. Slides were then incubated with 300 µL of primary antibody, 1:800 dilution of polyclonal rabbit phospho-Smad2 Ser465/467 (Cell Signaling, cat no. 3101), 1:200 dilution of polyclonal rabbit TAZ (Sigma-Aldrich HPA007415), or 1:100 dilution of monoclonal rabbit YAP (Cell Signaling, cat no. D8H1X) overnight at 4 °C. Slides were washed 3 times with TBST (2 min each) and incubated with biotinylated anti-rabbit IgG secondary antibody (Vector Laboratories Inc., Burlingame, CA) for one hour at room temperature. Slides were subsequently washed 3 times with TBST (2 min each) and incubated with the avidin-biotin complex (R.T.U VectaStain Kit Elite ABC Reagent, Vector Laboratories Inc., Burlingame, CA)

for one hour at room temperature. To detect immunolabelling, slides were washed 3 times with TBST (2 min each) and incubated with 2,2′-diaminobenzidine (DAB) substrate, prepared with the DAB substrate kit (Vector Laboratories, Burlington ON, Canada) for 1 min. Slides were immersed in deionized water to stop the reaction, counterstained in haematoxylin (Thermo Fisher Scientific, Waltham, MA, United States) and dehydrated with 3 washes in 100% isopropanol and 3 washes in xylene (2 min each). Slides were coverslipped using Richard-Allan Scientific Cytoseal XXL mounting media (Thermo Fisher Scientific, Waltham, MA, United States).

Tumour grading

Tumour grading was completed by a veterinary pathologist (C.R.S) using full-face tumour sections following the scoring system outlined by Kirpensteijn et al. [28] and Loukopoulos et al. [29] at 40X ($2.37~mm^2$) objective lens.

Immunohistochemistry Quantification & Statistical Analyses

The TMA was viewed and imaged with a Leica DM LM light Microscope (Leica Microsystems, Wetzlar, Germany) and each core was subsequently imaged using the QICAM digital camera and QCapture v.2.99.5 (QImaging, Surrey, Canada). Five images were taken randomly throughout each core of the TMA at 400X magnification in 8-bit format, which were used to score both nuclear Smad2 and total (nuclear plus cytoplasmic) TAZ and YAP immunoreactivity using the Allred method [54]. This method is based on two categories, the proportion score (PS) and the intensity score (IS), which are summed to the total score (TS), a maximum value of 8. The PS is based on percentage of positively stained cells 0–5 (0: 0%, 1: 0–1%, 2: 1–10%, 3: 10–33%, 4: 33–66% and 5: 67–100%) and IS ranges from 0 to 3 (0: absent, 1: weak, 2: intermediate, 3: strong). Initially, five cores (twenty-five images) were manually scored to obtain a PS, which was then compared to the PS obtained using the publicly available image processing software ImageJ v1.49 (http://imagej.nih.gov) with ImmunoRatio (Advanced Mode) plugin (http://jvsmicroscope.uta.fi). ImmunoRatio computes a "DAB/nuclear area" percentage that was then converted to a PS, as outlined by the Allred method above. As the PS determined by visual assessment and with ImageJ were found to be similar, ImageJ was used for the remainder of the quantification, while the IS was visually assessed. During this time, the observer was blinded to patient data until all quantification was performed. The TS was averaged for all fives images per core, resulting in a single score for each core. The TS was averaged for all cores on the TMA to establish the cut-off point of 6.00. All scores were compared to the established cut-off and were classified as high for pSmad2, TAZ and YAP expression if their TS were greater than or equal to 6.00, and conversely classified as low if less than 6.00 (Fig. 1a). Cores that were damaged during processing were excluded from analysis, such that 16 cases were available for TAZ and pSMAD2 and 14 were available for YAP analysis. Overall survival was defined as time from diagnosis to death, and time to metastasis was defined as the number of days from diagnosis to the confirmation (radiographic or postmortem examination) or strong suspicion (radiographic or clinical signs) of metastatic disease. Thus, dogs that died without confirmation of metastasis were censored from the analysis of time to metastasis and no dogs were assumed to have metastasis unless there was evidence for this. Dogs that died of causes unrelated to OSA were censored from overall survival analyses.

Associations of *TAZ/WWTR1* and *YAP* mRNA expression with metastasis and survival

Processed datasets (GSE14827, GSE32981, GSE39058 and GSE27217) and corresponding gene expression and clinical annotation files were downloaded from the Gene Expression Omnibus (GEO). Data was log2 transformed if needed, and in the case of microarrays with multiple probe sets mapping to a single gene, the probe set with the highest variance across samples was selected. To test the association of *TAZ/WWTR1* or *YAP* with metastasis, expression values were compared using Welch's t-test or ANOVA. For survival analysis, samples were split into High and Low expression groups using the median as a bifurcation point and Kaplan-Meier curves were compared using the log-rank test. All graphical and statistical analyses were performed using GraphPad Prism version 5.0 software (La Jolla, CA, USA).

Canine OSA cell lines and culture conditions

Four different canine osteosarcoma cell lines were used for these studies: the commercially available D17 (OSA lung metastases) and the OVC-cOSA series, OVC-cOSA-31 (OSA lung metastases), OVC-cOSA-75 (primary OSA, distal tibia) and OVC-cOSA-78 (primary OSA, proximal humerus). The OVC-cOSA series of cell lines were generated at GAW Laboratory (Department of Pathobiology, University of Guelph, Guelph, Canada). Cells were maintained as monolayers in HyClone™ DMEM/High Glucose media (Sigma Aldrich), supplemented with 10% FBS (Fisher Scientific) and HyClone™ 1% Penicillin/Streptomycin (Sigma Aldrich), and cultured at 37 °C in a humidified incubator, in the presence of 95% atmospheric air and 5% CO_2. Cells were passaged once monolayers reached 100% confluency. Monolayers were first washed with PBS (Sigma Aldrich) and then detached with 1X Trypsin-EDTA (Sigma Aldrich) diluted in PBS and neutralized with media. Cells were then re-plated into fresh media at 1:4 split ratio. Media was changed every 3–4 days.

Cell lysate collection and immunoblotting

Cells were lysed with lysis buffer containing the following components: 1X lysis buffer (Cell Signaling Technology), 1 mM PMSF (Sigma Aldrich), 2 µg/mL aprotinin (Sigma Aldrich), 1% Phosphatase Inhibitor Cocktail (Sigma Aldrich), and 1 mM sodium orthovanadate (New England BioLabs). To collect lysates, dishes were placed on ice, washed with PBS, and lysis buffer supplemented with inhibitors was added to the plate for five minutes and subsequently harvested and incubated for thirty minutes. Lysates were centrifuged at 15000 rpm for 20 min at 4 °C. The supernatant was aliquoted and stored at – 80 °C until further use. Protein concentration was determined prior to Western Blotting using a Bradford assay (Bio-Rad, Mississauga, ON, Canada). A standard Western Blot protocol was then used to determine the levels of proteins of interest. For this purpose, 25 µg – 30 µg of protein lysates were resolved in a 10% polyacrylamide gel (Bio-Rad, Mississauga, ON, Canada) and transferred to a PVDF membrane (Sigma Aldrich) by wet transfer at 100 V for 2 h. Membranes were washed briefly with Tris Buffered Saline + 0.01% Tween (pH = 7.6, TBST) and blocked with either 5% skim milk or 5% bovine serum albumin (BSA) prepared in TBST, according to manufacturer's recommendations, for one hour at room temperature with gentle rocking. Membranes were then incubated with primary antibody (see catalog # in first section of Methods) diluted in blocking solution at the following dilutions: TAZ (1:40,000), YAP (1:1000), β-actin (1:5000), pSmad2 (1:1000), Smad2 (1:2000), pSmad3 (1:3000), Smad3 (1:3000), TβRI (1:1000) and TβRII (1:500) overnight at 4 °C on a rocking platform. The next day, membranes were washed three times with TBST (10 min/wash) and incubated with HRP-secondary antibody for 1 h at room temperature with rocking. Membranes were washed again three times with TBST (10 min/wash) and then incubated with Luminata Forte Western HRP Substrate (Fisher Scientific) for two minutes before imaging with ChemiDoc (BioRad). Densitometry was performed with ImageLab v4.0.1 (BioRad). All bands were normalized to β-actin, or their respective native protein, in the case of phosphorylated proteins.

siRNAs and transfection

The siRNAs used were purchased from Integrated DNA Technologies (IDT) (Coralville, IA, USA). All sequences were custom designed using the DsiRNA design tool on the IDT website. The accession number for canine TAZ and YAP mRNA sequences were first obtained using NCBI BLAST and then inputted into the DsiRNA design tool on IDT's website. Sequences generated from the website were randomly selected and are shown in Additional file 4: Table S1. Before experimentation, oligos were resuspended in Nuclease-Free Duplex Buffer (catalogue no. 11–01–03-01, IDT) at a concentration of 5 µM according to manufacturer's protocol. Optimization experiments were performed to determine optimal concentrations before use.

For siRNA transfection, cells were seeded at a concentration of 275, 000 cells in 35 mm dishes (for the Transwell assay) or 25,000 cells in 8 well chamber slides (for immunofluorescence). siRNA transfection was completed with Lipofectamine® 3000 (Invitrogen) according to manufacturer's protocol using a total siRNA concentration previously optimized for each cell line. For TAZ, a total concentration of 24 nM (12 nM of Duplex 1 and 3) was used for OVC-cOSA-78, 30 nM (15 nM of Duplex 1 and 3) for OVC-cOSA-75 and D17, and 24 nM (12 nM of Duplex 1 and 2) for OVC-cOSA-31. For YAP, 30 nM (15 nM of Duplex 1 and 3) was used for all cell lines. Twenty-four hours post transfection, cells were serum-starved (0.2% FBS and 1% Pen/Strep) for 6 h and then treated with 5 ng/mL TGFβ for 24-h. Post TGFβ treatment and depending on the assay, cells were either seeded in transwells for migration analysis, or fixed for immunofluorescence-based analysis of cell proliferation via immunolabelling of phospho-Histone H3 (pHH3).

Cell viability assay and doxorubicin treatment

Cells were transfected with siRNA as described above and then counted and seeded in a 96-well plate at varying densities, which were previously optimized: 40,000 cells/mL (D17), 80,000 cells/mL (OVC-cOSA-31) or 50,000 cells/mL (OVC-cOSA-75). After cells were allowed to adhere, Doxorubicin (kept at a stock concentration of 2 mg/mL), was directly added to the plate at the respective IC50 doses previously calculated for each cell line: 30 µM (D17), 26 µM (OVC-cOSA-31) or 60 µM (OVC-cOSA-75); media alones was added to the control (non-Doxorubicin treated) cells. Twenty-four hours after treatment, 15 µL of a working solution of resazurin (5 mg/mL diluted in PBS; obtained from Sigma catalog no. R7017) was added to each well and allowed to incubate at 37 °C for 6 h. Fluorescence was measured at 530/590 nm using a BioTek Synergy HT plate reader and Gen5 software (BioTek). Values obtained were blank-corrected to the media only control. Experimental groups were plated in technical duplicate and two independent experiments were completed.

Transwell migration assay

Cells treated as described above were counted and seeded at 2×10^4 cells/200 µL of media in Corning™ 8 µm pore inserts (Fisher Scientific) and placed into a 24-well Corning™ companion plate (Fisher Scientific) containing regular growth media (10% FBS, 1% Pen/Strep). Cells were incubated for 24 h, after which the media was removed from the insert and non-migrated cells were removed from the

top of the insert with a Q-tip moistened in PBS. Migrated cells were stained with 1% crystal violet for 25 min at room temperature with gentle rocking. Inserts were then rinsed and allowed to dry overnight. The inserts were then imaged using an inverted light microscope at 4X objective lens. To quantify the degree of cell movement, crystal violet stain was extracted with 10% acetic acid diluted in de-ionized water with vigorous rocking for 15 min. The extracted dye was then read at 590 nm with a spectrophotometer. All readings were blank corrected with an insert containing no cells. All experimental groups were seeded in duplicate and extracted dye readings were performed in triplicate.

Immunofluorescence Staining & Quantification of nuclear pHH3

Cells were fixed with 4% paraformaldehyde diluted in PBS for 15 min at room temperature and subsequently washed with PBS. Cells were then permeabilized with ice-cold methanol for 15 min, washed 3 times with PBS and blocked with 5% normal donkey serum (Sigma) for 1 h at room temperature. Cells were then incubated with pHH3 antibody diluted in 5% normal donkey serum at the following dilutions: OVC-cOSA-75 (1:5000), OVC-cOSA-78 (1:10,000), D17 and OVC-cOSA-31 (1: 20,000) overnight at 4 °C. The following day, cells were washed with PBS, and incubated with Alexa-Fluor 488 (Invitrogen) at room temperature for 1 h in the dark. Cells were then washed with PBS and incubated with 0.3 µM DAPI (Fisher) for 10 min at room temperature. Following this, cells were washed with PBS, and slides mounted with Dako fluorescent mounting medium. Cells were visualized with an epifluorescent microscope and imaged at 20X objective magnification. The total number of cells in the image was determined by counting the number of DAPI-stained nuclei in a 20X image using Nucleus Counter (ImageJ) software. The number of pHH3 positive cells was assessed visually. The number of relative pHH3 positive cells was determined by dividing the number of pHH3 positive cells by the number of nuclei present in the field of the view and multiplying by 100 to determine the percentage of mitotic cells. Five images were taken per experimental group and the average percentage was calculated.

TGFβ receptor I inhibitor (LY2157299) experiments

D17 cells were siRNA-transfected as described above in either 35 mm dishes (for protein analysis) or 8 well chamber slides (for pHH3 staining). Twenty hours post transfection, cells were serum starved for 6 h and subjected to one of four treatments: 5 ng/mL TGFβ, 10 µM of the TGFβ receptor I inhibitor LY2157299 (LY), a combination of TGFβ and LY inhibitor, or serum starvation media (media plus 0.2% FBS) alone (control).

Twenty-four hours after treatment, protein lysates were extracted, or the immunofluorescence protocol explained above was performed.

Statistical analyses

Chi square test was used to assess the association between pSmad2, TAZ, YAP and histologic grade, metastasis and alkaline phosphatase (ALP) status using GraphPad Prism v6.0c. Kaplan-Meier plots and log-rank (Mantel-Cox) tests were used to determine the correlations of pSmad2, TAZ, and YAP levels and time to metastasis and overall survival using GraphPad Prism v6.0c. For these analyses, the number of days was calculated from the date of diagnosis with OSA (radiographic or histologic) to the endpoint of confirmation of clinical metastasis detection through radiography or clinical presentation (days to metastasis) or date of death due to OSA (overall survival). The endpoint of the study was June 12, 2018; if records did not indicate the patient experienced the event, they were censored accordingly. For in vitro studies assessing the effect of TGFβ on Smad activation, TAZ and YAP expression, significant differences in protein expression were determined using an independent t-test between control and TGFβ-treated cells. A two-way ANOVA and a Tukey-Kramer post hoc test were used to assess the effect of TGFβ and TAZ or YAP knockdown on cell migration and proliferation using GraphPad Prism v6.0c. For cell viability experiments, a one-way ANOVA Kruskal-Wallis test and a Dunn-Sidak post hoc was used to compare treatments to control within each, the minus Doxorubicin and the plus Doxorubicin group. All tests completed were two-sided, with a p-value < 0.05 considered statistically significant.

Additional files

Additional file 1: Figure S1. Immunoblotting of TAZ (WWTR1) and YAP in canine osteosarcoma cell lines to determine antibody specificity. TAZ antibody (cat no. HPA007415, Sigma-Aldrich) was used at a 1:80,000 dilution. The blot demonstrated a strong band at the predicted weight of 55 kDa (arrow) and slight reactivity to YAP. YAP antibody (cat no. D8H1X, Cell Signalling), used at a 1:1,000 dilution, identified a strong band at the predicted weight of 65 kDa (arrow).

Additional file 2: Figure S2. Representative immunoblots and densitometry demonstrating reduction in TAZ protein levels post siRNA transfection at 24 hours. TAZ levels were decreased with siRNA treatment by varying levels, as indicated by the percentages, when compared to the siRNA control (siCtrl), while YAP levels remained fairly consistent. Experimental groups were normalized to loading control β-actin. Graphs depict the average fold change in TAZ or YAP expression relative to siCtrl ± SEM from three independent experiments.

Additional file 3: Figure S3. Representative immunoblots and densitometry demonstrating reduction in YAP protein levels post siRNA transfection at 24 hours. YAP levels were decreased with siRNA treatment by varying levels, as indicated by the percentages, when compared to the siRNA control (siCtrl), while TAZ levels were not affected. Experimental groups were normalized to loading control β-actin. Graphs depict the average fold change in TAZ or YAP expression relative to siCtrl ± SEM from three independent experiments.

Additional file 4: Table S1. Duplex Sequences.

Abbreviations
ALP: Alkaline phosphatase; OSA: Osteosarcoma; SOC: Standard of care; TAZ: Transcriptional co-activator with a PDZ binding motif; TEAD: TEA domain DNA-binding family of transcription factors; TGFβ: Transforming growth factor beta; TMA: Tissue microarray; YAP: Yes associated protein

Acknowledgements
We dedicate this work to the late Helen Coates, for her invaluable advice during the optimization steps of the immunohistochemistry in this study and all the help she provided to our group over the years.

Funding
Authors would like to acknowledge financial support provided by OVC Pet Trust to A. M. Viloria-Petit (grant # 052655) and G. A. Wood (grant # 050411).

Authors' contributions
AKL drafted the manuscript and performed and analysed all experiments with the exception of the mRNA data set analysis, part of the doxorubicin treatment experiments, and the staining and quantification of the YAP TMA; CRS developed the TMA, performed histologic grading and organized all patient data; RJ performed all analyses with mRNA datasets; ACP performed the doxorubicin response experiments, analyzed the data generated, and provided advice for other experiments that were necessary to address reviewer's concerns; BG performed the IHC for the YAP TMA and imaged tissue samples; BG and RH both quantified tissue samples and performed the analyses. AJM provided reagents and expertise for doxorubicin response experiments; AVP created Figs. 3 and 4; BD, GAW and AVP provided the original idea for this study; GAW and AVP guided experimental design; all authors edited and revised the manuscript. All authors read and approved the final manuscript.

Consent for publication
Non-applicable.

Competing interests
The authors declare that they have no competing interests.

Author details
[1]Department of Biomedical Sciences, Ontario Veterinary College, University of Guelph, 50 Stone Road East, Guelph, ON N1G 2W1, Canada. [2]Department of Pathobiology, Ontario Veterinary College, University of Guelph, 50 Stone Road East, Guelph, ON N1G 2W1, Canada. [3]Medical City Forth Worth, HCA affiliated Hospital, 900 8th Ave, Fort Worth, TX 76104, USA.

References
1. Rowell JL, McCarthy DO, Alvarez CE. Dog models of naturally occurring cancer. Trends Mol Med. 2011;17(7):380–8.
2. Chun R, Kurzman ID, Couto CG, Klausner J, Henry C, MacEwen EG. Cisplatin and doxorubicin combination chemotherapy for the treatment of canine osteosarcoma: a pilot study. J Vet Intern Med. 2000;14(5):495–8.
3. McMahon M, Mathie T, Stingle N, Romansik E, Vail D, London C. Adjuvant carboplatin and gemcitabine combination chemotherapy postamputation in canine appendicular osteosarcoma. J Vet Intern Med. 2011;25(3):511–7.

4. Buijs JT, Stayrook KR, Guise TA. TGF-beta in the bone microenvironment: role in breast Cancer metastases. Cancer Microenviron. 2011;4(3):261–81.

5. Wu M, Chen G, Li YP. TGF-beta and BMP signaling in osteoblast, skeletal development, and bone formation, homeostasis and disease. Bone Res. 2016;4:16009.

6. Gilbert RWD, Vickaryous MK, Viloria-Petit AM. Signalling by Transforming. Growth Factor Beta Isoforms in Wound Healing and Tissue Regeneration. J Dev Biol. 2016;4(2):21.

7. Franchi A, Arganini L, Baroni G, Calzolari A, Capanna R, Campanacci D, Caldora P, Masi L, Brandi ML, Zampi G. Expression of transforming growth factor beta isoforms in osteosarcoma variants: association of TGF beta 1 with high-grade osteosarcomas. J Pathol. 1998;185(3):284–9.

8. Kloen P, Gebhardt MC, Perez-Atayde A, Rosenberg AE, Springfield DS, Gold LI, Mankin HJ. Expression of transforming growth factor-beta (TGF-beta) isoforms in osteosarcomas: TGF-beta3 is related to disease progression. Cancer. 1997;80(12):2230–9.

9. Chen Y, Guo Y, Yang H, Shi G, Xu G, Shi J, Yin N, Chen D. TRIM66 overexpresssion contributes to osteosarcoma carcinogenesis and indicates poor survival outcome. Oncotarget. 2015;6(27):23708–19.

10. Li F, Li S, Cheng T. TGF-beta1 promotes osteosarcoma cell migration and invasion through the miR-143-versican pathway. Cell Physiol Biochem. 2014; 34(6):2169–79.

11. Portela RF, Fadl-Alla BA, Pondenis HC, Byrum ML, Garrett LD, Wycislo KL, Borst LB, Fan TM. Pro-tumorigenic effects of transforming growth factor beta 1 in canine osteosarcoma. J Vet Intern Med. 2014;28(3):894–904.

12. Zhang H, Wu H, Zheng J, Yu P, Xu L, Jiang P, Gao J, Wang H, Zhang Y. Transforming growth factor beta1 signal is crucial for dedifferentiation of cancer cells to cancer stem cells in osteosarcoma. Stem Cells. 2013;31(3):433–46.

13. Singh A, Settleman J. EMT, cancer stem cells and drug resistance: an emerging axis of evil in the war on cancer. Oncogene. 2010;29(34):4741–51.

14. Varelas X, Sakuma R, Samavarchi-Tehrani P, Peerani R, Rao BM, Dembowy J, Yaffe MB, Zandstra PW, Wrana JL. TAZ controls Smad nucleocytoplasmic shuttling and regulates human embryonic stem-cell self-renewal. Nat Cell Biol. 2008;10(7):837–48.

15. Varelas X. The hippo pathway effectors TAZ and YAP in development, homeostasis and disease. Development. 2014;141(8):1614–26.

16. Cui CB, Cooper LF, Yang X, Karsenty G, Aukhil I. Transcriptional coactivation of bone-specific transcription factor Cbfa1 by TAZ. Mol Cell Biol. 2003; 23(3):1004–13.

17. Hong JH, Yaffe MB. TAZ: a beta-catenin-like molecule that regulates mesenchymal stem cell differentiation. Cell Cycle. 2006;5(2):176–9.

18. Zhao L, Jiang S, Hantash BM. Transforming growth factor beta1 induces osteogenic differentiation of murine bone marrow stromal cells. Tissue Eng Part A. 2010;16(2):725–33.

19. Hiemer SE, Varelas X. Stem cell regulation by the hippo pathway. Biochim Biophys Acta. 2013;1830(2):2323–34.

20. Bartucci M, Dattilo R, Moriconi C, Pagliuca A, Mottolese M, Federici G, Benedetto AD, Todaro M, Stassi G, Sperati F, et al. TAZ is required for metastatic activity and chemoresistance of breast cancer stem cells. Oncogene. 2015;34(6):681–90.

21. Cordenonsi M, Zanconato F, Azzolin L, Forcato M, Rosato A, Frasson C, Inui M, Montagner M, Parenti AR, Poletti A, et al. The hippo transducer TAZ confers cancer stem cell-related traits on breast cancer cells. Cell. 2011; 147(4):759–72.

22. Hiemer SE, Szymaniak AD, Varelas X. The transcriptional regulators TAZ and YAP direct transforming growth factor beta-induced tumorigenic phenotypes in breast cancer cells. J Biol Chem. 2014;289(19):13461–74.

23. Fullenkamp CA, Hall SL, Jaber OI, Pakalniskis BL, Savage EC, Savage JM, Ofori-Amanfo GK, Lambertz AM, Ivins SD, Stipp CS, et al. TAZ and YAP are frequently activated oncoproteins in sarcomas. Oncotarget. 2016; 7(21):30094–108.

24. Bouvier C, Macagno N, Nguyen Q, Loundou A, Jiguet-Jiglaire C, Gentet JC, Jouve JL, Rochwerger A, Mattei JC, Bouvard D, et al. Prognostic value of the hippo pathway transcriptional coactivators YAP/TAZ and beta1-integrin in conventional osteosarcoma. Oncotarget. 2016;7(40):64702–10.

25. Wang DY, Wu YN, Huang JQ, Wang W, Xu M, Jia JP, Han G, Mao BB, Bi WZ. Hippo/YAP signaling pathway is involved in osteosarcoma chemoresistance. Chin J Cancer. 2016;35:47.

26. Beffagna G, Sacchetto R, Cavicchioli L, Sammarco A, Mainenti M, Ferro S, Trez D, Zulpo M, Michieletto S, Cecchinato A, et al. A preliminary investigation of the role of the transcription co-activators YAP/TAZ of the

27. hippo signalling pathway in canine and feline mammary tumours. Vet J. 2016;207:105–11.

27. Guillemette S, Rico C, Godin P, Boerboom D, Paquet M. In vitro validation of the hippo pathway as a pharmacological target for canine mammary gland tumors. J Mammary Gland Biol Neoplasia. 2017;22(3):203–14.

28. Kirpensteijn J, Kik M, Rutteman GR, Teske E. Prognostic significance of a new histologic grading system for canine osteosarcoma. Vet Pathol. 2002;39(2): 240–6.

29. Loukopoulos P, Robinson WF. Clinicopathological relevance of tumour grading in canine osteosarcoma. J Comp Pathol. 2007;136(1):65–73.

30. Kobayashi E, Masuda M, Nakayama R, Ichikawa H, Satow R, Shitashige M, Honda K, Yamaguchi U, Shoji A, Tochigi N, et al. Reduced argininosuccinate synthetase is a predictive biomarker for the development of pulmonary metastasis in patients with osteosarcoma. Mol Cancer Ther. 2010;9(3):535–44.

31. Namlos HM, Kresse SH, Muller CR, Henriksen J, Holdhus R, Saeter G, Bruland OS, Bjerkehagen B, Steen VM, Myklebost O. Global gene expression profiling of human osteosarcomas reveals metastasis-associated chemokine pattern. Sarcoma. 2012;2012:639038.

32. Kelly AD, Haibe-Kains B, Janeway KA, Hill KE, Howe E, Goldsmith J, Kurek K, Perez-Atayde AR, Francoeur N, Fan JB, et al. MicroRNA paraffin-based studies in osteosarcoma reveal reproducible independent prognostic profiles at 14q32. Genome Med. 2013;5(1):2.

33. Scott MC, Sarver AL, Gavin KJ, Thayanithy V, Getzy DM, Newman RA, Cutter GR, Lindblad-Toh K, Kisseberth WC, Hunter LE, et al. Molecular subtypes of osteosarcoma identified by reducing tumor heterogeneity through an interspecies comparative approach. Bone. 2011;49(3):356–67.

34. Baglio SR, Lagerweij T, Perez-Lanzon M, Ho XD, Leveille N, Melo SA, Cleton-Jansen AM, Jordanova ES, Roncuzzi L, Greco M, et al. Blocking tumor-educated MSC paracrine activity halts osteosarcoma progression. Clin Cancer Res. 2017; 23(14):3721–33.

35. Lamora A, Talbot J, Bougras G, Amiaud J, Leduc M, Chesneau J, Taurelle J, Stresing V, Le Deley MC, Heymann MF, et al. Overexpression of smad7 blocks primary tumor growth and lung metastasis development in osteosarcoma. Clin Cancer Res. 2014;20(19):5097–112.

36. Yang R, Piperdi S, Zhang Y, Zhu Z, Neophytou N, Hoang BH, Mason G, Geller D, Dorfman H, Meyers PA, et al. Transcriptional profiling identifies the signaling axes of IGF and transforming growth factor-b as involved in the pathogenesis of osteosarcoma. Clin Orthop Relat Res. 2016;474(1):178–89.

37. Yu FX, Zhao B, Guan KL. Hippo pathway in organ size control, tissue homeostasis, and Cancer. Cell. 2015;163(4):811–28.

38. Schott CR, Tatiersky LJ, Foster RA, Wood GA. Histologic grade does not predict outcome in dogs with appendicular osteosarcoma receiving the standard of care. Vet Pathol. 2018;55(2):202–11.

39. Zhang YH, Li B, Shen L, Shen Y, Chen XD. The role and clinical significance of YES-associated protein 1 in human osteosarcoma. Int J Immunopathol Pharmacol. 2013;26(1):157–67.

40. Boerman I, Selvarajah GT, Nielen M, Kirpensteijn J. Prognostic factors in canine appendicular osteosarcoma - a meta-analysis. BMC Vet Res. 2012;8:56.

41. Garzotto CK, Berg J, Hoffmann WE, Rand WM. Prognostic significance of serum alkaline phosphatase activity in canine appendicular osteosarcoma. J Vet Intern Med. 2000;14(6):587–92.

42. Schmidt AF, Nielen M, Klungel OH, Hoes AW, de Boer A, Groenwold RH, Kirpensteijn J, Investigators VSSO. Prognostic factors of early metastasis and mortality in dogs with appendicular osteosarcoma after receiving surgery: an individual patient data meta-analysis. Prev Vet Med. 2013; 112(3–4):414–22.

43. Holmes KE, Thompson V, Piskun CM, Kohnken RA, Huelsmeyer MK, Fan TM, Stein TJ. Canine osteosarcoma cell lines from patients with differing serum alkaline phosphatase concentrations display no behavioural differences in vitro. Vet Comp Oncol. 2015;13(3):166–75.

44. Rodrigues LC, Holmes KE, Thompson V, Piskun CM, Lana SE, Newton MA, Stein TJ. Osteosarcoma tissues and cell lines from patients with differing serum alkaline phosphatase concentrations display minimal differences in gene expression patterns. Vet Comp Oncol. 2016;14(2):e58–69.

45. Selvarajah GT, Kirpensteijn J, van Wolferen ME, Rao NA, Fieten H, Mol JA. Gene expression profiling of canine osteosarcoma reveals genes associated with short and long survival times. Mol Cancer. 2009;8:72.

46. He M, Zhou Z, Shah AA, Hong Y, Chen Q, Wan Y. New insights into posttranslational modifications of hippo pathway in carcinogenesis and therapeutics. Cell Div. 2016;11:4.

47. Ehmer U, Sage J. Control of proliferation and Cancer growth by the hippo signaling pathway. Mol Cancer Res. 2016;14(2):127–40.
48. Zhang Y, Alexander PB, Wang XF. TGF-beta family signaling in the control of cell proliferation and survival. Cold Spring Harb Perspect Biol. 2017;9(4).
49. Yang Z, Zhang M, Xu K, Liu L, Hou WK, Cai YZ, Xu P, Yao JF. Knockdown of YAP1 inhibits the proliferation of osteosarcoma cells in vitro and in vivo. Oncol Rep. 2014;32(3):1265–72.
50. Shen S, Huang K, Wu Y, Ma Y, Wang J, Qin F, Ma J. A miR-135b-TAZ positive feedback loop promotes epithelial-mesenchymal transition (EMT) and tumorigenesis in osteosarcoma. Cancer Lett. 2017;407:32–44.
51. Ma J, Huang K, Ma Y, Zhou M, Fan S. The TAZ-miR-224-SMAD4 axis promotes tumorigenesis in osteosarcoma. Cell Death Dis. 2017;8(1):e2539.
52. Selmic LE, Burton JH, Thamm DH, Withrow SJ, Lana SE. Comparison of carboplatin and doxorubicin-based chemotherapy protocols in 470 dogs after amputation for treatment of appendicular osteosarcoma. J Vet Intern Med. 2014;28(2):554–63.
53. Chan SW, Lim CJ, Loo LS, Chong YF, Huang C, Hong W. TEADs mediate nuclear retention of TAZ to promote oncogenic transformation. J Biol Chem. 2009;284(21):14347–58.
54. Allred DC, Harvey JM, Berardo M, Clark GM. Prognostic and predictive factors in breast cancer by immunohistochemical analysis. Mod Pathol. 1998;11(2):155–68.

22

Notch2 signal is required for the maintenance of canine hemangiosarcoma cancer stem cell-like cells

Keisuke Aoshima*[iD], Yuki Fukui, Kevin Christian Montecillo Gulay, Ochbayar Erdemsurakh, Atsuya Morita, Atsushi Kobayashi and Takashi Kimura

Abstract

Background: Hemangiosarcoma (HSA) is a malignant tumor derived from endothelial cells which usually shows poor prognosis due to its high invasiveness, metastatic rate and severe hemorrhage from tumor ruptures. Since the pathogenesis of HSA is not yet complete, further understanding of its molecular basis is required.

Results: Here, we identified Notch2 signal as a key factor in maintaining canine HSA cancer stem cell (CSC)-like cells. We first cultured HSA cell lines in adherent serum-free condition and confirmed their CSC-like characteristics. Notch signal was upregulated in the CSC-like cells and Notch signal inhibition by a γ-secretase inhibitor significantly repressed their growth. Notch2, a Notch receptor, was highly expressed in the CSC-like cells. Constitutive activation of Notch2 increased clonogenicity and number of cells which were able to survive in serum-free condition. In contrast, inhibition of Notch2 activity showed opposite effects. These results suggest that Notch2 is an important factor for maintaining HSA CSC-like cells. Neoplastic cells in clinical cases also express Notch2 higher than endothelial cells in the normal blood vessels in the same slides.

Conclusion: This study provides foundation for further stem cell research in HSA and can provide a way to develop effective treatments to CSCs of endothelial tumors.

Keywords: Cancer stem cell-like cells, Hemangiosarcoma, Notch2, Oncology, Tumor Biology

Background

Hemangiosarcoma (HSA) is a malignant tumor derived from endothelial cells which commonly occurs in dogs (*Canis lupus familiaris*) [1]. Other animals and humans can have similar tumors but the occurrence is very rare [1, 2]. Most preferred sites in dogs are the liver, spleen, and right atrium of the heart [3–5]. Patients show poor prognosis due to its aggressive invasion to adjacent tissues, high metastatic rate, and blood loss from tumor ruptures [6, 7]. Surgical excision of tumor masses or affected organs and chemotherapy are the preferred treatment methods, however, survival time after treatment may not significantly increase [8, 9]. Furthermore, patients may suffer from severe side effects induced by chemotherapeutic drugs such as myelosuppression and cardiotoxicity, which can limit the survival time extension in treated humans and animals [10, 11]. Therefore, novel effective treatments which can selectively target neoplastic cells have been warranted for decades [9].

Tumors, in general, are composed of many types of cells at various differentiation states and form cellular hierarchy in which cancer stem cells (CSCs) are located at the top [12, 13]. CSCs are a source of neoplastic cells which form tumor masses and are also involved in tumor recurrence after surgical excision, chemotherapy, or radiotherapy [12, 13]. Therefore, CSCs can be a good therapeutic target to completely eliminate tumors [13–15]. Using adult stem cell markers for normal tissues, CSC-like cells have been identified from many types of cancers including leukemia, breast cancer, and melanoma [16–18]. CSCs of HSA, however, have not yet been

* Correspondence: k-aoshima@vetmed.hokudai.ac.jp
Laboratory of Comparative Pathology, Department of Clinical Veterinary Sciences, Faculty of Veterinary Medicine, Hokkaido University, Kita 18 Nishi 9, Kita-ku, Sapporo, Hokkaido 060-0818, Japan

identified and adult stem cell markers for endothelial cells are also still unknown.

Notch, a type I transmembrane protein, has four identified types (Notch1 to 4). Notch receives signals from neighboring cells expressing the ligands and transduces these signals by translocation of the intracellular domain into the nucleus [19, 20]. Notch signal is demonstrated to be highly involved in several biological events such as stem cell maintenance, cellular differentiation, angiogenesis, and tumorigenesis [21–24]. CSCs of several types of tumors use Notch signaling to communicate with tumor microenvironment in order to maintain their stemness [25–29]. Notch signal disruption has been reported to be associated with irregular vascular proliferation and vascular tumors in humans and mice [30–32]. Canine HSA is hypothesized to be regulated by the signal transduction, though the role of Notch in HSA has not yet been studied.

The aim of this study was to isolate CSC-like cells from canine HSA cell lines and investigate the role of Notch signaling in HSA CSC-like cells.

Methods
Cell culture
We used seven hemangiosarcoma cell lines (JuA1, JuB2, JuB4, Ud2, Ud6, Re12, and Re21) kindly given by Dr. Hiroki Sakai, Gifu University [33]. Human embryonic kidney 293 T cell line and HeLa cell line derived from human cervical cancer were purchased from RIKEN BioResource Research Center. These cells were cultured with Dulbecco's Modified Eagle's Medium (D-MEM; Wako, Osaka, Japan) supplemented with 10% fetal bovine serum (FBS; Biowest, UT, USA) and Penicillin/Streptomycin (Thermo Fisher Scientific, MA, USA). For serum free culture, cells were seeded in culture plates coated with 0.1% gelatin (Wako) and cultured with Dulbecco's Modified Eagle's Medium/ Nutrient Mixture F-12 Ham (Wako) supplemented with 10 ng/ml basic fibroblast growth factor (bFGF; Wako), 20 ng/ml epidermal growth factor (EGF; Thermo Fisher Scientific), NS Supplement (Wako) and Penicillin/Streptomycin [34–37]. Cells in both conditions were maintained at 37 °C with 5% CO_2 prior to use in experiments. Cells were maintained under serum-free condition at least 2 weeks prior to the experiments. Cells were stained with Trypan Blue (Thermo Fisher Scientific) to stain dead cells and only the unstained, viable cells were used for determining cell number.

Notch signal inhibition
A γ-secretase inhibitor, N-[N-(3,5-Difluorophenacetyl)--L-alanyl]-S-phenylglycine t-butyl estel (DAPT; Wako), was added to culture medium and dimethyl sulfoxide (DMSO) was used as the control. To find out the appropriate DAPT concentration, expression levels of Notch signal target genes (HES1 and HEY1) were analyzed in HSA cell lines treated with DAPT or DMSO for 48 h. To make the growth curves, 5×10^3 cells were seeded in 12-well plates in triplicate and were cultured in the medium containing 20 μM DAPT or DMSO. The cell numbers were counted at each passage point followed by reseeding of 5×10^3 cells into 12-well plates. This procedure was repeated three or four times and the relative cell number was counted as the cell number at each passage point normalized to the original seeding cell count.

Reverse transcription quantitative polymerase chain reaction (RT-qPCR)
Total RNA was extracted with TriPure Isolation Reagent (Roche, Basel, Switzerland) according to the manufacturer's instructions. Reverse transcription was performed using Primescript II 1st strand cDNA Synthesis Kit (Takara Bio, Kusatsu, Japan) according to the manufacturer's instructions after treatment with DNaseI (Thermo Fisher Scientific) for 15 mins at room temperature (RT) followed by EDTA treatment for 10 mins at 65 °C. Sample preparation for qPCR was performed using KAPA SYBR FAST qPCR Kit Master Mix (2×) ABI Prism (KAPA Biosystems, MA, USA). Reaction solution contains 1× KAPA SYBR FAST qPCR Master Mix, 200 nM forward and reverse primers, 1 μl cDNA and UltraPure DNase/RNase-free distilled water (UPDW, Thermo Fisher Scientific). The samples were applied in triplicate and analyzed by StepOne Real-time PCR system (Thermo Fisher Scientific). UPDW and no RT samples were used as negative controls. We confirmed that no signal was detected in the negative controls for all samples. Samples were denatured at 95 °C for 3 min followed by 40 cycles of 95 °C for 3 s and 60 ° C for 20 s. Results were normalized based on geometric mean of reference genes (GAPDH, ACTB, HMBS). Reference genes were selected from nine potential internal controls (GAPDH, ACTB, B2N, HMBS, HPRT1, RPL13A, RPL32, TBP, YWHAZ) by geNorm software [38, 39]. Primer sequences for qPCR are listed in Table 1. Ensembl and Primer3 softwares were used to design 80 to 150 bp primers which can target all splice variants and cross exon-exon junctions. The BLAST database and software were used to confirm that each primer sequence is not detected in other genes. The HES1 primer and potential internal control primer set sequences were obtained from a journal article published elsewhere [39, 40]. Primer efficiency was calculated based on the slope obtained from each standard curve and was confirmed to be more than 90% for all primer sequences (Additional files 1 and 2: Figures S1 and S2). Primer set specificity was evaluated by checking that each primer set have identical and singular peak in the melting curve.

Table 1 Primer list for RT-qPCR

Primer	Sequence		Gene ID and references	Efficiency (%)
	Forward primer	Reverse primer		
ERG	CAAACATGACCACGAACGAG	AGGCCGTATTCTTTCACTGC	ENSCAFG 00000009912	98.4
PROCR	GCAGGAACACAATGCTTCAA	AAGATGCCTACAGCCACACC	ENSCAFG 00000007945	95.5
SOX18	TGAACGCCTTCATGGTGTG	GGCGTCAGCTCCTTCCAC	ENSCAFG 00000029278	94.5
FLI1	TACTGAACAAAGGCCCCAAC	ACTGTCCGAGAGAAGCTCCA	ENSCAFG 00000032412	96.9
NOTCH1	TACCGGCCAGAACTGTGAGGAGAA	GGAGGGCAGCGGCAGTTGTAAGTA	ENSCAFG 00000019633	93.6
NOTCH2	TCGGGATAGCTATGAGCCCT	GGCATGTTGCTTTCCCCAAC	ENSCAFG 00000010476	93.6
NOTCH3	ACAACTGCCAGTGTCCTCCT	GTCCAGCCATTGACACACAC	ENSCAFG 00000016107	93.9
NOTCH4	AAGCCCTGTCCACACAATTC	CTGGCATAGGGAAGAAGCTG	ENSCAFG 00000000791	95.4
HEY1	GCGCGGATGAGAATGGAAAC	GTCGGCGCTTCTCAATGATG	ENSCAFG 00000008391	95.3
HEY2	CGGCGAGATCGGATAAATAA	CGCGTCGAAGTAGCCTTTAC	XM_541232.5 ENSCAFG 00000032212	96.4
HES1	CATCCAAGCCTATCATGGAGA	GTTCCGGAGGTGCTTCACT	Dailey DD et al.	95.5
HES6	CAGGCCAAGCTGGAGAAC	GCATGCACTGGATGTAGCC	ENSCAFG 00000012428	96.5
NRARP	TGAAGCTGCTGGTCAAGTTC	CTTGGCCTTGGTGATGAGAT	ENSCAFG 00000019445	94.5
FCER2	GAGGAGGTGGAGAAGCTGTG	CCTCGCCGAAGTAGTAGCAC	ENSCAFG 00000030055	97.5
GAPDH	ATTCCACGGCACAGTCAAG	TACTCAGCACCAGCATCACC	ENSCAFG 00000015077	99.5
ACTB	CCAGCAAGGATGAAGATCAAG	TCTGCTGGAAGGTGGACAG	ENSCAFG 00000016020 Peters IR. et al.	98.8
HMBS	TCACCATCGGAGCCATCT	GTTCCCACCACGCTCTTCT	ENSCAFG 00000012342 Peters IR. et al	95.8
RPL13A	GCCGGAAGGTTGTAGTCGT	GGAGGAAGGCCAGGTAATTC	ENSCAFG 00000029892 Peters IR. et al	98.2
RPL32	TGGTTACAGGAGCAACAAGAAA	GCACATCAGCAGCACTTCA	ENSCAFG 00000004871 Peters IR. et al	95.9
HPRT1	CACTGGGAAAACAATGCAGA	ACAAAGTCAGGTTTATAGCCAACA	ENSCAFG 00000018870 Peters IR. et al	95.7
B2M	ACGGAAAGGAGATGAAAGCA	CCTGCTCATTGGGAGTGAA	ENSCAFG 00000013633 Peters IR. et al	98.2
YWHAZ	CGAAGTTGCTGCTGGTGA	TTGCATTTCCTTTTTGCTGA	ENSCAFG 00000000580 Peters IR. et al	93.4
TBP	ATAAGAGAGCCCCGAACCAC	TTCACATCACAGCTCCCCAC	ENSCAFG 00000004119 Peters IR. et al	97.3

Colony formation assay (CFA)

One thousand cells were seeded in 6-well culture plates and were cultured until the diameter of the biggest colony reached 2 mm. Cells were fixed with 4% paraformaldehyde for 20 mins at RT and then stained with Crystal Violet (Sigma-Aldrich, MO, USA) for 30 mins at RT. After washing with phosphate buffered saline (PBS) and drying at RT, colonies were visualized using an inverted microscope (Eclipse TS100; Nikon, Tokyo, Japan) and colonies which have more than 50 cells were counted [41].

Chemoresistance assay

Three (normal culture) or five (serum-free culture) thousand cells seeded in 96-well culture plates and were treated with either DMSO, doxorubicin (Wako) or paclitaxel (Wako) at increasing concentrations the following day. Soon after the treatments, culture medium in each cell lines were collected and the absorbance at the time of treatment (Tz) was measured. Seventy-two hours after treatment, cell viability was analyzed using Cell Counting Kit-8 (Dojindo, Kumamoto, Japan) according to the manufacturer's instructions. The absorbance of each well 72 h after treatments (Ti) was measured at 450 nm using NanoDrop 2000 (Thermo Fisher Scientific). DMSO treated cells were used as the control (C). Growth inhibition rates were measured as: $[(Ti-Tz)/(C-Tz)] \times 100$ for concentrations in which $Ti >/= Tz$, $[(Ti-Tz)/Tz] \times 100$ for concentrations in which $Ti < Tz$ [42].

Aldehyde dehydrogenase (ALDH) assay

To analyze ALDH activity, ALDEFLUOR kit (STEMCELL technologies, Vancouver, Canada) was used according to the manufacturer's instructions. We stained 5×10^5 cells with ALDEFLUOR reagent for 50 mins at 37 °C. N,N-diethylaminobenzaldehyde (DEAB) was used to inhibit ALDH activity and DEAB treated cells were used as basis to gate ALDH positive population. The cells were analyzed using FACS-Verse (Becton Dickinson, NJ, USA) after excluding the dead cells which were positive for 7-aminoactinomycin D (Thermo Fisher Scientific). The data was analyzed using FACSuite software (Becton Dickinson).

Protein extraction and western blotting

Cells were lysed using Radioimmunoprecipitation buffer [RiPA buffer; 50 mM Tris-HCl (pH 8.0), 150 mM NaCl, 0.1% TritonX-100, 0.1% sodium dodecyl sulfate (SDS), 0.5% sodium deoxycholate, EDTA-free proteinase inhibitor cocktail (Sigma-Aldrich)]. Protein concentration was measured using Pierce BCA Protein Assay Kit (Thermo Fisher Scientific) according to the manufacturer's instruction. Samples were denatured by adding 1/4 volume of 4 × Sample buffer [200 mM Tris-HCl buffer (pH 6.8), 8% SDS, 40% Glycerol, 1% bromophenol blue, 20% 2-mercaptoethanol] to each sample followed by incubation at 98 °C for 5 mins. Ten

micrograms proteins were separated in 8% SDS polyacrylamide gels by electrophoresis and were transferred to polyvinylidene difluoride membrane (PVDF membrane: Merck Millipore, MA, USA) using Mini Trans-Blot Cell (BIO-RAD, CA, USA). Membranes were then blocked in 5% skim milk in Tris-buffered saline containing 0.05% Tween 20 (TBST) for 1 h at RT. Membranes were either incubated with anti-human Notch2 intracellular domain antibody (R&D systems, MN, USA; 1:2000), anti-FLAG M2 monoclonal antibody (Sigma-Aldrich; 1:1000) or anti-Actin antibody clone C4 (Merck Millipore; 1:10,000) overnight at 4 °C. After washing with TBST, membranes were incubated with donkey anti-goat IgG-HRP (Santa cruz, TX, USA; 1:5000) or ECL Mouse IgG HRP-linked whole antibody (GE Healthcare, IL, USA; 1:10,000) for 1 h at RT. After washing with TBST, signals were visualized with Immobilon Western Chemiluminescent HRP substrate (Merck Millipore) and detected by ImageQuant LAS 4000 mini (GE Healthcare). Images were processed with ImageJ software [43–45].

Plasmid construction

Canine NOTCH2 gene (ENSCAFG00000010476) cloned from the cDNA of Canine Aortic Endothelial Cells (CnAOEC; Cell Applications, CA, USA) was subcloned into a self-inactivating (SIN) lentiviral vector construct, CSII-CMV-MCS-IRES2-Bsd. To make the dominant negative form and constitutive active form of Notch2, 1–5343 bp and 5161–7413 bp of NOTCH2 were amplified from full length NOTCH2 gene, respectively [46]. These two mutants were also subcloned into the SIN lentiviral vector construct. FLAG sequences were added at the C-terminus of full length and mutant Notch2 constructs by inverse PCR.

Lentivirus infection

We seeded 8×10^5 293 T cells in a 6 cm dish and cultured in antibiotic-free medium. Cells were transfected, using Lipofectamine 3000 (Thermo Fisher Scientific) according to the manufacturer's instructions, with three constructs; a packaging construct (pCAG-HIVgp), a VSV-G and Rev expressing construct (pCMV-VSV-G-RSV-Rec) and SIN lentiviral vector constructs. Forty-eight hours after transfection, culture media containing the produced viruses were collected in 15 mL tubes and centrifuged at 6000 g for 16 h at 4 °C. Pellets were resuspended in normal culture medium and used as virus reagent. Cells were cultured in the virus reagent with 8 μg/ml Polybrene (Sigma-Aldrich). Eight hours after infection, the medium in cell culture wells was replaced with a fresh medium without the viruses. Forty-eight hours later, culture medium was changed to normal medium supplemented with 10 μg/ml Blasticidin for selection and the cells were maintained for future experiments.

Immunohistochemistry (IHC)

Twelve canine HSA cases collected from Hokkaido University Veterinary Teaching Hospital were used for IHC. These cases were derived from the spleen, liver, kidney and thoracic cavity (Table 2). Tissue samples were processed routinely as described previously [47]. The slides were immersed in 10 mM sodium citrate buffer (pH 6.0), boiled for 15 mins in a microwave for antigen retrieval and then cooled down to RT. After washing with PBS, sections were treated with 0.3% H_2O_2 in methanol for 15 mins at RT to inactivate endogenous peroxidases followed by blocking with 10% rabbit normal serum (Nichirei biosciences, Tokyo, Japan) for 1 h at RT. Sections were incubated with anti-human Notch2 intracellular domain antibody (R&D systems; 1:40) for overnight at 4 °C. PBS instead of the primary antibody was added to the negative controls. After washing with PBS, sections were treated with biotinylated anti-goat IgG (Nichirei biosciences) for 1 h at RT followed by incubation with peroxidase conjugated streptavidin (Nichirei biosciences) for 10 mins at RT. After washing with PBS, signal detection was carried out by submerging the sections in freshly prepared solution of 3,3′-diaminobenzidine tetrahydrochloride (Dojindo, Kumamoto, Japan) for 5 mins, and the sections were counterstained with hematoxylin for 1 min and then dehydrated and mounted with cover glasses. Signals were captured with BX63 microscope (Olympus, Tokyo, Japan) and processed with ImageJ software.

Statistical analyses

For the comparison of gene expression between two samples, Student's t test was performed. Dunnett's test was used in comparing the effects of Notch2 and Notch2 mutant expressions with empty vector-infected cells as the control.

Table 2 Case information

Case No.	Breed	Age	Sex	Location
1	Labrador retriever	10y	Spayed female	Spleen, Liver
2	Border Collie	13y	Male	Spleen
3	Maltese	10y	Male	Spleen
4	Scottish terrier	10y	Spayed female	Thoracic cavity
5	Miniature dachshund	11y	Female	Spleen, Liver
6	Golden retriever	9y	Spayed female	Spleen
7	Miniature schnauzer	11y	Male	Spleen
8	Golden retriever	9y	Castrated Male	Liver
9	Bichon frise	8y	Spayed female	Kidney
10	Labrador retriever	10y	Male	Spleen
11	Great pyrenees	10y	Castrated Male	Spleen
12	Golden retriever	9y	Male	Spleen

Results

HSA cell lines in serum-free culture condition have CSC-like characteristics

To isolate CSC-like cells from HSA cell lines, we cultured HSA cell lines in adherent serum-free (SF) culture condition in gelatin-coated cell culture plates. Approximately 70–90% Ju and Ud cells died within 2 days after culturing and surviving cells proliferated slowly. On the other hand, Re cells did not survive in this condition. Next, we checked expression levels of undifferentiated endothelial cell-related genes: *ERG*, *PROCR*, *SOX18* and *FLI1* (Fig. 1a) [48–50]. Prior to qPCR analysis, reference gene sets were selected from nine potential internal controls (*GAPDH*, *ACTB*, *B2M*, *HMBS*, *HPRT1*, *RPL13A*, *RPL32*, *TBP*, *YWHAZ*) using geNorm software (Additional file 3: Figure S3) [38, 39]. Based on the analysis, three reference genes (*GAPDH*, *ACTB*, *HMBS*) were selected and the geometrical mean of the expression levels of these genes was used as a control for normalization. *ERG* and *PROCR* were upregulated in all cell lines except for *PROCR* in JuA1. *SOX18* was highly expressed in JuB4, Ud2 and Ud6. *FLI1* was upregulated in JuB4 and Ud6. No significant repression of these genes was detected in SF condition except for *PROCR* in JuA1. We also analyzed the clonogenicity of HSA cells in serum-free condition using CFA. All cell lines cultured in SF condition had significantly increased number of colonies compared to cell lines cultured in normal condition (Fig. 1b).

Since cancer stem cells have higher resistance to anti-cancer drugs, we analyzed sensitivities of HSA cell lines to doxorubicin and paclitaxel in normal and SF conditions [12, 13]. All cell lines cultured in SF condition had significantly higher resistance to both chemotherapeutic drugs although the extents vary between cell lines (Fig. 2). ALDH is known as one of the CSC markers highly associated with drug resistance capability, hence, ALDH activities were analyzed [51, 52]. Flow cytometry analysis revealed that the percentage of ALDH positive cells were significantly increased in SF condition except for Ud2 (Fig. 3).

These results suggest that HSA cells isolated by our SF culture method have CSC-like characteristics.

Notch2 signal is required for HSA CSC-like cell survival in serum-free culture condition

We succeeded in isolating CSC-like cells from HSA cell lines but the genes nor the factors which are important for these cells' survival were still unclear. Notch signal has been previously reported as a necessary signal transduction for tumor development, stem cell maintenance including CSCs, and angiogenesis [19–28]. Dysregulation of Notch signal has been associated with vascular tumors in humans and mice [30–32]. Thus, we tried to

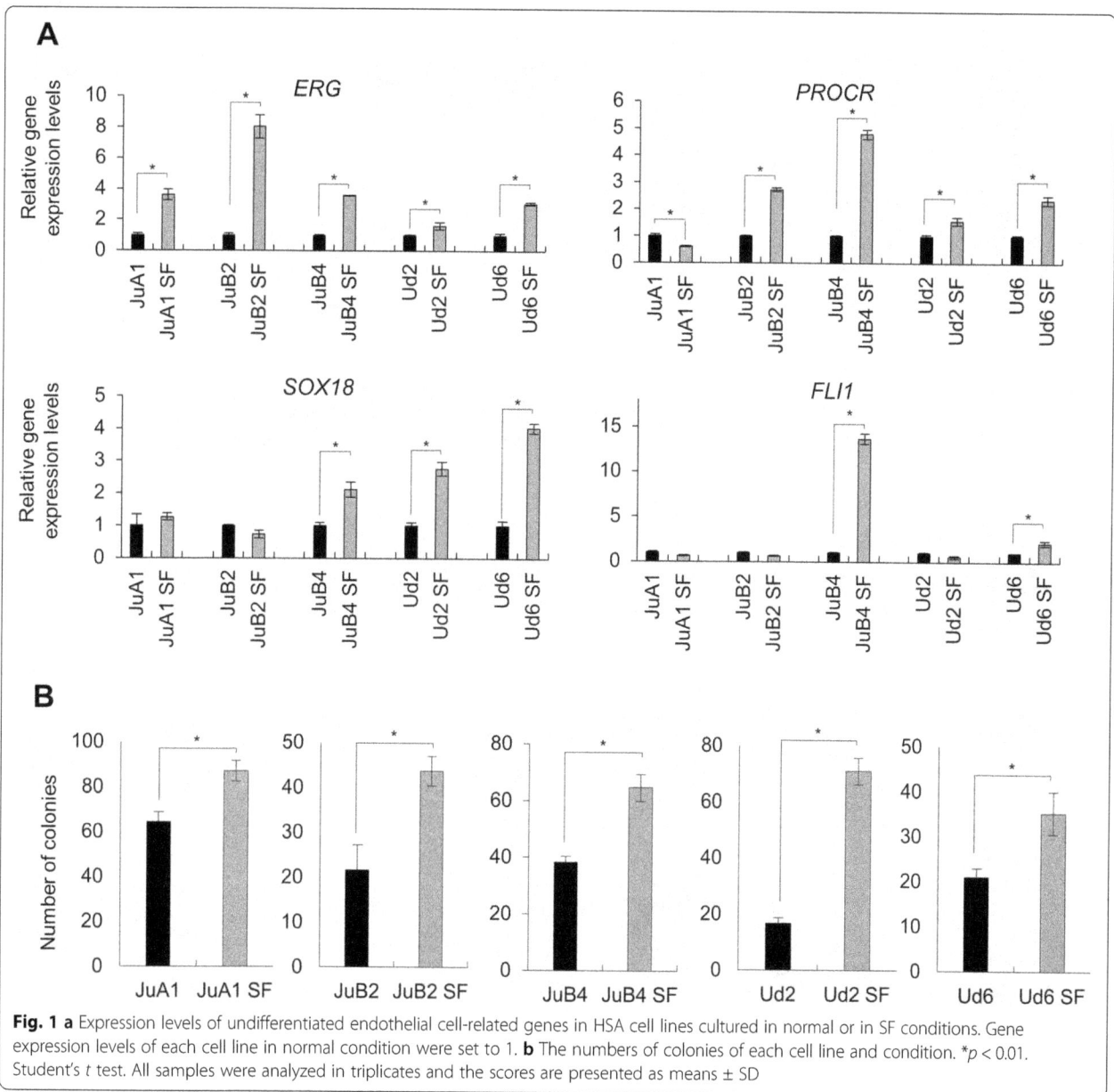

Fig. 1 a Expression levels of undifferentiated endothelial cell-related genes in HSA cell lines cultured in normal or in SF conditions. Gene expression levels of each cell line in normal condition were set to 1. **b** The numbers of colonies of each cell line and condition. *p < 0.01. Student's t test. All samples were analyzed in triplicates and the scores are presented as means ± SD

investigate its function in HSA cell lines. First, we analyzed gene expression levels of Notch receptors (*NOTCH1*, *NOTCH2*, *NOTCH3* and *NOTCH4*) and Notch target genes (*NRARP*, *HEY2*, *HES6* and *FCER2*) in normal and in SF conditions. *NOTCH2* and *NOTCH4* were upregulated in SF condition in all cell lines except for *NOTCH2* in Ud6, in addition, at least two target genes were expressed higher in SF condition than normal condition (Fig. 4a and b). To check the Notch2 function in HSA cell growth, we tried to inhibit the function with a γ-secretase inhibitor, DAPT. We tested DAPT for HSA cell lines at several concentration and found out that 20 μM DAPT was enough to repress Notch signal target gene expression (Additional file 4:

Figure S4) and was therefore used for further experiments. In normal condition, all cell lines except for JuB2 did not show any significant decrease in growth rate after DAPT treatment when compared to the control (Fig. 5a). In contrast, all cell lines in SF condition had dramatically decreased growth rate after treatment with DAPT (Fig. 5a and b). These results suggest that Notch signal is required for HSA cell survival in SF condition.

Although *NOTCH2* and *NOTCH4* were upregulated in SF condition (Fig. 4a), $2^{-\Delta Ct}$ values of *NOTCH2* was much higher than that of *NOTCH4* (Table 3). In addition, Notch2 specific target *FCER2* was upregulated, which encouraged us to analyze the effects of Notch2 in HSA cell lines. Prior to examining Notch2 protein

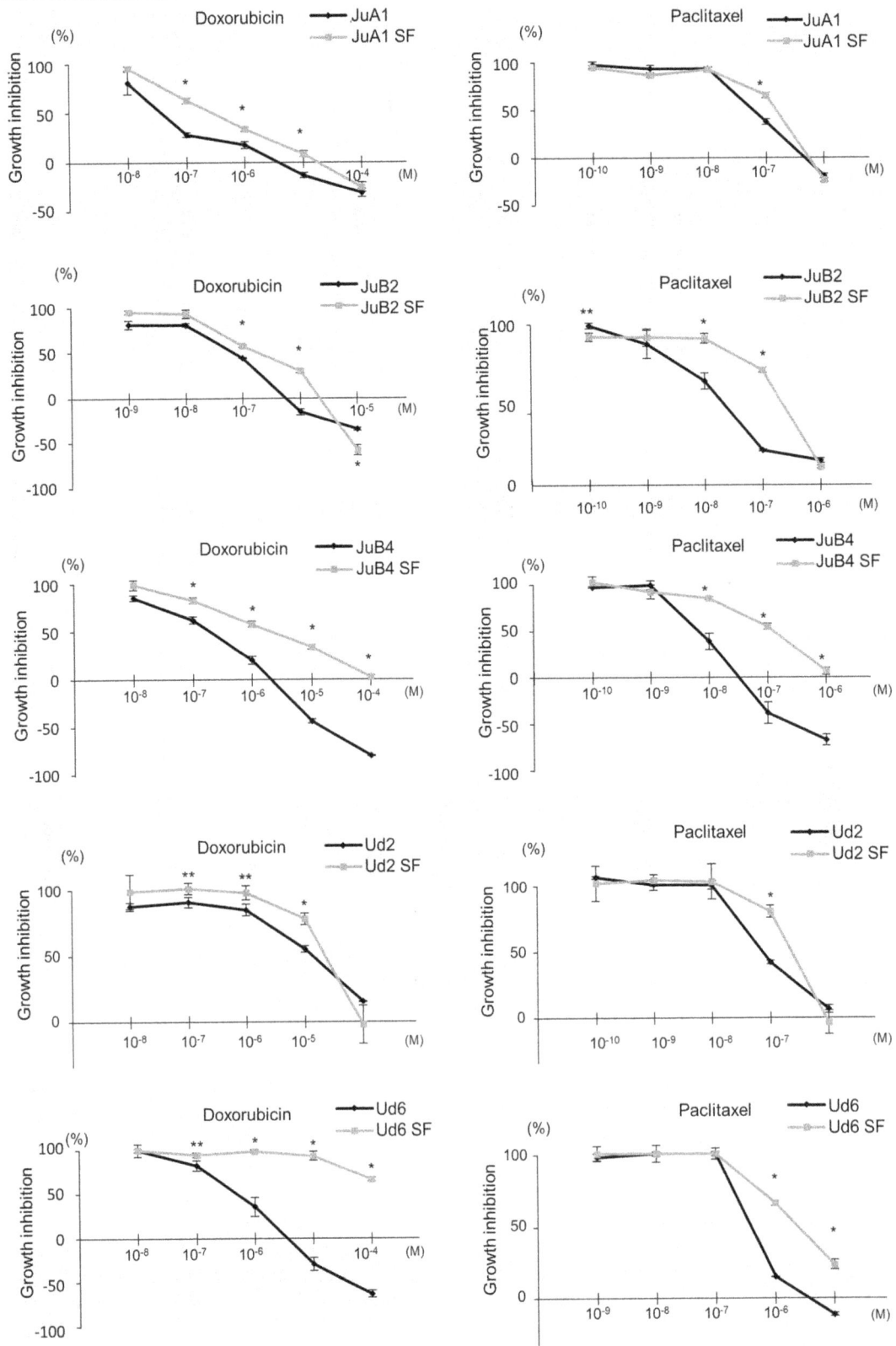

Fig. 2 Survival rate of HSA cell lines treated with doxorubicin or paclitaxel. *$p < 0.01$. **$p < 0.05$. Student's t test. All samples were analyzed in triplicates. Survival curves are plotted as average percentages ± SD

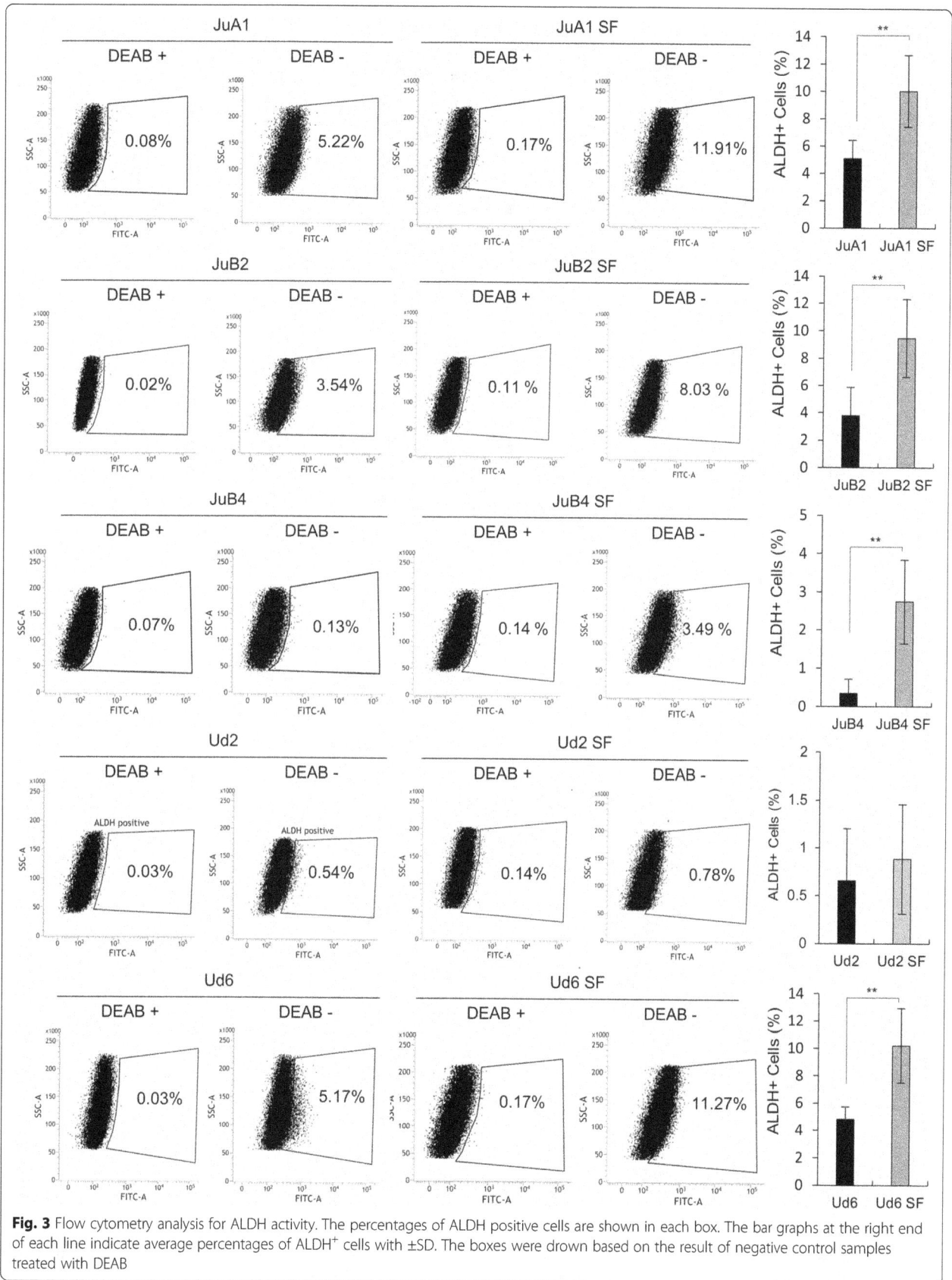

Fig. 3 Flow cytometry analysis for ALDH activity. The percentages of ALDH positive cells are shown in each box. The bar graphs at the right end of each line indicate average percentages of ALDH⁺ cells with ±SD. The boxes were drown based on the result of negative control samples treated with DEAB

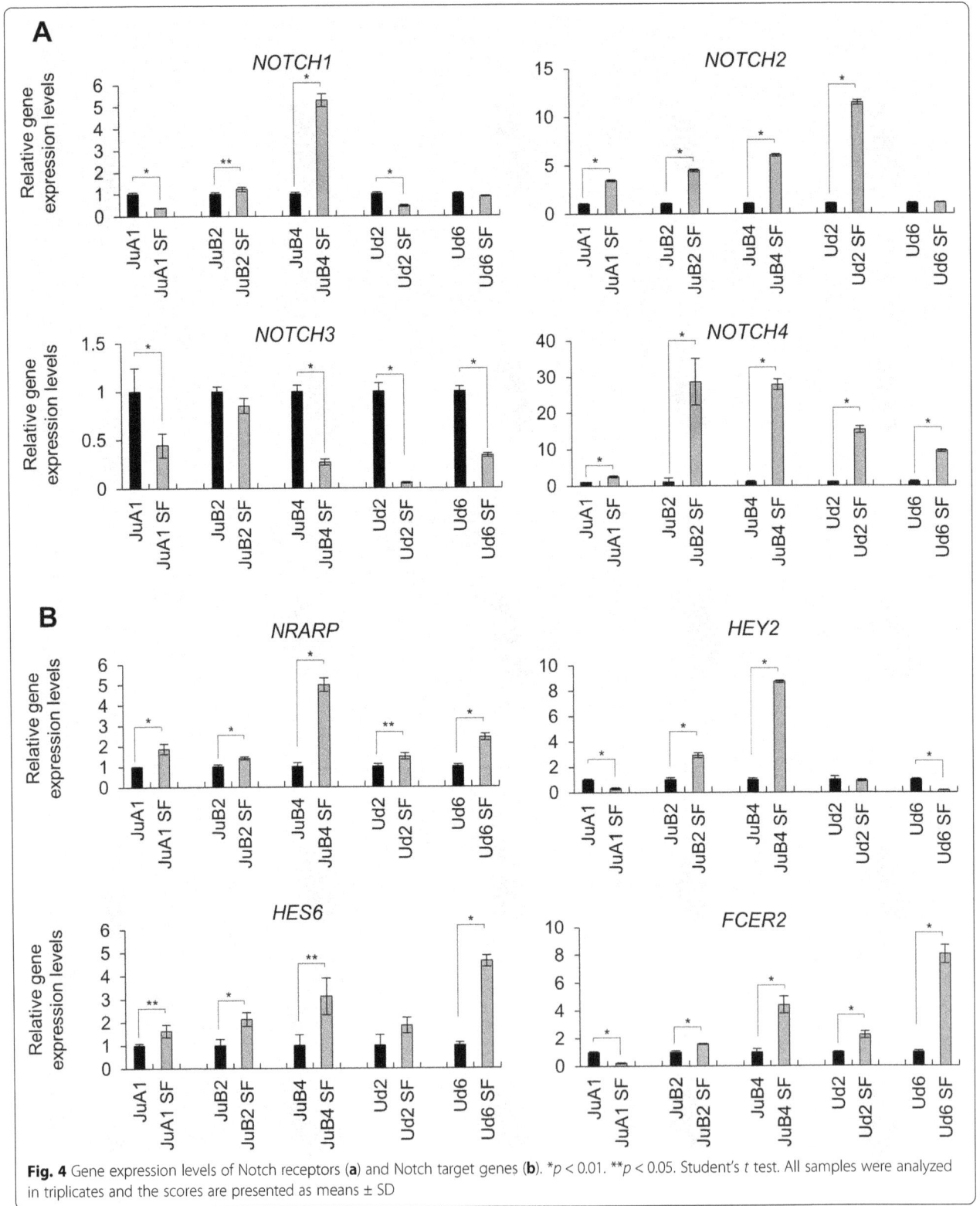

Fig. 4 Gene expression levels of Notch receptors (**a**) and Notch target genes (**b**). *$p < 0.01$. **$p < 0.05$. Student's t test. All samples were analyzed in triplicates and the scores are presented as means ± SD

expression, we confirmed that anti-human Notch2 antibody can cross-react with canine Notch2 (Fig. 6a). Notch2 protein expression was higher in SF condition than the normal condition (Fig. 6b). Based on previous

research, we constructed lentiviral vectors to stably express Notch2 full length form (FL), dominant negative form (Ex) and constitutive active form (In) in JuB2, Ud6, and Re12 in normal culture condition (Fig. 6c) [46].

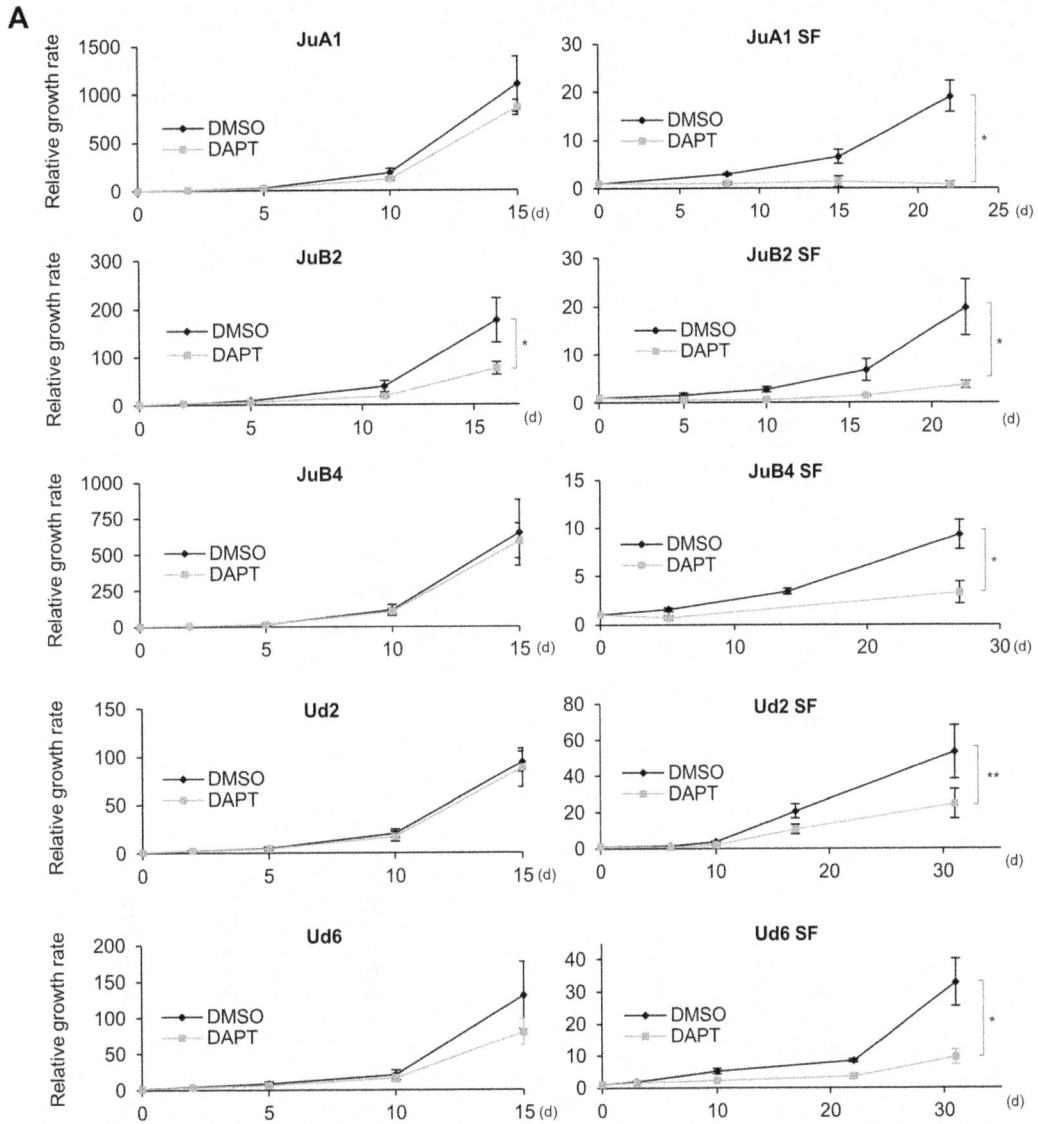

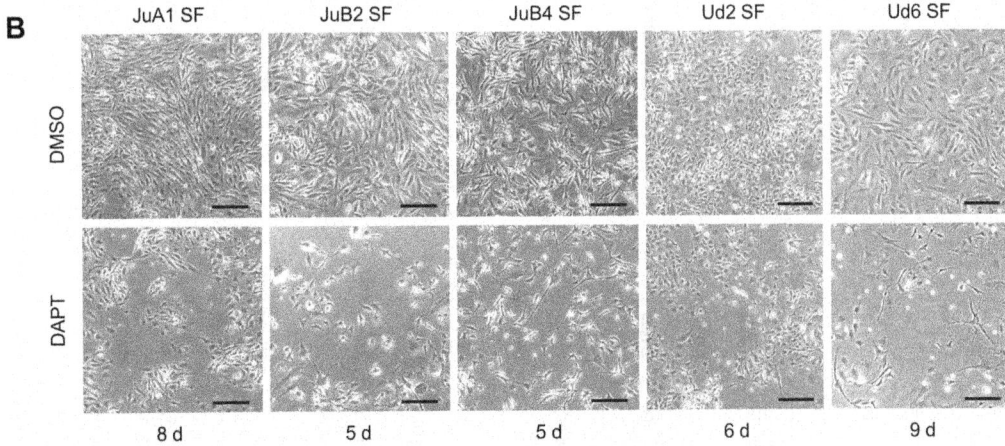

Fig. 5 a Relative growth rate of HSA cell lines cultured in normal or SF condition treated with DMSO or DAPT. *$p < 0.01$. **$p < 0.05$. Student's *t* test. All samples were analyzed in triplicates and growth curves are presented as means ± SD. **b** Representative images of HSA cell lines in serum-free condition treated with DAPT or not. Bars = 100 μm

Table 3 $2^{-\Delta Ct}$ values of *NOTCH2* and *NOTCH4*

$2^{-\Delta Ct}$	JuA1	JuA1 SF	JuB2	JuB2 SF	JuB4	JuB4 SF	Ud2	Ud2 SF	Ud6	Ud6 SF
NOTCH2	0.0179	0.0618	0.2430	1.0862	0.2346	1.4135	0.0828	0.9478	0.9553	1.0772
NOTCH4	0.0606	0.1553	0.0002	0.0053	0.0009	0.0240	0.0052	0.0801	0.0009	0.0084

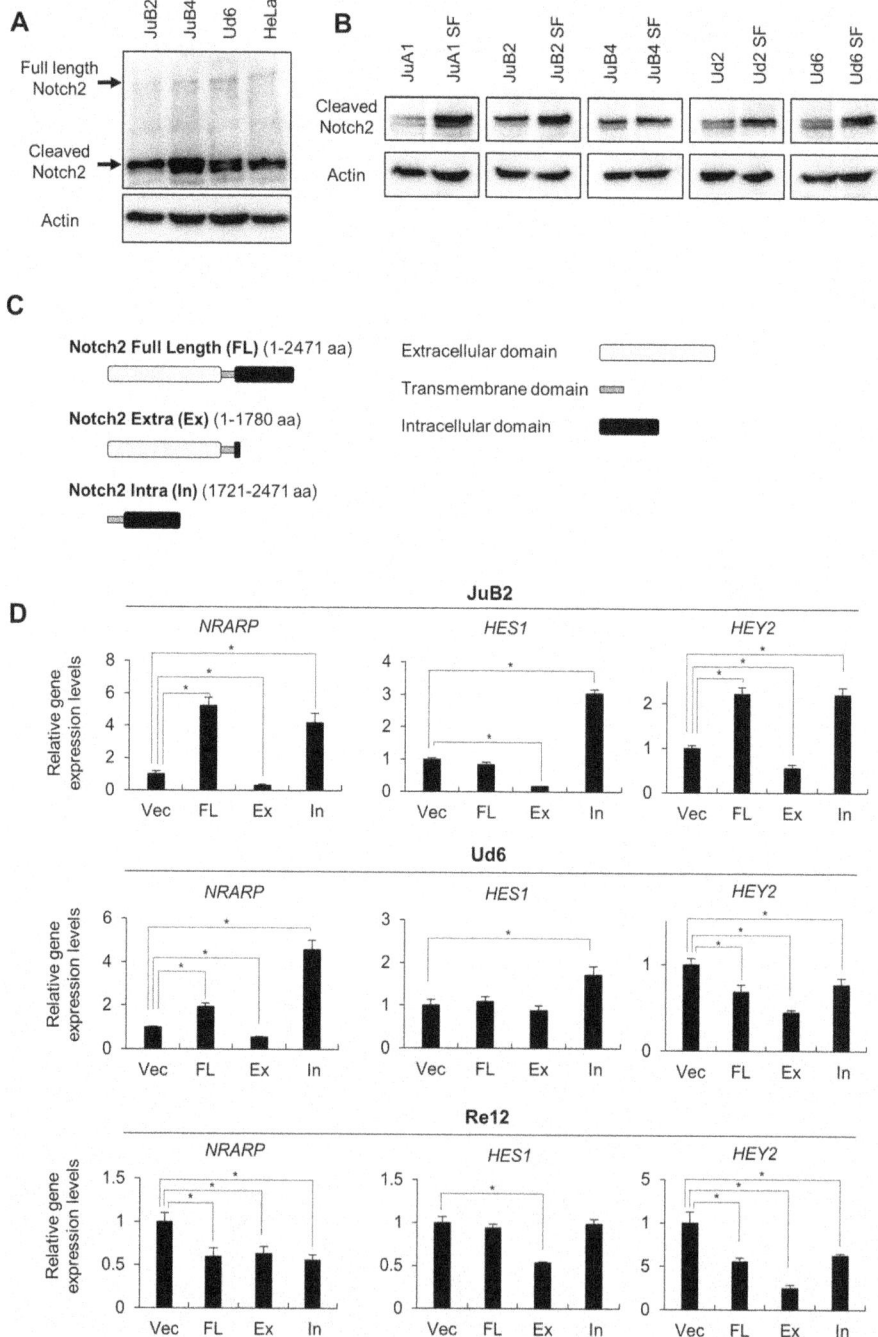

Fig. 6 a Western blot analysis using anti-human Notch2 antibody. HeLa cell line was used as a positive control. **b** Notch2 protein expression levels in HSA cell lines cultured under the normal or serum-free condition, **c** Conceptual diagram of Notch2 protein and its mutants. **d** Gene expression levels of Notch target genes. Vec = cells transfected the empty vector. FL = cells overexpressing full length of Notch2. Ex = cells overexpressing dominant negative form of Notch2. In = cells overexpressing constitutive active form of Notch2. Gene expression levels of Vec were set to 1. *$p < 0.01$. **$p < 0.05$. Dunnett's test. Samples for gene expression analysis were analyzed in triplicates and the scores are presented as means ± SD

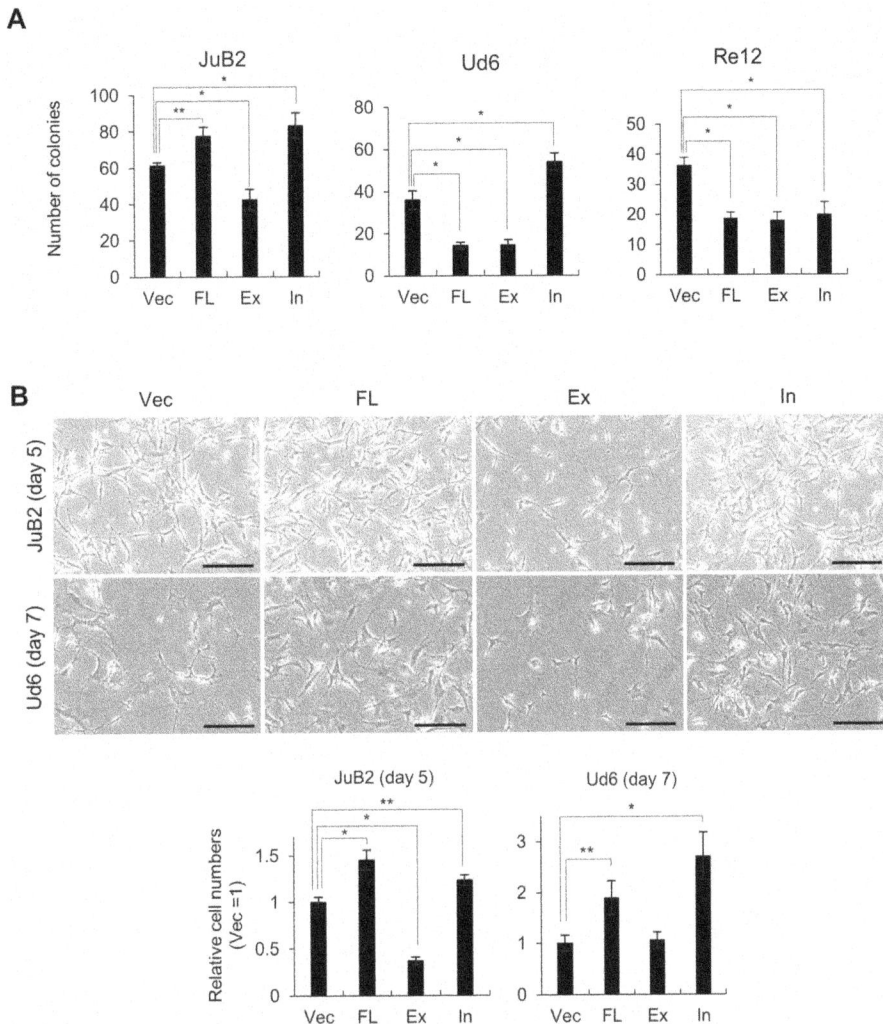

Fig. 7 a Colony numbers of HSA cell lines overexpressing Notch2 vector constructs. **b** (Top) Representative images of JuB2 and Ud6, 5 and 7 days after starting serum-free culture, respectively. Bars = 100 μm. (Bottom) Relative cell numbers of JuB2 and Ud6. Number of Vec was set to 1. *$p < 0.01$. **$p < 0.05$. Dunnett's test. The scores are presented as means ± SD

Notch2 expression from these constructs were confirmed using anti-FLAG antibody and anti-Notch2 antibody (Additional file 5: Figure S5). After establishment of stable cell lines, we analyzed Notch signal target genes, *NRARP, HES1* and *HEY2* to confirm the functions of wild type and mutant Notch2 in stable cell lines. JuB2 and Ud6, where we succeeded in isolating CSC-like cells with SF culture, showed significantly higher expressions of these target genes in cells overexpressing FL and In, and significantly lower expressions in cells overexpressing Ex compared to vector controls (Vec) (Fig. 6d). In contrast, Re12 did not show any upregulation of the target genes' expression in cells overexpressing FL and In although Ex overexpression in Re12 repressed them. Next, we checked the effects of Notch2 on clonogenicity using CFA, which resulted in the significant increase of colony numbers in In-overexpressing cells and significant decrease in Ex-overexpressing cells in both JuB2

and Ud6 cells, on the other hand, the colony formation was significantly decreased in Re12 overexpressing any types of Notch2 (Fig. 7a). Lastly, we checked whether Notch2 inhibition or activation affected CSC-like cell numbers after changing culture condition from normal to SF. As a result, Notch2 inhibition by Ex overexpression significantly decreased the number of viable cells in JuB2, while, Notch2 activation by FL- and In-overexpression resulted to significantly increased number of viable cells in JuB2 and Ud6 cell lines (Fig. 7b). These results suggest that Notch2 signal is required for the maintenance of HSA CSC-like cells.

Notch2 is highly expressed in clinical HSA cases

We analyzed Notch2 expression in clinical HSA cases with IHC. Twelve HSA cases were tested and all cases were positive for anti-Notch2 antibody (Fig. 8). Stronger staining intensities were observed in neoplastic cells

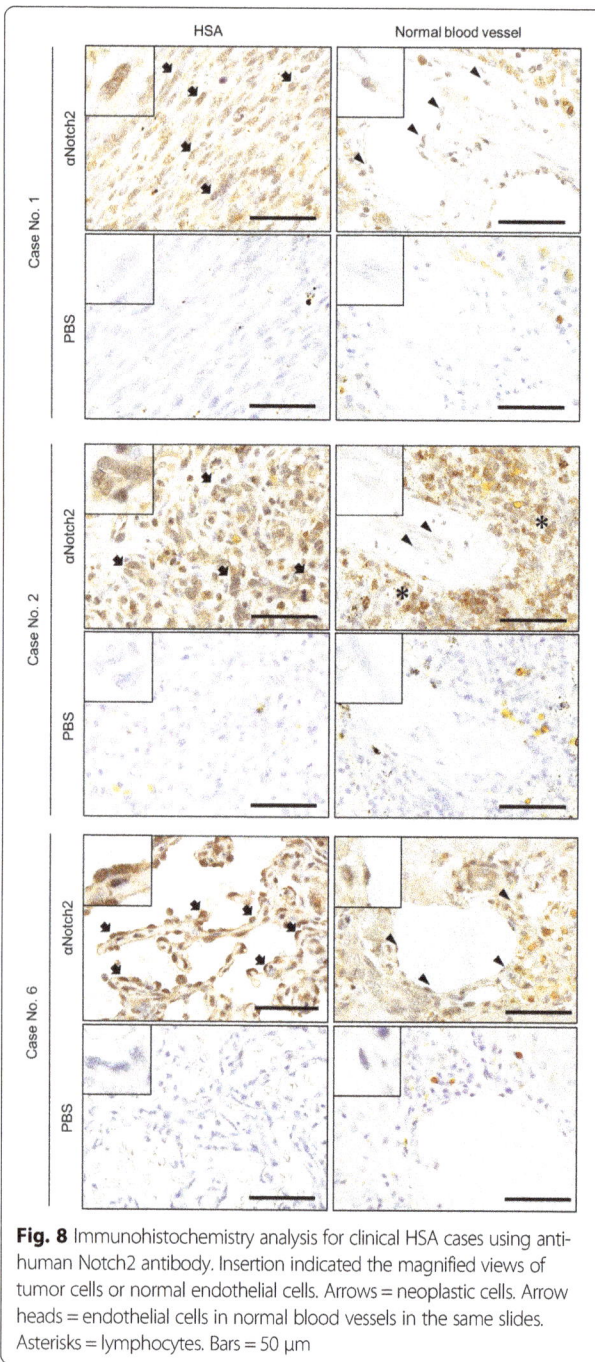

Fig. 8 Immunohistochemistry analysis for clinical HSA cases using anti-human Notch2 antibody. Insertion indicated the magnified views of tumor cells or normal endothelial cells. Arrows = neoplastic cells. Arrow heads = endothelial cells in normal blood vessels in the same slides. Asterisks = lymphocytes. Bars = 50 μm

compared to the endothelial cells of normal blood vessels in the same slide. The staining intensities of tumor cells were at the same level with lymphocytes, a positive control for Notch2 (Fig. 8 case No.2). These results suggest that Notch2 is also active in clinical HSA cases.

Discussion

In this study, we found that Notch2 is a key factor for the maintenance of HSA CSC-like cells. Isolated cells from our serum-free culture method had CSC-like

characteristics such as upregulation of undifferentiated endothelial cell markers, high clonogenicity, high drug resistance, and increased ALDH$^+$ cell population. Constitutive activation of Notch2 resulted to an increase of the number of cells with high clonogenicity in normal culture condition and cells which can survive in SF condition, while Notch2 inhibition caused opposite effects. Furthermore, Notch2 was found to be highly expressed and active in clinical HSA cases.

We succeeded in culturing CSC-like cells from Ju and Ud cell lines but, unfortunately, we were not able to isolate CSC-like cells from Re cell lines (Re12 and Re21). Furthermore, any types of Notch2 overexpression in Re12 repressed downstream gene expressions and colony formation. Re cell lines were derived from HSA in the right atrium of the heart of a Golden retriever [33, 53]. Several reports have indicated that HSA of Golden retrievers has different characteristics from those of other breeds [54–56]. Tamburini et al. have demonstrated that significant upregulation of VEGFR1 was observed in HSA from Golden retrievers compared to other breeds [54]. Vegfr1 is a tyrosine kinase receptor which can bind to an angiogenic factor Vegfa. It was thought as a decoy receptor for Vegfr2 which has higher tyrosine kinase activity than Vegfr1 and works as a major transducer of Vegfa. However, it has recently been reported that Vegfr1 can also transduce signals and stimulates tumor growth and metastasis [57]. Vegfr2 has different signal transductions from Vegfr1 and induces angiogenesis specifically by regulating Ets1 transcription factor [58]. Those different signal transductions and transcriptional regulation probably give different characteristics to HSA in Golden Retrievers. Further research comparing the molecular biology of HSA from Golden Retrievers and other breeds is required.

Notch2 is one of the Notch signal receptors and has been reported as an important factor both for tumorigenesis and stem cell maintenance. Active mutations in NOTCH2 are involved in developments of diffuse large B cell lymphoma and marginal zone B-cell lymphoma [59–62]. In human hepatocellular carcinoma, Notch2 regulates the stemness of liver CSCs via upregulation of NRARP, HES1 and HES6 [63]. Notch2 is also highly upregulated in pancreatic cancer-stem cells [64]. In our study, activation of Notch2 by FL and In in JuB2 increased the number of colonies observed in CFA and survival cell numbers in SF condition, and Notch signal inhibition by Ex indicated opposite effects. Ud6 overexpressing In had similar results with JuB2, but Ud6 cells overexpressing FL or Ex showed different results wherein the cells overexpressing FL had decreased number of colonies while those overexpressing Ex showed no difference with vector control even after changing to SF culture medium. The discrepancy between JuB2 and

Ud6 both of which expressed FL is probably resulted from the difference in the amount of ligands which can trigger Notch signals. In, the constitutive active form, overexpression showed increase in number of colonies and survival of cells in either experiment. There may not be enough number of cells secreting ligands in Ud6 in normal cell culture condition. Negative feedback system of Notch signaling may also be related [65]. In Ud6 cells over-expressing Ex, other factors such as other Notch receptors may compensate for the loss of function of Notch2 in SF condition. Notch2 may be important for stemness mainten-ance in HSA, however, we could not identify its responsible ligands and direct targets. Further experiments which focus on the targets of Notch2 to maintain stemness in HSA are warranted. Also, since *NOTCH4* was also highly upregu-lated in SF condition, it is worth analyzing its function for cell survival in SF condition.

Although we can't exclude the possibility that Notch signal was just artificially activated by stimulating the Fgf pathway and gelatin coating, we speculate that our culture condition imitates the microenvironment for hemangiosarcoma cancer stem cells. In general, micro-environment is required to maintain stem cells in their undifferentiated state by transducing signals and/or by providing cytokines. Neoplastic cells can be differenti-ated when they go out of the microenvironment [12]. Based on this nature, imitating suitable microenviron-ment is necessary to culture cancer stem cell-like cells even in vitro condition. However, further experiments to analyze Fgf pathway activity including Fgf receptor and ligand expression in tumor cells and in microenviron-ment components such as inflammatory cells and fibro-blasts are required.

Conclusions

In conclusion, we succeeded in isolating CSC-like cells in HSA using our own method, and demonstrated that Notch2 is a key factor for the maintenance of HSA CSC-like cells. Our study can encourage further stem cell research in HSA and may provide a way to develop effective treatments targeting CSCs.

Additional files

Additional file 1: Figure S1. Standard curves for each primer. Slope was used to calculate primer efficiencies. (TIF 801 kb)

Additional file 2: Figure S2. Standard curves for each primer. Slope was used to calculate primer efficiencies. (TIF 794 kb)

Additional file 3: Figure S3. Results of geNorm analysis for reference gene candidates. To determine optimal number of reference genes, 0.15 *V* value was used as the cut-off value as Vandesompele et al. [38] recommended.

Additional file 4: Figure S4. Gene expression levels of Notch signal target genes. HSA cells treated with DMSO were set to 1. *$p < 0.01$. **$p < 0.05$. Dunnett's test.

Additional file 5 Figure S5. Western blot analysis to detect Notch2 constructs expressions using anti-FLAG antibody (A) and anti-Notch2 anti-body (B). Since anti-Notch2 antibody that we used can detect the Notch2 intracellular domain, the Notch2 Ex was not detected. Vec = cells trans-fected the empty vector. FL = cells overexpressing full length of Notch2. Ex = cells overexpressing dominant negative form of Notch2. In = cells overexpressing constitutive active form of Notch2.

Abbreviations
ALDH: Aldehyde dehydrogenase; bFGF: Basic fibroblast growth factor; CFA: Colony formation assay; CnAOEC: Canine Aortic Endothelial Cells; CSCs: Cancer stem cells; DAPT: N-[N-(3,5-Difluorophenacetyl)-L-alanyl]-S-phenylglycine t-butyl estel; DEAB: N,N-diethylaminobenzaldehyde; D-MEM: Dulbecco's Modified Eagle's Medium; DMSO: Dimethyl sulfoxide; EGF: Epidermal growth factor; Ex: Notch2 dominant negative form; FL: Notch2 full length form; HSA: Hemangiosarcoma; IHC: Immunohistochemistry; In: Notch2 constitutive active form; PBS: Phosphate buffered saline; PCR: Polymerase chain reaction; PVDF: Polyvinylidene difluoride membrane; RiPA buffer: Radioimmunoprecipitation buffer; RT: Room temperature; RT-qPCR: Reverse transcription quantitative polymerase chain reaction; SDS: Sodium dodecyl sulfate; SF: Serum-free; SIN: Self-inactivating; TBST: Tris-buffered saline containing 0.05% Tween 20; UPDW: UltraPure DNase/RNase-free distilled water

Acknowledgements
We would like to extend our sincerest gratitude to Dr. Hiroki Sakai (Gifu University) for providing canine hemangiosarcoma cell lines, and to Dr. Hiroyuki Miyoshi (RIKEN BioResource Research Center) for providing lentiviral vector constructs. We also acknowledge the efforts of Dr. Jumpei Yamazaki and Mr. Shinichi Onishi for giving useful pieces of advice and constructive discussion. We are grateful to all the members of the Laboratory of Comparative Pathology, Faculty of Veterinary Medicine, Hokkaido University for their helpful discussions, encouragements, and support.

Funding
This research was supported by JSPS KAKENHI Grant-in-Aid for Young Scien-tist (Number 18K14575), a Grants-in-Aid for Regional R&D Proposal-Based Pro-gram from Northern Advancement Center for Science & Technology of Hokkaido, Japan and a grant from The Akiyama Life Science Foundation.

Authors' contributions
KA conceived and designed the experiments. KA, YF, OE and AM performed experiments and analyzed the data. KA, KCMG, AK and TK wrote the manuscripts. All authors read and approved the final manuscript.

Consent for publication
Not applicable.

Competing interests
The authors declare that they have no competing interests.

References

1. Meuten DJ. Tumors in domestic animals. 5th ed. Ames: Wiley/Blackwell; 2017.
2. Young RJ, Brown NJ, Reed MW, Hughes D, Woll PJ. Angiosarcoma. Lancet Oncol. 2010;11(10):983–91.
3. Brown NO, Patnaik AK, MacEwen EG. Canine hemangiosarcoma: retrospective analysis of 104 cases. J Am Vet Med Assoc. 1985;186(1):56–8.
4. Kim JH, Graef AJ, Dickerson EB, Modiano JF. Pathobiology of Hemangiosarcoma in Dogs: Research Advances and Future Perspectives. Vet Sci. 2015;2(4):388–405.
5. Pearson GR, Head KW. Malignant haemangioendothelioma (angiosarcoma) in the dog. J Small Anim Pract. 1976;17(11):737–45.
6. Goritz M, Muller K, Krastel D, Staudacher G, Schmidt P, Kuhn M, Nickel R, Schoon HA. Canine splenic haemangiosarcoma: influence of metastases, chemotherapy and growth pattern on post-splenectomy survival and expression of angiogenic factors. J Comp Pathol. 2013;149(1):30–9.
7. Smith AN. Hemangiosarcoma in dogs and cats. Vet Clin North Am Small Anim Pract. 2003;33(3):533–52 vi.
8. Ogilvie GK, Powers BE, Mallinckrodt CH, Withrow SJ. Surgery and doxorubicin in dogs with hemangiosarcoma. J Vet Intern Med. 1996;10(6): 379–84.
9. Wendelburg KM, Price LL, Burgess KE, Lyons JA, Lew FH, Berg J. Survival time of dogs with splenic hemangiosarcoma treated by splenectomy with or without adjuvant chemotherapy: 208 cases (2001-2012). J Am Vet Med Assoc. 2015;247(4):393–403.
10. Olson RD, Mushlin PS, Brenner DE, Fleischer S, Cusack BJ, Chang BK, Boucek RJ Jr. Doxorubicin cardiotoxicity may be caused by its metabolite, doxorubicinol. Proc Natl Acad Sci U S A. 1988;85(10):3585–9.
11. Hammer AS, Couto CG, Filppi J, Getzy D, Shank K. Efficacy and toxicity of VAC chemotherapy (vincristine, doxorubicin, and cyclophosphamide) in dogs with hemangiosarcoma. J Vet Intern Med. 1991;5(3):160–6.
12. Batlle E, Clevers H. Cancer stem cells revisited. Nat Med. 2017;23(10):1124–34.
13. Jin X, Jin X, Kim H. Cancer stem cells and differentiation therapy. Tumour Biol. 2017;39(10):1010428317729933.
14. Chen K, Huang YH, Chen JL. Understanding and targeting cancer stem cells: therapeutic implications and challenges. Acta Pharmacol Sin. 2013;34(6): 732–40.
15. Dragu DL, Necula LG, Bleotu C, Diaconu CC, Chivu-Economescu M. Therapies targeting cancer stem cells: Current trends and future challenges. World J Stem Cells. 2015;7(9):1185–201.
16. Bonnet D, Dick JE. Human acute myeloid leukemia is organized as a hierarchy that originates from a primitive hematopoietic cell. Nat Med. 1997;3(7):730–7.
17. Al-Hajj M, Wicha MS, Benito-Hernandez A, Morrison SJ, Clarke MF. Prospective identification of tumorigenic breast cancer cells. Proc Natl Acad Sci U S A. 2003;100(7):3983–8.
18. Fang D, Nguyen TK, Leishear K, Finko R, Kulp AN, Hotz S, Van Belle PA, Xu X, Elder DE, Herlyn M. A tumorigenic subpopulation with stem cell properties in melanomas. Cancer Res. 2005;65(20):9328–37.
19. Artavanis-Tsakonas S, Rand MD, Lake RJ. Notch signaling: cell fate control and signal integration in development. Science. 1999;284(5415):770–6.
20. Hori K, Sen A, Artavanis-Tsakonas S. Notch signaling at a glance. J Cell Sci. 2013;126(Pt 10):2135–40.
21. Serra H, Chivite I, Angulo-Urarte A, Soler A, Sutherland JD, Arruabarrena-Aristorena A, Ragab A, Lim R, Malumbres M, Fruttiger M, et al. PTEN mediates Notch-dependent stalk cell arrest in angiogenesis. Nat Commun. 2015;6:7935.
22. Xiao W, Gao Z, Duan Y, Yuan W, Ke Y. Notch signaling plays a crucial role in cancer stem-like cells maintaining stemness and mediating chemotaxis in renal cell carcinoma. J Exp Clin Cancer Res. 2017;36(1):41.
23. Klinakis A, Lobry C, Abdel-Wahab O, Oh P, Haeno H, Buonamici S, van De Walle I, Cathelin S, Trimarchi T, Araldi E, et al. A novel tumour-suppressor function for the Notch pathway in myeloid leukaemia. Nature. 2011; 473(7346):230–3.
24. Kopan R, Ilagan MX. The canonical Notch signaling pathway: unfolding the activation mechanism. Cell. 2009;137(2):216–33.
25. Yamamoto M, Taguchi Y, Ito-Kureha T, Semba K, Yamaguchi N, Inoue J. NF-kappaB non-cell-autonomously regulates cancer stem cell populations in the basal-like breast cancer subtype. Nat Commun. 2013;4:2299.
26. Gonzalez ME, Moore HM, Li X, Toy KA, Huang W, Sabel MS, Kidwell KM, Kleer CG. EZH2 expands breast stem cells through activation of NOTCH1 signaling. Proc Natl Acad Sci U S A. 2014;111(8):3098–103.

27. Hovinga KE, Shimizu F, Wang R, Panagiotakos G, Van Der Heijden M, Moayedpardazi H, Correia AS, Soulet D, Major T, Menon J, et al. Inhibition of notch signaling in glioblastoma targets cancer stem cells via an endothelial cell intermediate. Stem Cells. 2010;28(6):1019–29.
28. Su Q, Xin L. Notch signaling in prostate cancer: refining a therapeutic opportunity. Histol Histopathol. 2016;31(2):149–57.
29. Baghdadi MB, Castel D, Machado L, Fukada SI, Birk DE, Relaix F, Tajbakhsh S, Mourikis P. Reciprocal signalling by Notch-Collagen V-CALCR retains muscle stem cells in their niche. Nature. 2018;557(7707):714–8.
30. Dill MT, Rothweiler S, Djonov V, Hlushchuk R, Tornillo L, Terracciano L, Meili-Butz S, Radtke F, Heim MH, Semela D. Disruption of Notch1 induces vascular remodeling, intussusceptive angiogenesis, and angiosarcomas in livers of mice. Gastroenterology. 2012;142(4):967–977.e2.
31. Kluk MJ, Ashworth T, Wang H, Knoechel B, Mason EF, Morgan EA, Dorfman D, Pinkus G, Weigert O, Hornick JL, et al. Gauging NOTCH1 Activation in Cancer Using Immunohistochemistry. PLoS One. 2013;8(6):e67306.
32. Panse G, Chrisinger JS, Leung CH, Ingram DR, Khan S, Wani K, Lin H, Lazar AJ, Wang WL. Clinicopathological analysis of ATRX, DAXX and NOTCH receptor expression in angiosarcomas. Histopathology. 2018;72(2):239–47.
33. Murai A, Asa SA, Kodama A, Hirata A, Yanai T, Sakai H. Constitutive phosphorylation of the mTORC2/Akt/4E-BP1 pathway in newly derived canine hemangiosarcoma cell lines. BMC Vet Res. 2012;8:128.
34. Pollard SM, Yoshikawa K, Clarke ID, Danovi D, Stricker S, Russell R, Bayani J, Head R, Lee M, Bernstein M, et al. Glioma stem cell lines expanded in adherent culture have tumor-specific phenotypes and are suitable for chemical and genetic screens. Cell Stem Cell. 2009;4(6):568–80.
35. Scheel C, Eaton EN, Li SH, Chaffer CL, Reinhardt F, Kah KJ, Bell G, Guo W, Rubin J, Richardson AL, et al. Paracrine and autocrine signals induce and maintain mesenchymal and stem cell states in the breast. Cell. 2011;145(6):926–40.
36. Kobayashi S, Yamada-Okabe H, Suzuki M, Natori O, Kato A, Matsubara K, Jau Chen Y, Yamazaki M, Funahashi S, Yoshida K, et al. LGR5-positive colon cancer stem cells interconvert with drug-resistant LGR5-negative cells and are capable of tumor reconstitution. Stem Cells. 2012;30(12):2631–44.
37. Kimura T, Wang L, Tabu K, Tsuda M, Tanino M, Maekawa A, Nishihara H, Hiraga H, Taga T, Oda Y, et al. Identification and analysis of CXCR4-positive synovial sarcoma-initiating cells. Oncogene. 2016;35(30):3932–43.
38. Vandesompele J, De Preter K, Pattyn F, Poppe B, Van Roy N, De Paepe A, Speleman F. Accurate normalization of real-time quantitative RT-PCR data by geometric averaging of multiple internal control genes. Genome Biol. 2002;3(7):RESEARCH0034.
39. Peters IR, Peeters D, Helps CR, Day MJ. Development and application of multiple internal reference (housekeeper) gene assays for accurate normalisation of canine gene expression studies. Vet Immunol Immunopathol. 2007;117(1–2):55–66.
40. Dailey DD, Anfinsen KP, Pfaff LE, Ehrhart EJ, Charles JB, Bonsdorff TB, Thamm DH, Powers BE, Jonasdottir TJ, Duval DL. HES1, a target of Notch signaling, is elevated in canine osteosarcoma, but reduced in the most aggressive tumors. BMC Vet Res. 2013;9:130.
41. Rafehi H, Orlowski C, Georgiadis GT, Ververis K, El-Osta A, Karagiannis TC. Clonogenic assay: adherent cells. J Vis Exp. 2011;(49):2573.
42. NCI-60 Screening Methodology. Discovery & Development Services | DTP. https://dtp.cancer.gov/discovery_development/nci-60/methodology.htm. Accessed 31 Jan 2018.
43. Schneider CA, Rasband WS, Eliceiri KW. NIH Image to ImageJ: 25 years of image analysis. Nat Methods. 2012;9(7):671–5.
44. Schindelin J, Arganda-Carreras I, Frise E, Kaynig V, Longair M, Pietzsch T, Preibisch S, Rueden C, Saalfeld S, Schmid B, et al. Fiji: an open-source platform for biological-image analysis. Nat Methods. 2012;9(7):676–82.
45. Rueden CT, Schindelin J, Hiner MC, DeZonia BE, Walter AE, Arena ET, Eliceiri KW. ImageJ2: ImageJ for the next generation of scientific image data. BMC Bioinformatics. 2017;18(1):529.
46. Zeuner A, Francescangeli F, Signore M, Venneri MA, Pedini F, Felli N, Pagliuca A, Conticello C, De Maria R. The Notch2-Jagged1 interaction mediates stem cell factor signaling in erythropoiesis. Cell Death Differ. 2011;18(2):371–80.
47. Maharani A, Aoshima K, Onishi S, Gulay KCM, Kobayashi A, Kimura T. Cellular atypia is negatively correlated with immunohistochemical reactivity of CD31 and vWF expression levels in canine hemangiosarcoma. J Vet Med Sci. 2018; 80(2):213–8.
48. Ginsberg M, James D, Ding BS, Nolan D, Geng F, Butler JM, Schachterle W, Pulijaal VR, Mathew S, Chasen ST, et al. Efficient direct reprogramming of mature amniotic cells into endothelial cells by ETS factors and TGFbeta

suppression. Cell. 2012;151(3):559–75.

49. Yu QC, Song W, Wang D, Zeng YA. Identification of blood vascular endothelial stem cells by the expression of protein C receptor. Cell Res. 2016;26(10):1079–98.

50. Kanki Y, Nakaki R, Shimamura T, Matsunaga T, Yamamizu K, Katayama S, Suehiro JI, Osawa T, Aburatani H, Kodama T, et al. Dynamically and epigenetically coordinated GATA/ETS/SOX transcription factor expression is indispensable for endothelial cell differentiation. Nucleic Acids Res. 2017; 45(8):4344–58.

51. Korkaya H, Paulson A, Iovino F, Wicha MS. HER2 regulates the mammary stem/progenitor cell population driving tumorigenesis and invasion. Oncogene. 2008;27(47):6120–30.

52. Croker AK, Goodale D, Chu J, Postenka C, Hedley BD, Hess DA, Allan AL. High aldehyde dehydrogenase and expression of cancer stem cell markers selects for breast cancer cells with enhanced malignant and metastatic ability. J Cell Mol Med. 2009;13(8B):2236–52.

53. Kodama A, Sakai H, Matsuura S, Murakami M, Murai A, Mori T, Maruo K, Kimura T, Masegi T, Yanai T. Establishment of canine hemangiosarcoma xenograft models expressing endothelial growth factors, their receptors, and angiogenesis-associated homeobox genes. BMC Cancer. 2009;9:363.

54. Tamburini BA, Trapp S, Phang TL, Schappa JT, Hunter LE, Modiano JF. Gene expression profiles of sporadic canine hemangiosarcoma are uniquely associated with breed. PLoS One. 2009;4(5):e5549.

55. Tamburini BA, Phang TL, Fosmire SP, Scott MC, Trapp SC, Duckett MM, Robinson SR, Slansky JE, Sharkey LC, Cutter GR, et al. Gene expression profiling identifies inflammation and angiogenesis as distinguishing features of canine hemangiosarcoma. BMC Cancer. 2010;10:619.

56. Tonomura N, Elvers I, Thomas R, Megquier K, Turner-Maier J, Howald C, Sarver AL, Swofford R, Frantz AM, Ito D, et al. Genome-wide association study identifies shared risk loci common to two malignancies in golden retrievers. PLoS Genet. 2015;11(2):e1004922.

57. Shibuya M. Involvement of Flt-1 (VEGF receptor-1) in cancer and preeclampsia. Proc Jpn Acad Ser B Phys Biol Sci. 2011;87(4):167–78.

58. Koch S, Claesson-Welsh L. Signal transduction by vascular endothelial growth factor receptors. Cold Spring Harb Perspect Med. 2012;2(7):a006502.

59. Lee SY, Kumano K, Nakazaki K, Sanada M, Matsumoto A, Yamamoto G, Nannya Y, Suzuki R, Ota S, Ota Y, et al. Gain-of-function mutations and copy number increases of Notch2 in diffuse large B-cell lymphoma. Cancer Sci. 2009;100(5):920–6.

60. Rossi D, Trifonov V, Fangazio M, Bruscaggin A, Rasi S, Spina V, Monti S, Vaisitti T, Arruga F, Fama R, et al. The coding genome of splenic marginal zone lymphoma: activation of NOTCH2 and other pathways regulating marginal zone development. J Exp Med. 2012;209(9):1537–51.

61. Arcaini L, Rossi D, Lucioni M, Nicola M, Bruscaggin A, Fiaccadori V, Riboni R, Ramponi A, Ferretti VV, Cresta S, et al. The NOTCH pathway is recurrently mutated in diffuse large B-cell lymphoma associated with hepatitis C virus infection. Haematologica. 2015;100(2):246–52.

62. Kiel MJ, Velusamy T, Betz BL, Zhao L, Weigelin HG, Chiang MY, Huebner-Chan DR, Bailey NG, Yang DT, Bhagat G, et al. Whole-genome sequencing identifies recurrent somatic NOTCH2 mutations in splenic marginal zone lymphoma. J Exp Med. 2012;209(9):1553–65.

63. Zhu P, Wang Y, Du Y, He L, Huang G, Zhang G, Yan X, Fan Z. C8orf4 negatively regulates self-renewal of liver cancer stem cells via suppression of NOTCH2 signalling. Nat Commun. 2015;6:7122.

64. Zhou ZC, Dong QG, Fu DL, Gong YY, Ni QX. Characteristics of Notch2(+) pancreatic cancer stem-like cells and the relationship with centroacinar cells. Cell Biol Int. 2013;37(8):805–11.

65. Lamar E, Deblandre G, Wettstein D, Gawantka V, Pollet N, Niehrs C, Kintner C. Nrarp is a novel intracellular component of the Notch signaling pathway. Genes Dev. 2001;15(15):1885–99.

PERMISSIONS

LIST OF CONTRIBUTORS

Fernanda B. Mantovani
Department of Clinical Studies, Ontario Veterinary College, University of Guelph, Guelph, Ontario, Canada

Anthony J. Mutsaers
Department of Clinical Studies, Ontario Veterinary College, University of Guelph, Guelph, Ontario, Canada
Department of Biomedical Sciences, Ontario Veterinary College, University of Guelph, Guelph, Ontario, Canada

Jodi A. Morrison
Department of Biomedical Sciences, Ontario Veterinary College, University of Guelph, Guelph, Ontario, Canada

SER Lovell
Animal Referral Centre, Auckland, New Zealand

RK Burchell and A Gal
Institute of Veterinary, Animal and Biomedical Sciences, Massey University, Palmerston North 4442, New Zealand

PJ Roady and RL Fredrickson
Veterinary Diagnostic Laboratory, University of Illinois at Urbana-Champaign, Springfield, IL, USA

Hyun-Ji Choi, Sungwoong Jang, Jae-Eun Ryu, Hyo-Ju Lee, Han-Byul Lee, Woo-Sung Ahn and Woo-Chan Son
Asan Institute for Life Sciences, Asan Medical Center, Seoul, Republic of Korea
Department of Pathology, University of Ulsan College of Medicine, Asan Medical Center, 88 Olympic-ro 43-gil, Songpa-gu, Seoul 138-736, South Korea

Hye-Jin Kim, Hyo-Jin Lee, Hee Jin Lee and Gyung-Yub Gong
Department of Pathology, University of Ulsan College of Medicine, Asan Medical Center, 88 Olympic-ro 43-gil, Songpa-gu, Seoul 138-736, South Korea

Romy M. Heilmann
College of Veterinary Medicine, University of Leipzig, An den Tierkliniken 23, DE-04103 Leipzig, Germany

Gastrointestinal Laboratory, Texas A&M University, TAMU 4474, College Station, TX 77843 4474, USA

Jörg M. Steiner, David J. Lanerie and Jan S. Suchodolski
Gastrointestinal Laboratory, Texas A&M University, TAMU 4474, College Station, TX 77843-4474, USA

Elizabeth A. Mc Niel
Cummings School of Veterinary Medicine, Tufts University, 200 Westboro Rd, North Grafton, MA 01536, USA
College of Veterinary Medicine, Michigan State University, 784 Wilson Rd, East Lansing, MI 48824, USA

Niels Grützner
Farm Animal ClinicVetsuisse Faculty, University of Bern, Bremgartenstrasse 109a, CH-3012 Bern, BE, Switzerland
Gastrointestinal Laboratory, Texas A&M University, TAMU 4474, College Station, TX 77843-4474, USA

Yang Li, Shuai Cui, Yixin Wang, Zhizhong Cui, Peng Zhao and Shuang Chang
College of Veterinary Medicine, Shandong Agricultural University, Tai'an 271018, China

Weihua Li
China Animal Health and Epidemiology Center, Qingdao 266032, China

Milan Milovancev, Stuart C. Helfand, Kevin Marley, Cheri P. Goodall and Shay Bracha
Department of Clinical Sciences, College of Veterinary Medicine, Oregon State University, Corvallis, OR 97331, USA

Christiane V. Löhr
Department of Biomedical Sciences, College of Veterinary Medicine, Oregon State University, Corvallis, OR 97331, USA

Floor A. S. Bonestroo, Elpetra P. M. Timmermans Sprang, Jolle Kirpensteijn and Jan A. Mol
Department of Clinical Sciences of Companion Animals, Faculty of Veterinary Medicine, University of Utrecht, Yalelaan 104, 3584, CM, Utrecht, The Netherlands

Gayathri Thevi Selvarajah
Department of Clinical Sciences of Companion Animals, Faculty of Veterinary Medicine, University of Utrecht, Yalelaan 104, 3584, CM, Utrecht, The Netherlands
Department of Veterinary Clinical Studies, Faculty of Veterinary Medicine, University Putra Malaysia, UPM, 43400 Serdang, Malaysia

Eun Jung Park, Seok-Hee Lee, Young-Kwang Jo, Sang-Eun Hahn and Byeong-Chun Lee
Laboratory of Theriogenology & Biotechnology, College of Veterinary Medicine and the Research Institute of Veterinary Science, Seoul National University, Kwanak-ro 1, Daehak-Dong, Kwanak-Gu, Seoul 08826, Republic of Korea
Veterinary Teaching Hospital, College of Veterinary Medicine and the Research Institute of Veterinary Science, Seoul National University, Seoul 08826, Republic of Korea

Goo Jang
Laboratory of Theriogenology & Biotechnology, College of Veterinary Medicine and the Research Institute of Veterinary Science, Seoul National University, Kwanak-ro 1, Daehak-Dong, Kwanak-Gu, Seoul 08826, Republic of Korea
Veterinary Teaching Hospital, College of Veterinary Medicine and the Research Institute of Veterinary Science, Seoul National University, Seoul 08826, Republic of Korea
Emergence Center for Food-Medicine Personalized Therapy System, Advanced Institutes of Convergence Technology, Seoul National University, Gyeonggi-do 443-270, Republic of Korea

Do-Min Go and Su-Hyung Lee
Veterinary Pathology, College of Veterinary Medicine and the Research Institute of Veterinary Science, Seoul National University, Seoul 08826, Republic of Korea

Darja Pavlin and Ana Nemec
University of Ljubljana, Veterinary faculty, Small Animal Clinic, Gerbičeva, 60 Ljubljana, Slovenia

Tamara Dolenšek and Tanja Švara
University of Ljubljana, Veterinary faculty, Institute of Pathology, Wild Animals, Fish and Bees, Gerbičeva, 60 Ljubljana, Slovenia

Cristian M. Suárez-Santana, Carolina Fernández-Maldonado, Josué Díaz-Delgado, Manuel Arbelo, Alejandro Suárez-Bonnet, Antonio Espinosa de los Monteros, Nakita Câmara, Eva Sierra and Antonio Fernández
Division of Histology and Animal Pathology, Institute for Animal Health and Food Security, Veterinary School, University of Las Palmas de Gran Canaria, C/Transmontana, 35413 Canary Islands, Spain

Manuela Martano, Brunella Restucci, Maria Ester De Biase, Giuseppe Borzacchiello and Paola Maiolino
Department of Veterinary Medicine and Animal Productions, Naples University "Federico II", Via F. Delpino 1, 80137 Naples, Italy

Annunziata Corteggio
Institute of Protein Biochemistry (IBP) National Research Council (CNR), Via Pietro Castellino 111, 80131 Naples, Italy

Amy E. De Clue and Yan Zhang
Department of Veterinary Medicine and Surgery, Comparative Internal Medicine Laboratory, University of Missouri, College of Veterinary Medicine, 900 E. Campus Dr, Columbia, MO 65203, USA

Jeffrey N. Bryan and Sandra M. Axiak-Bechtel
Department of Veterinary Medicine and Surgery, Comparative Oncology Radiobiology and Epigenetics Laboratory, University of Missouri, College of Veterinary Medicine, 900 E. Campus Dr, Columbia, MO 65203, USA

Saurabh Saha, Linping Zhang and David D. Tung
Biomed Valley Discoveries, 4435 Main Street, Suite 550, Kansas City, MO 64111, USA

Elena Pagani, Massimiliano Tursi, Chiara Lorenzi, Alberto Tarducci, Barbara Bruno and Renato Zanatta
Department of Veterinary Sciences, University of Turin, Largo Paolo Braccini 2-5, 10095 Grugliasco, TO, Italy

Enrico Corrado Borgogno Mondino
Department of Agriculture, Forest and Food Sciences, University of Turin, L. Paolo Braccini, 2, 10095 Grugliasco, TO, Italy

Simon Rütten and Getu Abraham
Institute of Pharmacology, Pharmacy and Toxicology, Faculty of Veterinary Medicine, Leipzig University, An den Tierkliniken 15, 04103 Leipzig, Germany

Gerald F. Schusser
Department of Large Animal Medicine, Faculty of Veterinary Medicine, Leipzig University, An den Tierkliniken 11, 04103 Leipzig, Germany

Wieland Schröd
Institute of Bacteriology and Mycology, Faculty of Veterinary Medicine, Leipzig University, An den Tierkliniken 29, 04103 Leipzig, Germany

Elisa Baioni, Rosanna Desiato, Silvia Bertolini, Cristiana Maurella and Giuseppe Ru
Biostatistics, Epidemiology and Risk Analysis Unit, Istituto Zooprofilattico Sperimentale del Piemonte, Liguria e Valle d'Aosta, Via Bologna 148, 10154 Torino, Italy

Eugenio Scanziani
Department of Veterinary Science and Veterinary Public Health, Università degli Studi di Milano, Milan, Italy

Maria Claudia Vincenti
Azienda Sanitaria Locale Valle d'Aosta, Aosta, Italy

Mauro Leschiera
Azienda Sanitaria Locale TO4, Ivrea, Turin, Italy

Elena Bozzetta and Marzia Pezzolato
Histopathology Unit, Istituto Zooprofilattico Sperimentale del Piemonte, Liguria e Valle d'Aosta, Torino, Italy

Yi-Chen Chen
Department of Veterinary Medicine, College of Veterinary Medicine, National Chung Hsing University, 250 Kuo-Kuang Road, Taichung 40227, Taiwan
Graduate Institute of Veterinary Pathobiology, College of Veterinary Medicine, National Chung Hsing University, 250 Kuo-Kuang Road, Taichung 40227, Taiwan

Shih-Chieh Chang
Department of Veterinary Medicine, College of Veterinary Medicine, National Chung Hsing University, 250 Kuo-Kuang Road, Taichung 40227, Taiwan
Veterinary Medical Teaching Hospital, College of Veterinary Medicine, National Chung Hsing University, 250 Kuo-Kuang Road, Taichung 40227, Taiwan

Jiunn-Wang Liao
Graduate Institute of Veterinary Pathobiology, College of Veterinary Medicine, National Chung Hsing University, 250 Kuo-Kuang Road, Taichung 40227, Taiwan

Wei-Li Hsu
Graduate Institute of Microbiology and Public Health, College of Veterinary Medicine, National Chung Hsing University, 250 Kuo-Kuang Road, Taichung 40227, Taiwan

Jung-Hyun Kim and Hee-Jin Kim
Department of Veterinary Internal Medicine, Konkuk University Veterinary Medical Teaching Hospital, #120 Neungdong-ro, Gwangjin-gu, Seoul 143-701, Korea

Sung-Jun Lee and Hun-Young Yoon
Department of Veterinary Surgery, College of Veterinary Medicine, Konkuk University, #120 Neungdong-ro, Gwangjin-gu, Seoul 143-701, Korea

Radu Andrei Baisan and Vasile Vulpe
Department of Clinics, University of Agricultural Sciences and Veterinary Medicine "Ion Ionescu de la Brad", Aleea M. Sadoveanu no. 8, 700489 Iaşi, Romania

Mircea Lazăr and Sorin Aurelian Paşca
Department of Pathology, University of Agricultural Sciences and Veterinary Medicine "Ion Ionescu de la Brad, Iaşi, Romania

Tommaso Banzato and Alessandro Zotti
Department of Animal Medicine, Production and Health, University of Padua, Viale dell'Università 16, AGRIPOLIS, Legnaro, 35020 Padua, Italy

Marco Bernardini
Department of Animal Medicine, Production and Health, University of Padua, Viale dell'Università 16, AGRIPOLIS, Legnaro, 35020 Padua, Italy
Portoni Rossi Veterinary Hospital, Via Roma 57, Zola Predosa, 40069 Bologna, Italy

Giunio B. Cherubini
Dick White Referrals, Six Mile Bottom, Cambridgeshire CB8 0UH, UK

Silvia Sabattini, Andrea Renzi, Marco Fantinati, Antonella Rigillo and Giuliano Bettini
Department of Veterinary Medical Sciences, Alma Mater Studiorum University of Bologna, Via Tolara di Sopra, 50, 40064 Ozzano Emilia, (BO), Italy

Francesco Albanese, Maria Massaro, Teresa Bruna Pagano and Giovanni Tortorella
"La Vallonea" laboratory, Via Giuseppe Sirtori, 9, 20017 Rho, MI), Italy

Francesca Abramo
Department of Veterinary Sciences, University of Pisa, Viale delle Piagge, 1, 56124 Pisa, Italy

Raimondo Tornago
"Città di Bolzano" veterinary clinic, Via Resia, 20, 39100 Bolzano, Italy

Julia Buchholz
Radiation Oncology Consultant, Unterrenggstrasse 36, CH-8135 Langnau am Albis, Switzerland

Anita K. Luu, Robert Jones, Andrew C. Poon, Brandon Golding, Roa'a Hamed, Anthony Mutsaers and Alicia M. Viloria-Petit
Department of Biomedical Sciences, Ontario Veterinary College, University of Guelph, 50 Stone Road East, Guelph, ON N1G 2W1, Canada

Courtney R. Schott and Geoffrey A. Wood
Department of Pathobiology, Ontario Veterinary College, University of Guelph, 50 Stone Road East, Guelph, ON N1G 2W1, Canada

Benjamin Deheshi
Medical City Forth Worth, HCA affiliated Hospital, 900 8th Ave, Fort Worth, TX 76104, USA

Keisuke Aoshima, Yuki Fukui, Kevin Christian Montecillo Gulay, Ochbayar Erdemsurakh, Atsuya Morita, Atsushi Kobayashi and Takashi Kimura
Laboratory of Comparative Pathology, Department of Clinical Veterinary Sciences, Faculty of Veterinary Medicine, Hokkaido University, Kita 18 Nishi 9, Kita-ku, Sapporo, Hokkaido 060-0818, Japan

Index

www.ingramcontent.com/pod-product-compliance
Lightning Source LLC
Chambersburg PA
CBHW082024190326
41458CB00010B/3266